PATHS AND PRACTICES FOR BALANCE AND WHOLENESS

Healing and Awakening, Timeless teachings from Wisdom Traditions

Zen Master Doshin
Michael Nelson
Rev Shikyo Jiryu Janel Houton

IZ Publishing

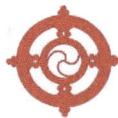

Dedicated to the healing and awakening of all beings. Special thanks to not only all of the teachers, but everyone who has supported Integral Zen, Doshin Roshi and Rev Shikyo, which has led to the publication of this book. May this bring benefit to you, and all beings whom you are connected to.

CONTENTS

CONTENTS

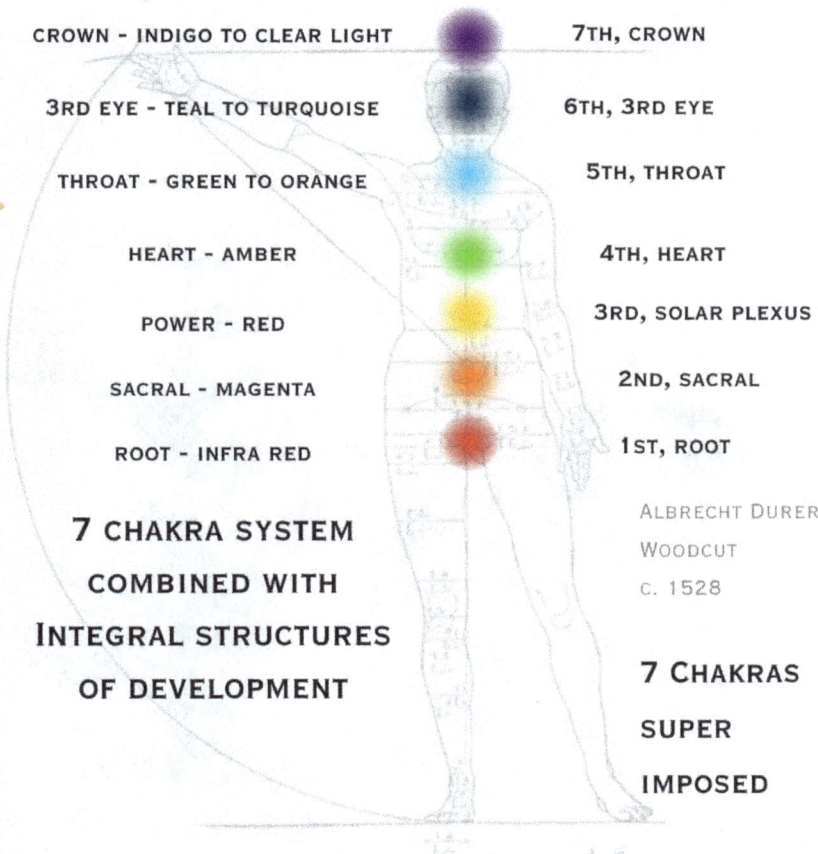

CROWN - INDIGO TO CLEAR LIGHT   7TH, CROWN

3RD EYE - TEAL TO TURQUOISE   6TH, 3RD EYE

THROAT - GREEN TO ORANGE   5TH, THROAT

HEART - AMBER   4TH, HEART

POWER - RED   3RD, SOLAR PLEXUS

SACRAL - MAGENTA   2ND, SACRAL

ROOT - INFRA RED   1ST, ROOT

7 CHAKRA SYSTEM COMBINED WITH INTEGRAL STRUCTURES OF DEVELOPMENT

ALBRECHT DURER
WOODCUT
C. 1528

7 CHAKRAS SUPER IMPOSED

PREFACE

Doshin Michael Nelson

My intention in this preface is to tell a story that creates a personal and collective context which will help you understand how the emphasis on something so simple as healing and awakening arose and became a cornerstone of a new Integral Zen Framework. Then we will point to ways that this might be helpful to you and benefit all beings. My life's work seems to be integrating the Depth Psychology of Carl Jung, the Integral Theory of Ken Wilber, and the intuitive noble wisdom of Zen and Buddhism. This story is a creation story. It is the story of the creation of a new perspective, which began with a realization and articulation of the inter-dynamics of both healing and awakening that includes the practice of Conflict Liberation and the Wilber's method of Kosmic Addressing.

In his first sermon after awakening, the Buddha allegedly described the four noble truths and the eightfold path. The first noble truth is: There is suffering in the world. The second is: There is a cause to the suffering. The third is: If there is a cause to the suffering, then there's a way to end the suffering. And the fourth noble truth is: The way to end suffering is to follow the eightfold path.

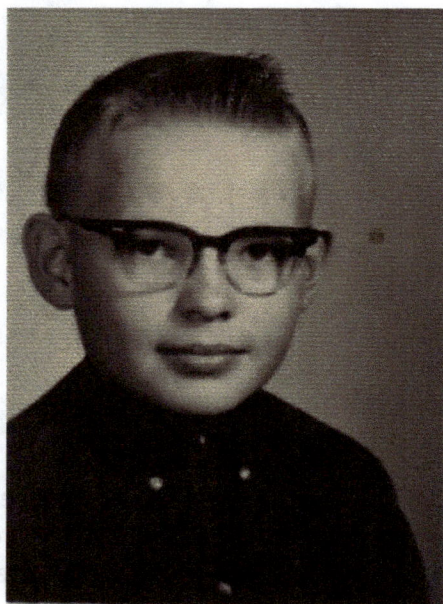

Young Michael Nelson

As a lineage holder in Rinzai Zen, a so-called Zen master and the Abbot of Integral Zen, my intention is to remove obstructions that limit our individual and collective views that obscure the vast, open infinite space, so that a possible 4th turning of Buddhism might emerge. One interpretation of the four noble truths that adds a more integral perspective is: There are conflicts in the world; There is a cause to these conflicts; if there is a cause to the conflicts, then there's a way to end the conflicts; and the way to end conflicts is for the individual to follow a practice path of conflict liberation. The cause of suffering is conflict, and irresolvable collective conflicts are the cause of war. Each turning of Buddhism describes how conflicts are caused by the three poisons of desire/greed, anger/hatred, and ignorance/delusion/unconsciousness. In Integral Zen, we differentiate the conflicts of individual human beings from the collective conflicts of groups of human beings (in Integral terms, we differentiate the conflicts of individual holons from those of social holons).

This is the first book in a series of books, in which we will attempt to bring the integration of ancient wisdom traditions and post-postmodern integral teachings into the lives of those who are interested and desperate for something practical and new, which brings some relief from the intensifying suffering of these crazy times where everything seems to be falling apart. In this modern age after so many religious paths have been blocked, and ancient wisdom teachings have been negated and rejected, the bar for awakening has changed. It is no longer enough just to awaken. In this modern world, it is impossible to awaken without healing, and it is impossible to heal without awakening.

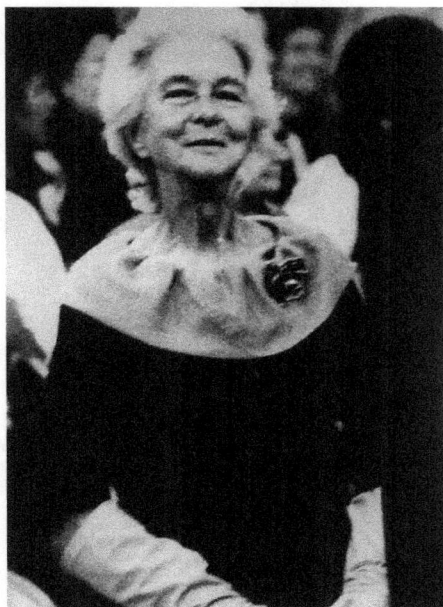

At 17, Doshin's best friend invited him to meet Mary Nevin, a teacher who changed his life

Focusing on this simple truth that healing and awakening are not two, we will present a place where you could enter a path of liberating yourself from the cause of your own personal and collective conflicts. A path that can be followed for a lifetime, perhaps many lifetimes. A path that will not only benefit you but all beings. Be warned that it will not always be easy, pleasant, kind or without suffering, and don't expect any shortcuts. I always remember something that Mary Nevin said to me.

She was the first great teacher I had the good fortune to meet, who changed the course of my life. She said: "The best things in life come unbeknownst to you." They can't be found, discovered, created, forced or engineered. You can't make them happen. They come unbeknownst to you and in the readiness of time.

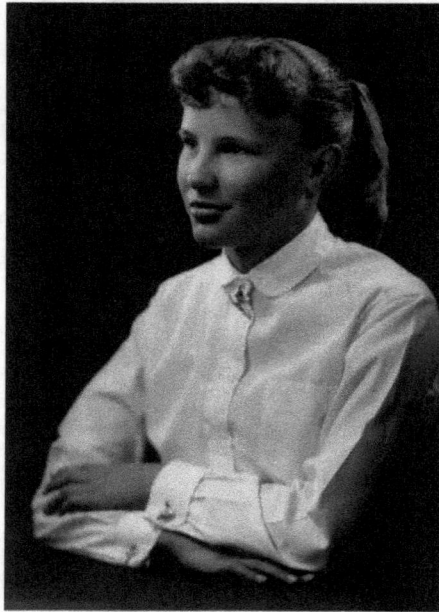

Jo Nelson, Doshin's sister

Long before I had ever heard the word Zen about the age of five or six, unbeknownst to me, I innocently experienced my first Zen Koan. My sister was studying for a spelling bee. She was five years older than I. As she was practicing, I would watch her and listen intently. She would pronounce a word and then spell it. If I didn't understand the meaning of the word, I would ask her what it meant, and she would tell me. She was very kind, extremely smart, and was always patient with me. This would often go on for hours. I loved learning new words. One day she pronounced the word infinity and spelled it. I asked her what it meant. She said that infinity means unending time and space. Something that goes on forever and ever without beginning or end. That didn't make any sense to me. It deeply disturbed my young rational mind, which was just beginning to form.

My mother told me that counting sheep would help me fall asleep, but I found that was boring, so I would think myself to sleep. The more I thought about infinity, the more disturbed I got. I thought and thought about never ending space and time. The more I thought about it, the more exhausted my innocent thinking mind became. Until finally, thinking tied itself into a knot and just stopped. Suddenly there was a profound direct experience of the emptiness of thought and time. A great inexplicable void appeared beyond thought, beyond space and time. Timeless, spaceless, thoughtless infinity opened and continued opening without end. That experience lasted for hours and the perfume of it I can still smell. It had a profound impact on me. It foreshadowed what was to become my life path.

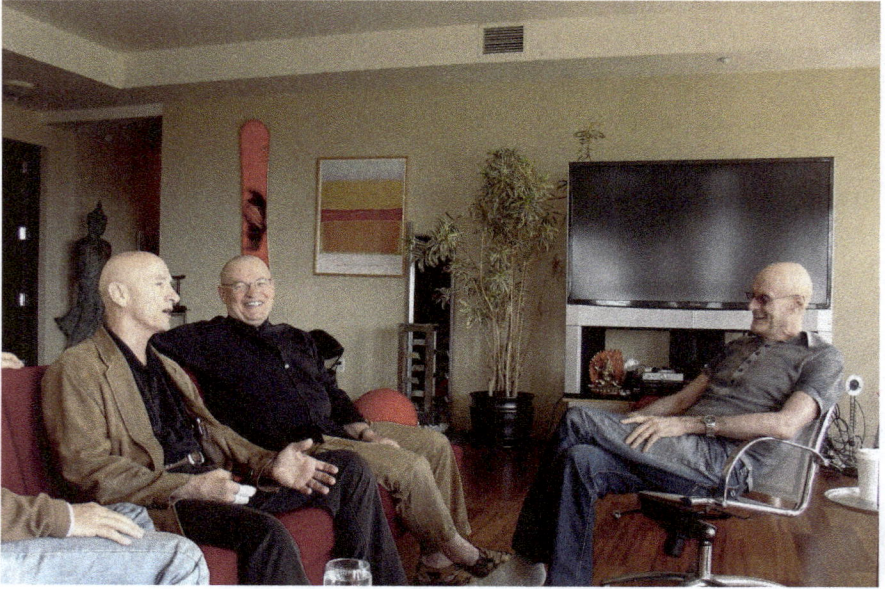

JunPo Kelly Roshi, Doshin Roshi and Ken Wilber in Ken's loft

O f course, now after many years of practicing meditation, teaching Zen, and working with koans, I now recognize that such an experience of vast empty silence, beyond the noise of any emotions, feelings, thoughts, opinions, beliefs and even stories, is what in Zen we call an insight, or perhaps if it is deep enough, a kensho—a temporary peak experience of awakened mind that is empty of self, or more specifically empty of any self-referencing, self-reactivity, or any individual self-contamination or any socio/cultural pollution of collective biases. Empty of any biases for or against anything that contaminate the purity of raw naked awareness.

My lifetime journey began in earnest when I was 17. That was the year that a very angry, troubled, rebellious teenager had three profound experiences that changed the course of his life. First, I met a girl who was a meditator, and I started meditating. This blossomed into a very stable and devoted mediation practice. Second, I was introduced to Mrs. Nevin, who deeply inspired me and turned my life "right-side-up." And third, I was in a serious automobile accident where a good friend was killed, and I almost died. These experiences continued to ripen for many years. The consistent meditation practice provided a more stable ground than I had ever known. I developed a deep thirst for what Mrs. Nevin had inspired me to study. I began reading Carl Jung, Erich Neumann, Joseph Campbell, Herman Hesse, D.T. Suzuki and J. Krishnamurti voraciously. The death of my friend and my own brush with death was a Dharma gate that made me re-prioritize everything and ask a new question, "what is the most important thing." The rebellious teenage dream began to fade, as I was being reborn into a new life–the life of a more determined, but still troubled and confused young man.

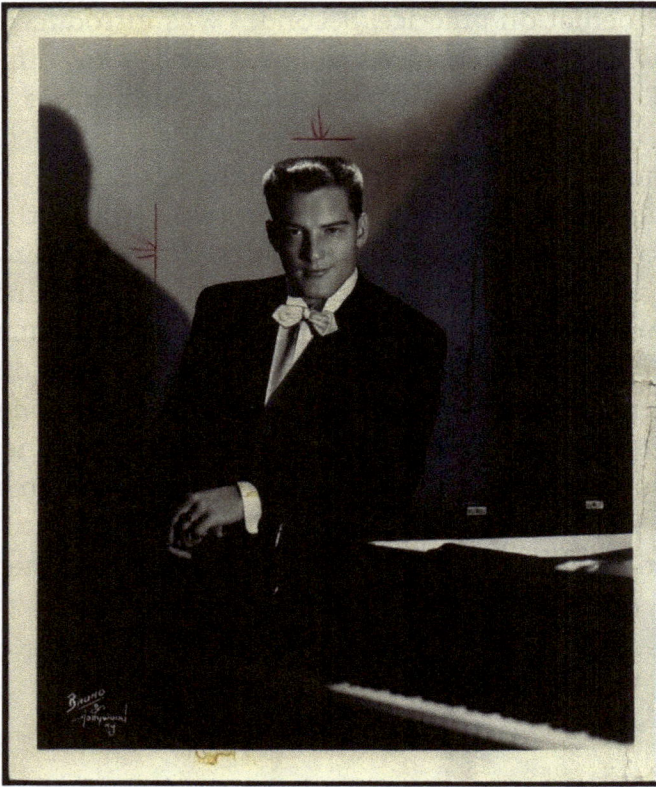

Doshin's cousin Jerry Mackey who gave up a promising career as a pianist trained at Juliard, to run a chain of Karate schools in New York, where Doshin worked

I worked many jobs, loved excitement and moved around a lot seeking new adventures. I was deeply drawn to and began Gestalt Therapy and Jungian Analysis. One day, I decided to take off with only the clothes on my back and 10 cents in my pocket. I spent a year hitch hiking and riding freight trains all over the country. There were many adventures, many endings and new beginnings for the next 10 years.

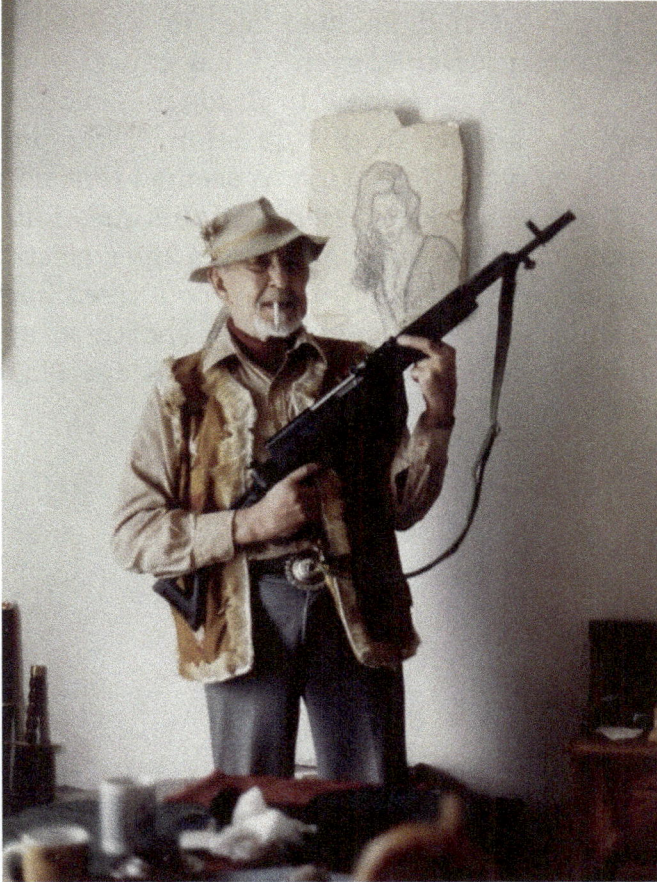

Tony Shearer, an Urban Shaman who opened Doshin's heart to the spirituality of the Lakota and Native Americans. Photo by Doshin

I needed all those experiences, and considerable therapy to become stable enough to go back and finish my studies at the university and go on to graduate school.

In graduate school, I entered a program that allowed me to pursue a master's degree in the social sciences. This gave me the freedom to study anything I wanted within any branch of the social sciences, at least theoretically. I entered graduate school with a clear intention of finding the answer to a question that had haunted me for as long as I can remember, perhaps even longer. "What causes war?" I had naively hoped that somewhere in Graduate School someone would have the answer to this question. I was profoundly disappointed by two things. First, it seemed that no one had considered, nor were they interested in this question. Second, I was astounded by how many individual and collective biases for and against almost everything I encountered in graduate school. I withdrew from the university shortly after I wrote the following poem patterned after William Blake's, The Garden of Love.

The Castle Of Knowledge

I went to the castle of knowledge,
To see what I never had learned,
The bricks and the mortar were crumbling,
In hearts where compassion once burned.

But the minds of professors seemed open
And "Know Thy Self" hung over the door.
So, I entered the castle of knowledge
And I asked them what causes war?

Then I saw it was filled with fools
Opinions where insights should be.
Good doctors in college were blinded by knowledge,
Eschewing my queries with second-hand theories.

– Michael Nelson

P ersonal computers had just emerged upon the scene, and I had purchased one in order to write my master's thesis. I discovered that I had an innate ability to intuitively resolve computer problems. When I left the university, I took all the energy that I had applied to my studies in graduate school and applied it to learning about computers. I entered what some would call the real world and became a self-taught network engineer, working for a large company. I spent the next 17 years wandering in what I call the orange spiritual desert of corporate America. Right on schedule around the age of 50 something began to die and something new was born, that was not so compatible with the so-called, "real world.

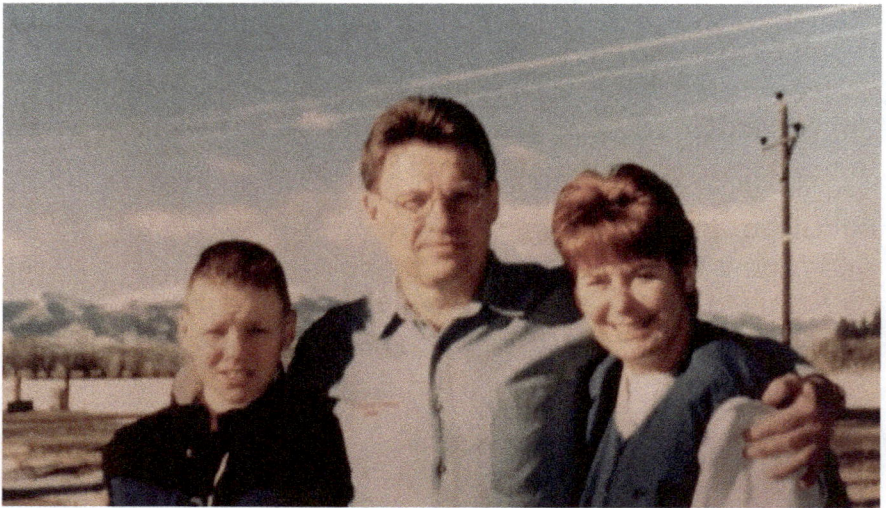
Michael Nelson, and his wife Patty, and son Preston

Over a period of several years, my modern orange friends who were mainly interested in making money and improving their status began to fall away, and I began to meet new postmodern green friends who were interested in seeing themselves and being seen by others as living more meaningful lives. My friends, life and interests all began to change. I began a new phase of self-exploration, hoping to find, or perhaps develop, a more authentic, more meaningful self. I have always been hypersensitive to lies, duplicity, hypocrisy and partial truths.

As I began looking more deeply inward, at myself and my relationships, I soon discovered that I had many more hidden blind spots and shadows than the Jungian analysis had revealed. They were causing great suffering for myself and others, for my family and all beings. I began looking fervently for new, more effective ways of doing shadow work that I could learn and master. It was at the beginning of this new phase of my life that I met my root Zen teacher JunPo Denis Kelly Roshi.

I realized immediately that he was my perfect teacher. About the same time, I discovered the work of Ken Wilber and began ardently reading about Integral Theory. As this new postmodern phase of my life was maturing and beginning to grow old, another deeper and more complex transformation simultaneously began. This one was bigger and would require more time to take root and bear fruit.

As I was becoming more conscious of my shadows and disowned selves and deepening my understanding of Jung, my religious devotion to practicing Zen and my fascination with Integral Theory both intensified.

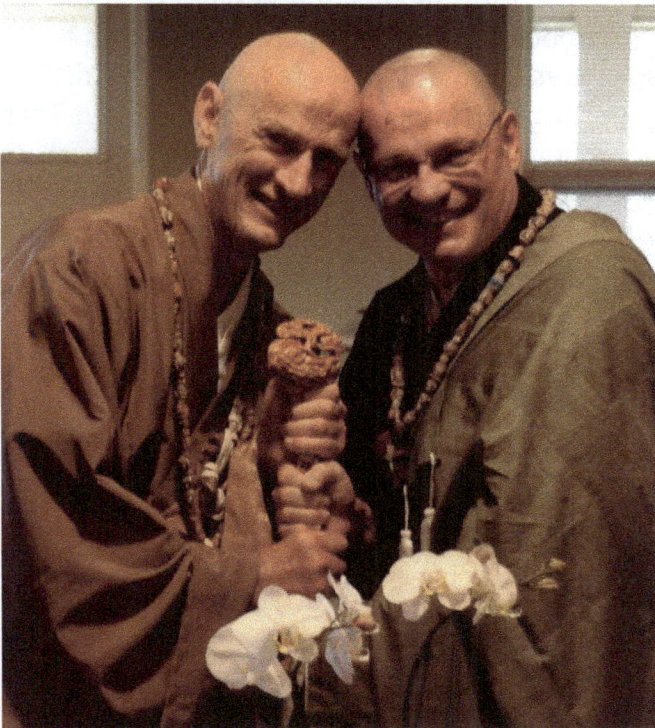

JunPo Kelly Roshi and Doshin Roshi

I met Ken Wilber and began to meet with him whenever the opportunity presented itself. I was invited to a group that met in Ken's loft every week. I consider himto be one of the "great teachers" who changed the course of my life. The insights of Jung, Wilber and Zen began coming together within my heart-mind, and a coherent Integral Zen Framework began very slowly to emerge. It was a framework that didn't argue with or negate anything in Jung, Wilber or Zen Buddhism. It enriched and complemented them all. It seems inevitable that those who are passionate "true believers" in any one of these three schools, will most likely strongly disagree with my perspective and find this framework threatening to some of their precious personal and collective moral values and ideological beliefs. This is worth mentioning now but will not be addressed in this introductory book. This book will focus more on healing from the perspectives of many lineage wisdom traditions, while slowly beginning to introduce the Integral Zen Framework. Healing is a more gentle point to enter Integral Zen, than Rinzai Zen. Most people are interested in healing, while few in this postmodern age will be able to tolerate the discipline, devotion and intensity of Samurai Zen.

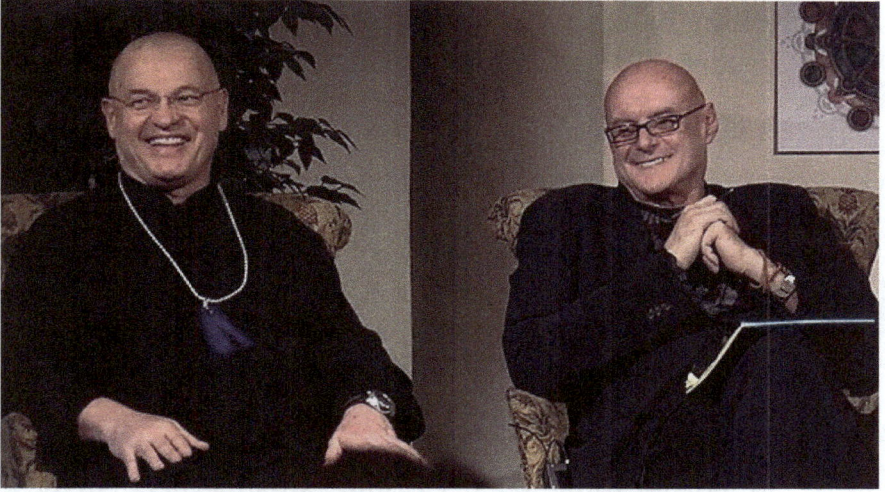
Doshin and Ken Wilber at the Fourth Turning of Buddhism Event

Some of my students and others who were familiar with my work began calling me the *Shadow Roshi*. I had known for some time that many who were attracted to Zen, desperately needed psychotherapy and shadow work. I often told new students that they needed to do some serious psychotherapy before I would consider accepting them as a student. I strongly encouraged, and if I'm honest, required that everyone in the sangha do shadow work. In addition to my studies of Jung and the experience of analysis and therapy, I had ardently sought out, studied and practiced about twenty different forms of shadow work. After years of study and practice, I achieved mastery of many of them. I intuitively knew that in spite of all this deep personal work, the years of therapy, and the intense shadow work I had done on myself and with others, I still had some deeper hidden dysfunctions that interfered with my ability to skillfully help my students and benefit all beings.

It seems that it might be helpful to some to briefly tell the story of how Janel and I met and came to work together, around 2019. About seven years before Janel showed up I had encountered the best trauma therapist I've ever had the good fortune to meet and asked him if he could help some of the students that I couldn't seem to reach. He did, and I was inspired to begin some deep trauma work with him. I also began working with several other trauma therapists. This opened the door to the considerable amount of preverbal trauma that I had experienced but which had remained below the threshold of consciousness. As I slowly began to become conscious of the extent of my own trauma, I began to study many different types of trauma work and insecure attachment issues. Intuitively I knew that it was not my karma to become a trauma therapist, so I left that work to a few carefully chosen professionals who had earned my trust and respect. JunPo supported some, what I would call superficial shadow work, but was not open at all to letting trauma work into his Hollow Bones sangha. I knew from experiences of trying to get him to see the value of Integral Theory and the need for deeper shadow work, that arguing wasn't helpful, so I tried something else. I knew that his wife was more than open to the deep need many of us have for trauma work, so I quietly sent her a book: *The Body Keeps the Score*, by Bessel van der Kolk M.D. The barrier was removed and the closed door suddenly opened.

J anel showed up on my radar when her husband gave her as a gift, a package of shadow sessions. We began to work together. I tried using many of the different shadow work methods I had mastered with her. None of them seemed to really resonate deeply with her. This got my attention, and I was extremely curious why that was. I became fascinated with her dreams. She dreamed almost every night and vividly remembered them. I encouraged her to write them down and begin a dream journal. When she attended her first Zen retreat, she had already been studying Vajrayana Buddhism for a number of years. As we continued working on her dreams it became evident to me that she was a natural born healer. As she continued attending Zen retreats, I urged her to continue deepening her Vajrayana practice and continue refining her healing skills. We began to explore trauma work and healing in the context of an integral perspective. We started using the chakras in the same way that Ken Wilber did, correlating them with the structures of ego development. When she decided to enroll in a two year intensive Sowa Rigpa Tibetan Healing Program, I encouraged her, and Integral Zen helped her with the tuition. She is a quick learner and took on many of the new integral ideas and perspectives, integrating them into the traditional healing methods she already knew and was learning.

At the same time, I was becoming conscious that Integral Zen was well on its way to falling into a familiar karmic groove that I have experienced many times in other organizations I have belonged to. It is a very predictable pattern that begins to emerge when the founder of an organization starts aging and is no longer able to hold the sharp edge they held during the beginning and early stages of the organization's growth. Be warned that I am about to use some Integral language, that many haven't been exposed to and most won't understand. Relax and don't worry if you don't understand it, just take it in. An organization is a social holon. Holons are both a whole and a part at the same time. Each holon is a whole that is made of parts that are also wholes. Organizations are made of individuals and other groups. They are all parts of the organization, and they are both parts and wholes at the same time. Each individual is a whole individual holon, and each group is a whole social holon. They are all parts of a bigger social holon of the organization. For example, you and I both are individual holons that are composed of other holons such as organs, cells, molecules and atoms. Individual holons are significantly different from social holons. This may sound strange and confusing at first, but when studied and digested, it exponentially expands our capacity to understand the complexity and interdynamics of many conflicts that are hidden without it. In order to fully grasp this, it all needs to be studied and applied in real world circumstances over a period of time guided by a qualified teacher. I learned this directly from Ken Wilber himself and it has taken me years to understand and digest it. Unfortunately, such teachers who have really mastered this are very rare and hard to find, even in the so-called integral community, which seems to have changed into more of a mass movement. Understanding this and mastering the application of this in real life circumstances creates a foundation that must be built in order to understand much more deeply what is really going on within organizations as they undergo changes that are hidden in the individual and collective shadows of the individuals and groups that are part of the inter-dynamics of organizations. This foundation does not yet exist in modern or postmodern science or in any of the traditional noble wisdom traditions.

Now let me describe organizational change in a story format that speaks more directly to the heart without the new Integral language. An organization is born, and it goes through a life cycle like any other form that comes into being and therefore ceases to be in the same form that exists now. It is a creation story of a circle, a cycle of life told by the right hemisphere of the brain, what I would call "Big Mind." It is a very different articulation than what the left hemisphere of the brain might postulate as a progression, a linear line progressing from a lower point to a higher point. This is a view from what I would call "Little Mind." The organization forms in response to circumstances that arise in the world. It goes through a youthful stage and then matures and approaches a zenith. After the peak, it begins to decline. It is usually here that two separate groups form within the organization. One group wants the organization to stay the same as it is and the other group wants the organization to change. If the organization continues to decline the polarization between these two different groups with different agendas grows more intense. They begin to polarize. This internal conflict is often complicated by external individuals and groups which share a similar agenda and align with one of the polarizing groups. I have lived through this cycle with multiple organizations that I belonged to and believed in. These inter-dynamics were previously hidden to me, and I was left confused by what I didn't understand because it made no sense to me.

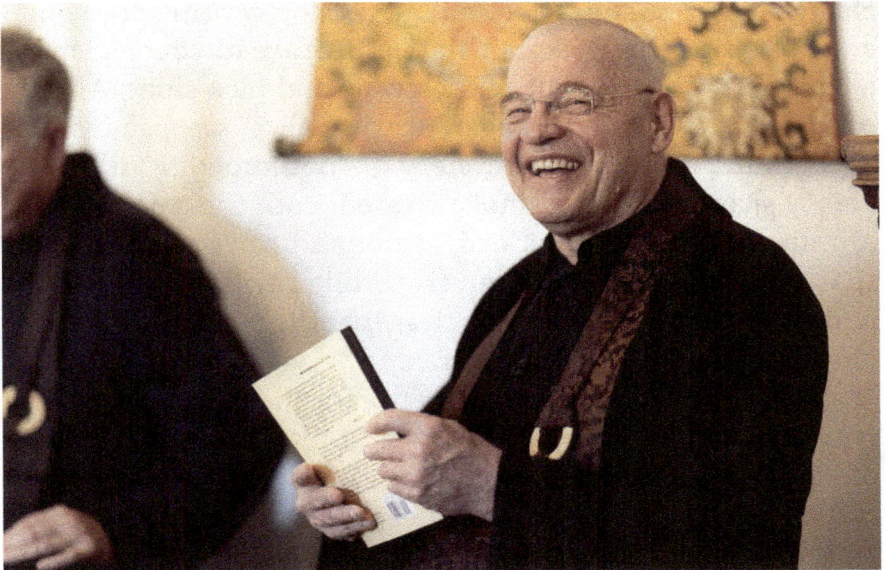

Doshin teaching on retreat in Arizona

It wasn't until Ken Wilber invited me to participate in a group where he laid this out with very specific examples in a very skillful way that slowly began to make sense. It has been profoundly useful to me and has enabled me to understand many things that I couldn't possibly understand before. Things like what causes war, for example.I intuitively knew that something needed to change radically in Integral

Zen. We had fallen into a familiar karmic groove. Something needed to die so something new could rise like a phoenix out of the ashes. On one very intense retreat, the energetic glue that was holding "US" together was loosening. The old "WE" was unraveling and falling apart. I could feel the tension rising like two opposing forces in the sangha, and I simply bore witness to what was unfolding. And unfold it did. Things began unraveling right along hidden fault lines that had not been visible before. I could now see that there were several factions aligning into two separate groups with different agendas. Each group had very different ideas of what should or shouldn't change in the organization. As the tension continued to build and polarize, I stood back and let nature take its course. I made a conscious decision not to intervene and pick sides. A sense of curiosity and wonder began to arise. As "I" stepped into the background a numinous mystery of "not knowing" filled the empty space. After the smoke cleared, both the "me" and the numinous mystery remained, although I can't truthfully say that we became one. All I can truthfully say is we are not one and we are not two. It became clear that the organization could change, could be symbolically reborn.

Another life cycle very naturally began, and it was my karmic responsibility as a lineage holder; to maintain the integrity of the lineage by keeping it pure. It is the lineage holder's responsibility to keep the lineage teachings from being polluted and poisoned by the individual and collective agendas and delusions of all beings. After the smoke cleared, neither of the opposing group's collective agendas and delusions were fulfilled and the individuals who were strongly identified with and invested in those agendas eventually chose to leave the organization, which saddened me deeply. As my Zen teacher said: "Things are as they are because they can be no different." As one of my Dharma heirs said after becoming a lineage holder: "The sangha is not a family." It is not a place to resolve your family karma. That is a hidden agenda and delusion. This sangha is a place, a sacred space that supports the healing and awakening of all beings. Both healing and awakening are two of *the best things in life that will come unbeknownst to you.* You, me or we cannot make them happen or know when or if they will happen. Only not-knowing, knows.

T he organization of Integral Zen slowly re-focused on **healing and awakening** in a fresh new way. A new "WE" began to emerge. Remember that each "ME" and "WE" will come and go, and even the karmic patterns will change, though much more slowly like the mountains and the seas. Only nothing, the Vast Empty Silence is always the same, never changing.

Over the last few years it has gradually become clear to me that the expression in Integral Theory about Growing Up, Waking Up, Cleaning Up and Showing Up, which I had adopted from Ken and had been dogmatically repeating, had become a meaningless platitude. It was too abstract and had lost its aliveness. It needed to be simplified in a more Zen-like way, and that was the beginning of a fresh new Integral Zen Framework: *It is impossible to fully awaken without healing, and it is impossible to fully heal without awakening.* So, with all this in mind, let it "fall like rain on a hot tin roof." Let it enter your heart.

Healing involves many, many lifetimes. We are not just healing ourselves, we are also healing the wounds of our ancestors and purifying the karma of all beings. After modernity, healing must also include deep trauma and shadow work, as well as knowledge from science and deep insight from authentic lineage wisdom traditions. This and Kosmic Addressing is part of what I learned directly from Wilber and what I am calling *inter-holonic inter-dynamics.* Awakening is not a half-hearted casual affair; it is a whole-hearted commitment, which almost always requires a disciplined investment of 40,000 hours of serious religious practice inspired not by religious beliefs but by religious devotion that leads to a causal state vantage point and beyond.

W hen modern science negated religion, it closed the door to the traditional paths of Noble Wisdom. Now more than ever in the history of the human race, we need that door to reopen and the ancient noble wisdom paths to re-appear; the lineage paths that have been successfully followed by millions of human beings for thousands of years. We need to transcend the limitations of left brain science and re-include not just wisdom but the "noble wisdom" of right brain legitimate lineage traditions. We need both a new version of science and a new version of religions, and they need to be integrated into something that doesn't yet exist. The religious function of human beings can be negated but never eliminated. We are religious animals. Karma enters the individual human being at conception. There is nothing in modern western psychology that can help us heal or purify karma. This requires the religious function and devotional religious practices. Modernity at least in the West has negated religion and devalued religious practices. Postmodernity proclaims the possibility of being spiritual but not religious. This however is a fallacy that causes harm by breeding a false sense of spirituality which has little if any integrity. Is it even possible to be truly spiritual without being religious? This is a profound question that hasn't yet even been asked.

Janel is a gifted healer and trained scholar who provides a wonderful overview of some of the powerful original teachings of deep lineage traditions where healing and awakening have not yet been split into two and separated from nature. And I am an old fool who relentlessly talks about nothing, which is the only water that can quench our deepest thirst, so our deepest wounds can finally heal. What enables us to work together to benefit all beings is our unique hypersensitivities which arose out of our karmic wounds. She has a gift for seeing and feeling imbalances, and I have a gift for smelling and intuiting lies, shadows and hypocrisy. By working together for the benefit of all beings, we are also creating space for our own healing and awakening to continue its karmic unfolding.

May you find something useful in this book and the books to follow that helps you lead a richer life and benefit more beings, especially yourself on your own sacred path of healing and awakening.

INTRODUCTION

Reverend Shikyo Jiryu Janel Houton

I n the midst of midlife confusion (when unresolved experiences rear their head, calling for healing), feeling driven by restless, disruptive energies, internal strife, unsure of what was happening and also simply experiencing a lengthy sense of unease, I clearly remember wondering, *is it actually really possible, to experience mostly ease, to be content, at peace within, and with what is*? Maybe a decade later, I am learning that the answer is yes, it is possible, to heal, to live more *in* peace than *out* of peace, and to experience profound trust in the ground of just being. Doshin Roshi and I share the intention to describe in this book what we have found most helpful, in creating what you could call "sign posts", towards paths, for healing and awakening.

My individual path to self-awareness was slow to start, and yet, it is a path most people will simply never embark on. While now I see many synchronicities within the trajectory of my life, it was many years before any clarity began to dawn, or before I was even ready to be introduced to Buddhist *right view*. Only with time, gradual practice, and experience could I start appreciating the entirety of my life, of what I was *born into*. So today with gratitude, I acknowledge the incredible blessings that have led to the present moment, and the love and support of so many people, my family, teachers, people I work with, and other beings, present and past.

O n a cold, clear New England January day, walking outside, I suddenly remembered close to 50 years ago, being with my mother at the allergy doctor.

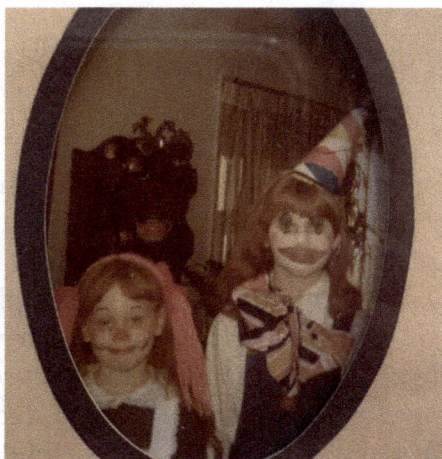

Janel the clown on the right with her sister, during some of the worst of her asthma, around the age 9 or 10

I remembered him telling her that the best thing for my health would be to move to the dry Southwestern US. Why was I remembering this so many years later? I quickly realized that that particular moment was likely the first time I became aware that there are multifaceted influences on health. I was maybe nine years old, and while I was acutely aware of the discomfort of my allergies, asthma, insomnia, and knew that I desperately did not want to feel like this, I also recall that this statement piqued my curiosity, along with sadness and helplessness, since almost certainly, my family could not pick up and leave everything just for my illness. At the time I wondered, and feared, if from now on *I would just always be sick.*

This was a hard time, and for a few years, I was quite sick. I remember constantly throughout the fall from the age nine to thirteen being caught in cycles of strong allergies, moderate to significant asthma attacks, taking steroid medications with side effects, adrenal activation and exhaustion, (having no idea why) insomnia, falling asleep in school, always tired. During this time I was told and hoped that I might grow out of the acute phase, which around the age of fourteen, I finally did.

Of course now as an adult, aware of interdependence, seeing the horror of children and families suffering in so many places in the world filled with poverty, strife, or those in the path of destructive climate chaos, I count my blessings to have only experienced what I did. At the same time just as I tell the people I support, one should not dismiss one's experiences, because our experiences greatly impact our development (children don't have the capacity to understand what is happening the way adults do), our lifelong relationship and quality of health, experiences, beliefs, patterns, and karma. Our early experiences impact the whole of life. As children, even in families where there was enough to eat and shelter was not threatened, there can be illness, physical, emotional pain and suffering for many reasons, that almost always have precedents, and interdependent contexts of what led to those conditions. What appears evident is that unprocessed trauma, loss, abuse, grief, unhealthy attachment patterns, do not simply disappear as new generations come along. On many levels, what is not addressed, healed or integrated, continues on, more often unconsciously than consciously, until or unless it is faced, healed, accepted, integrated and allowed–given permission–to metaphorically see the light of day. These are the times we very much live in, where so much of what

I have just described keeps being passed on, by and large unconsciously, individually and collectively. The unresolved pain of the past lives on in the energy and unconscious lives of its descendents: how this is frequently revealed is where relatively small triggers activate what can feel like life threatening levels of fear, and reactivity.

As I say this everyday I see the patterns I'm describing laid out in people's lives. We all are born into family "karmic" (cause and effect) constellations that greatly shape our experience and conditioning internally, while on the surface, external aspects of life can appear relatively "normal", so that what is hidden is temporarily masked. While Western (European and American life) has been for much of the world in the 20th century a model of living standards, under the surface, life for many, is not as happy and neat as it appears. Parents and grandparents of adults living today in Western countries, for example, may have left lives in strife-filled countries or experienced prior wars, great hardship, which dramatically impacted them, and thus, following generations this continues on often below the surface. People all over the world obviously still experience crisis situations now, and will be dealing with the impact of it, for further generations. Relatively "successful" families carry the karma of both how the success was generated, (most obviously for example families with legacies of slaveholding) and intergenerational pressure to live up to past standards, as well as maintaining the power, money and control over what was gained. Another problem with intergenerational wealth and success is the not uncommon neglect and abuse of children, often resulting from the karma of wealth and the privileges, indulgences, and addictions it invites. From what I observe, wealth rarely fosters ideal caregiving environments for children. Educational opportunities may often be more highly prioritized, but nurturance and attunement is often more complicated, and more frequently done by hired nannies.[1]

Tragedies that are personal or collective, are often buried by people, in an attempt to start anew, or from the fear of revealing vulnerability or weaknesses. Pogroms, religious and political persecution, war (victims of war, perpetrators/victims of being aggressors of war), starvation, just as well interpersonal trauma, simple *bad luck*, people tend to wish to forget events that were not that long ago... and yet, the effects of these histories run deep, in ways that we are only beginning to understand or acknowledge. Survivors of these experiences often masked and mask their trauma, self-medicating through addiction, or may have trouble with violence, keeping secrets, may have been the victims of and also perpetrating incest, mental illness; some of these being more easily hidden than others. *I see this in every single family history I review.* All of this carries down to the current generation, in our bodies, our psyches, our personal and collective unconscious, our health. This does not even cover the victims of wide scale persecution, due to race, religion, ethnicity, etc.. where there is deep moral injury, and families have struggled to even meet the most basic needs, with little or no opportunity for internal exploration or healing.

Most of Western medicine and healthcare is blind to the nuances of these legacies, although symptomatically, clinically there are often signs, and medicine is changing. Meanwhile it is spiritual, traditional, indigenous, wisdom traditions, where a wider perspective and framework can often provide a context of looking at cause and effect (karma), the impact on health, physical, emotional, mental and spiritual, as well as the environment and all the life systems contained, which cannot be excluded, and point to pathways for healing. Most of these systems however do not include an *Integral Framework*, which for understanding the contemporary world's conflicts and polarization, is critical.

Returning to today, from my childhood perspective, getting through the worst of my health as a child, reaching the age of fifty-six and walking outside in the stark Massachusetts cold, I greatly appreciate having arrived at the present moment, this age, my life. The recall of this early experience taught me to *never, ever, take my health for granted*, as anyone who has experienced challenging health conditions comes to know.

This only touches on the seemingly endless interdependencies, which support health (and likewise, disease, or the imbalances that lead to disease). Further health problems as an adult for me, would point to having originated from karmic causes from my early life, and my family's struggles, which were the basis for what would unfold in my own life, and health. Only in my studies of introductory Tibetan Medicine, would it become (finally!) glaringly apparent, that karmic, interdependent factors were dynamically impacting health, and specifically, my health, as a child, that has carried throughout my life.

I realized that my early health problems didn't start with my own life...Eastern medicine recognizes that the lungs store grief, not just my grief, but my family's grief. I did not have memories of struggles breathing or hospitalization as a two year old, where my mother said I was "very very angry" at being left alone. I had no early knowledge of the genetic predisposition of my Italian American grandfather's asthma (whose mother suffered a terrible tragic loss of her young mother, in his early life around the age of 2 or 3).

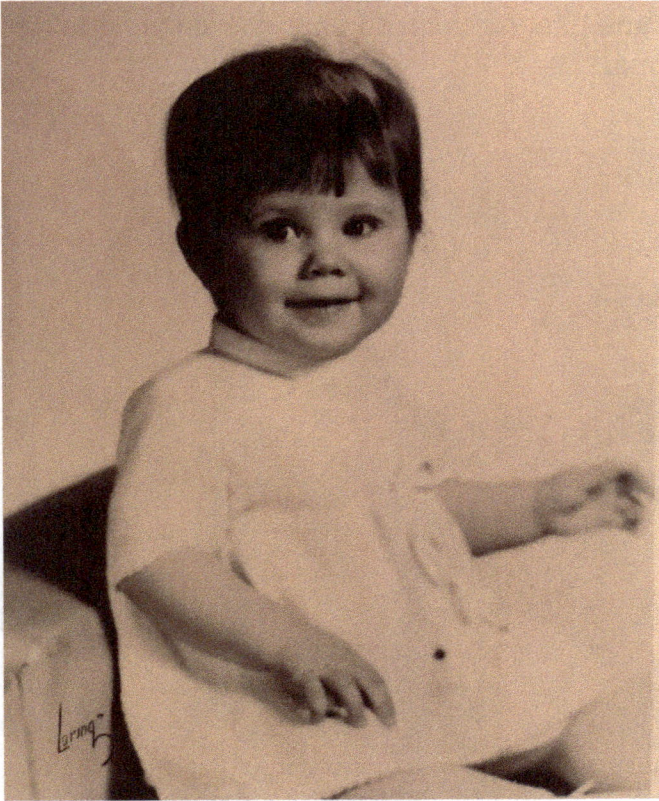

Young Janel

I would learn that he and I had a karmic connection with our lung health, and family tragedies that took place at approximately the same age for us. As a two year old I experienced the effects of this family tragedy my own father was involved in, something I would have no knowledge of for another 45 years, when my father's increasing dementia led him to mention something that had been long buried, leading me to discover this history. What I uncovered was a tragic accident that threw my parents into great distress, guilt, public shame, and fear, while my mother was pregnant with my sister, and I was two. At this young age I could not have understood in any rational way, but experienced viscerally, and would have experienced my parents changing in an instant, and likely activated in me, the (epigenetic) propensity for asthma.

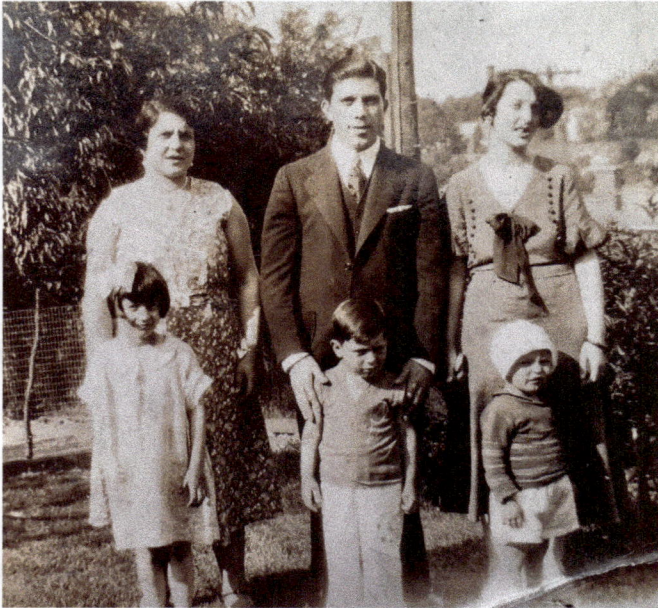

Janel's Italian American family, grandfather George in the center of the picture as a child, with her Great Grandparents to the right

My family of relatively recent immigrants struggled to establish themselves in America, a suffering common in the US in the early 20th century. Deadly childhood illness, pre-antibiotics, premature deaths, the toll and sacrifices of fighting in wars, accidental death due to poor reproductive care, sexual trauma, alcoholism, mental illness all impacted my family and many others of these generations. Higher mortality was common before antibiotics and improved health care.

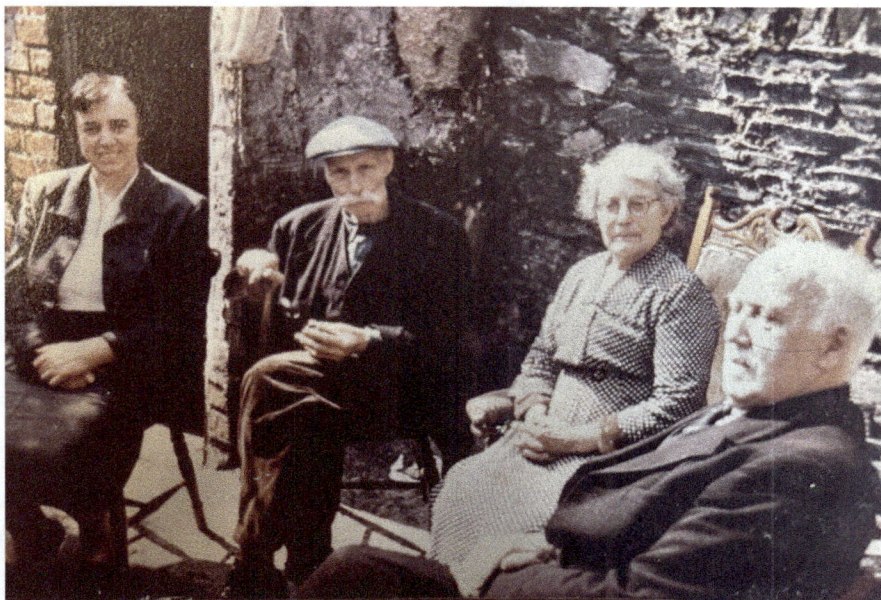

Janel's paternal grandmother on the left, and Great grandparents next to her in Ireland

All of these factors I would come to realize, to a large extent-- like everyone I do healing work with–I was "born into." Only now could I weave together the patches and pieces, and with a devoted daily spiritual practice, come to acceptance, first starting to see my own imbalances, which have settled gradually over time, and then start to see how I could facilitate and support others, towards healing and balance.

M y early life set me off towards seeking health and healing, though this did not become conscious for some time. I remember my mother searching for healing remedies through nutrition, in addition to weekly anti-allergy shots, and her exploring what were called "health foods" in the 1970s. I remember an early tofu egg salad sandwich (not successful), gagging on cold yeast drinks, cod liver oil, and vitamins.

Now I meet with people from vastly different backgrounds, ages, life experiences, to explore what they were born into. Over time we revisit their ancestry, family, cultures, histories, health, spiritual development, so that I can help provide guidance and identify karmic patterns that people unconsciously repeat, that are hard to see on our own. It is a dynamic process that everyone isn't ready for, and I adapt as needed to support integration, healing, and also if they are inclined, directing them towards spiritual development by encouraging meditation and spiritual practices. This is where working with Doshin Roshi has been so transformative. This is also where his own healing journey, crossed paths with mine, coming together and evolving now to create frameworks and possibilities for the many people we encounter and work with, towards healing and awakening.

Back to Christmas of 2018, my husband gave me a gift of shadow work sessions with Doshin Roshi. I think I first became aware of Doshin through some of his interviews with spiritual teacher Andrew Cohen in a documentary, since my husband had lived in, and left, Andrew's community after following him as a student for many years.

Doshin and I had started meeting at a time when I was feeling a lot of imbalance, fear, confusion and angst as I have described, but now I recognize was a storm of unseen, unacknowledged and unresolved generational and early childhood trauma coming to the surface.

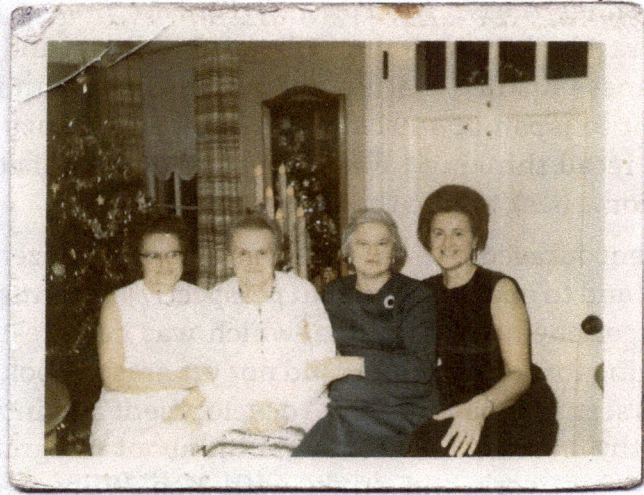

Janel's Polish American grandmother on the right, from the left her Great Aunt, then Janel's Great Grandmother from Poland, and other Great Aunt

Both sides of my parent's families mostly immigrated to the US in the mid to late and early 20th centuries, (my great great grandparents were the first Polish emigrants to become US citizens), a small number earlier, bringing with them as immigrants do, a variety of struggles in establishing themselves in a new country, along with the Depression, wars and all the impacts of living in such times (and the situations they all left in Europe). But perhaps what I see now was the lingering impacts in particular of the *known* traumas.

Doshin worked one-on-one with me initially much through dream exploration, and my prolific dreams, and my struggling to find the right direction spiritually, that really started around 2006 when challenges in my life and health arose during the process of adopting my daughter, after I lived in Japan for ten years. At that time I found Buddhism the only source from which I could make sense of what I was experiencing, and one book in particular I read devotedly and carried with me everywhere by the Dalai

Lama: *Healing Anger: The Power of Patience from a Buddhist Perspective.* I had studied some Tibetan Buddhism and Chinese and Japanese history, culture and art in college, and when I first went to Japan in 1991 I read a book by DT Suzuki about Zen and recall thinking I was not yet ready for this then but that I'd come back to it in the future.

Doshin encouraged me to establish a regular Zazen sitting practice, and to open to a Jungian perspective in terms of what I was experiencing at the time, which was deep restlessness and longing for something I could not yet grasp. (Looking back now this seems to have been the development and integration of a healthy *animus*). He also taught me about Integral Theory based on his work and study with Ken Wilber, and as I started volunteering for Integral Zen, I gradually shifted out of my disturbance, into a context of understanding what I was experiencing, and identifying and integrating, gradually, what was helpful for my stabilization, healing and practice, and what was not.

Following a retreat in the fall of 2021 at the Aryaloka Buddhist Center in New Hampshire, Doshin shared more about own needs for healing, having experienced significant Pediatric Medical Trauma (PMT) as a child. Doshin had been describing to me some of his experience in somatic healing through breathwork, and the dramatic unleashing and (re)traumatization he experienced in what he described as doing too much too fast, resulting in overwhelming dysregulation, what happens when the arising of trauma is not properly titrated/ paced.

Having attended school for Massage Therapy in 2009 (I had prior degrees in Art History and Historic Documentation and Research), and past work as a massage therapist, and having explored many alternative health options, practicing yoga, and an interest in wider contexts for viewing healing and my own energetic healing capacities, I started reviewing old references, looking at connections between Hindu chakra systems and developmental histories, with trauma, and health in general. As I worked with him reigniting my prior explorations, before I knew it, we were using Integral theory, the teachings of Carl Jung, and Zen, to form a method to work with people, piecing and weaving together both Eastern and Western approaches I had engaged with throughout my life. From my time and work in Japan I had a foundation of cultural knowledge, working in healthcare and religious settings for another decade (a Boston Cancer Hospital, a Healthcare provider, four different ministers, and Shambhala Boston), I then started studying Tibetan Medicine with the Sowa Rigpa Institute and Dr. Nida Chenagtsang and Dr. Caroline van Damme in their Sowa Rigpa Counseling program. Combining basic Tibetan Medicine, Buddhist healing history and training, and Western health and Psychology (Dr. Caroline is a Belgian Psychiatrist), this helped me further refine a method to support my own and others' healing, holistic balance, and wholeness.

In 2023 after a few years of introducing healing, teaching, and using a technique from Chinese Meridian and Acupressure systems, along with Buddhist healing methods at our live retreats, Doshin Roshi and I began an online series of Courses, called *Introduction to Integral Zen Healing*, Integral Chakras. 2023 was our first Introduction Course, and in 2024 we taught two more, first was *Foundations, the early Chakras,* and then the *Heart Chakra*. In the fall of 2025 our final course in the series is planned, for the throat to the crown chakras (*The Upper Chakras - Gateways to Transcendence and Liberation*).

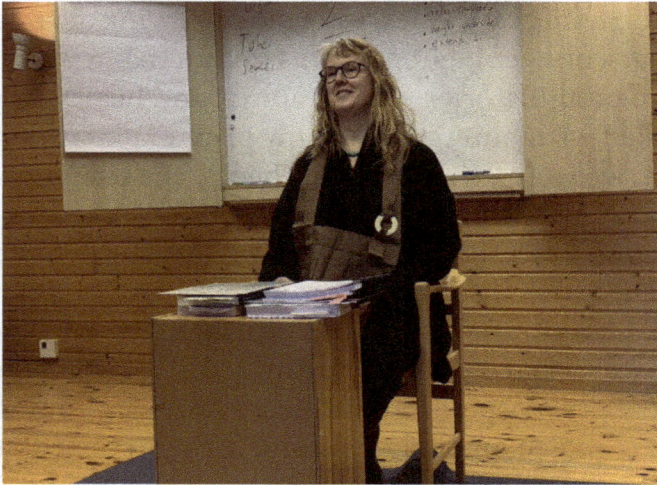

Janel teaching in Sweden, 2025

What the courses present is our unique perspective on healing and awakening, which is summarily, a system offering perspectives including Eastern and Western practices, methodologies, modalities and approaches, for returning to balance to wholeness, including acceptance and preparation for death, and ending our wars, within.

What we lay out are *potentials*, emphasizing that what works must be discovered by the individual, as the Buddha supposedly said, that *the heart knows the way, when the foot touches the ground*. Why we are writing this book is so that we may share our approach wider, and also offer a reference for all of the people we work with and support. Doshin and I have seen remarkable healing in the work we do with others, and living during a time where people are constantly flooded with overwhelming, distorted, chaotic, fragmented information, often from unknown and thus questionable sources (made more confusing by AI), we feel it is important to point back to the many Wisdom Traditions which have supported humans for not just thousands, but tens if not hundreds of thousands of years. Great confidence is available when one establishes a trust that balance, freedom, healing, liberation, and unreasonable joy, are accessible to anyone, and can be (re)discovered within. As Dr. Nida Chenagtsang says, the teacher just reminds the student of what is already there. So let us share with you, what has been so healing for us, and many others.

Lastly, I want to acknowledge all of those who have supported me in this work and development, more than anyone Doshin Roshi who took the time to work with me from where I was when we met, and support my evolution and healing, and also the guidance of the great mystery, available to us all. Dreams directed me towards meeting Doshin, led me to find Dr. Nida, and the training and guidance on how to assist in people's healing. Also the people, sources and other Wisdom Tradition teachers that have shared additional precious methods for healing, instruction where people need help most in their health, and the methods that will be most effective. To the individuals and divine forces that guide us, I bow.

The following is adapted and edited from transcripts of the *Introduction to Integral Zen Healing* Course, from 2023, with Doshin Roshi and Rev Shikyo Janel Houton.

PATHS AND PRACTICES FOR BALANCE AND WHOLENESS

CHAPTER 1, THE ROOT CHAKRA

Doshin Roshi

Here we are. Let's begin with the teachers.[2] There are a bunch of troublemakers, some lineage holders and some incredible teachers. Many of these are teachers of mine and many of them Janel's. Let's just take a moment, and really show them some deep respect, and devotion. As Daniel P. Brown used to say, "let's call in the retinue." The retinue of teachers and teachings, the presence of generations and generations of teachers and their teachings. A living stream of lineage holders, each realizing the deepest truth of who they are. A lineage that flows down from timeless time into the present moment that is now. Looking out from this pure awareness realized by each lineage holder, this present moment is not separate from the past, not separate from the future. It is all here now. It is just this, naked isness that just is. It is "What Is." Just this, Buddha Nature, before human nature adds anything to "what is" or takes anything away from it. Before anything is filtered out or projected in. This is the teaching that has been perpetually taught and received. A teacher accepts students, who study until some become teachers. And they accept other students, who study until they become teachers. This is the living stream of purified, realized, embodied awareness. Let's just be silent and still for a few moments, and call in this sacred retinue.

Janel

I hope that people will reflect on their own teachers. I suppose you may do this, but that's part of my practice every night, is gratitude for all the teachers I have and have had, and teachers who didn't necessarily know they were teachers. Some very humble people.

Doshin

All the bodhisattvas, all the human beings who have triggered me. All of my teachers who have encouraged me to face a part of myself I didn't want to face. Deepest bows to all of you. So what's this introduction, Janel?

Janel

So we're going to outline a bit how each class is going to be. Doshin is going to teach parts of each section. In this course we will introduce some variations of chakra systems and how we are using them; we're going to talk about a variety of views and systems of subtle energy, almost all traditional systems originating from Asia and India. We will introduce each of the chakras, and do exercises. Some exercises will be on your own, then group ones, as well as ideas you can explore on your own. We'll do an introduction to the Tibetan Medicine Buddha lineage, Five Element theory and the Sowa Rigpa framework. Here and there, I'll introduce some varieties of Buddhist and other selected Asian lineage healing methods. It's not just talking about it historically, we are doing exercises and explorations. The more we talk about this, the more you'll see the interconnectedness, and then in further courses we'll explore this introductory ground in greater depth and detail. Also, I just want to state that my knowledge is very limited, and as I paraphrase the wisdom of another teacher, anything that will be presented to you that comes through, is due to the transmission, blessings and wisdom from the lineages and teachers I have studied with. That which is incorrect, is due to my limitations.

Doshin

That is really taking ownership of all of our limitations and giving homage to all the teachers and teachings. If we could all just do that, we would be further on the path to "just getting along." By practicing, by cultivating respect and humility, we each can contribute to the world being a better place. To this I bow, let's all bow together. Thank you, Janel.

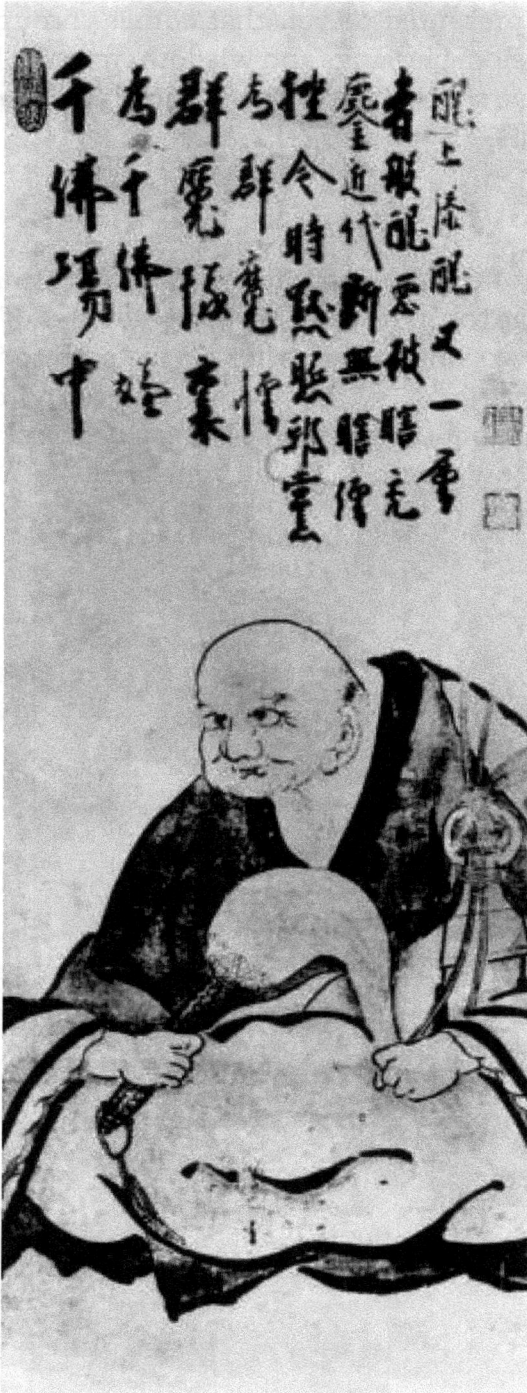

Hakuin Eikaku, (1686–1769) Self-portrait, Edo period (1603–1867), Public Domain

Zen Master Hakuin Eikaku, 1686 – 1769

Hakuin was born in the 1600s in Japan; his career extended into the 1700s into the 18th century. He entered the Zen lineage at a time when Rinzai Zen (Linchi Zen), Samurai Zen, had almost completely died. Hakuin was a real troublemaker; he took no prisoners and produced 80 some Dharma heirs. Then, he got sick, with an incurable disease which some might call Zen disease. Studying so intensely had disturbed the delicate balance of his health, radically disturbed it. Several had indicated that his condition was incurable. Because of this disease, many had written Hakuin off. But, he knew that there were some teachers out there with mysterious healing powers that could heal him. He heard of an old Taoist master who lived in the forest named Hakuyu. He went high into the mountains to find him and begged him to teach him how he could heal. Hakuyu was part of an ancient oral tradition that had been passed on from teacher to teacher for many generations. The old Daoist master was able to heal Hakuin's Zen disease. Hakuin brought these healing practices into the Rinzai Zen school where they still remain to this day.

I find this story particularly moving because at a certain point in time I found that I was suffering from the same disease, Zen disease. I also went around looking for cures, I did all this shadow work, I did all this Trauma work, I did all this insecure attachment work, all this psychotherapy. I investigated many kinds of different healing methodologies, and finally, one of my students suggested that before I lose the ability to move my body that I go see this Chinese Tai Chi master. That was two years ago. The arthritis that I was suffering from, as well as many other things have completely disappeared. Then, at the same time, Janel showed up. She showed up with a discovery of some other healing methods that were part of Soto Zen, which had been brought from Japan to North America and northern Europe. I found these particularly useful for many of the health issues that I was facing, both physically, mentally and spiritually. We began adding these ancient healing methods and practices to Integral Zen, which was already an integration of Carl Jung, Ken Wilber and Zen. This is what we are beginning to present, this new integration in this course. I realized that it is impossible to fully heal without awakening. I've always known that, but what I really didn't understand is that it is also impossible to fully awaken without healing.

The most difficult thing to heal is karma. There is absolutely nothing that I've found in Western medicine or psychotherapy that will even touch the karma. For this, we have to turn to the East. We have to go into the ancient lineage religions and uncover these precious practices and practice them. We have to not only practice them, we have to integrate them into the inner and outer world that we live in. This course is the beginning of this integration, which I fully expect will take many generations before it's even adequately complete. So this is just the first step in this long path. Thank you, Hakuin.

I have been deeply influenced, of course, by Zen, as a lineage holder in Rinzai Zen. I have also been deeply influenced by the Depth psychology of Carl Jung and the direct teachings of Ken Wilber and his Integral theory.

Wilber's Four Quadrants

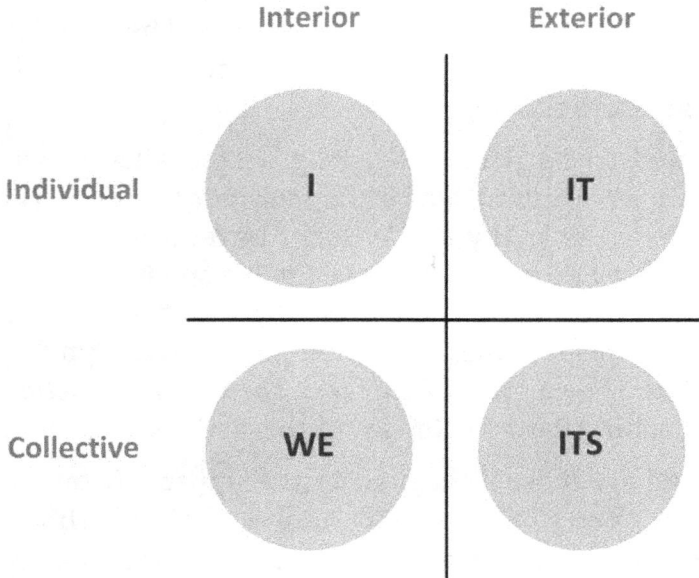

	Interior	Exterior
Individual	I	IT
Collective	WE	ITS

One of Wilber's primary teachings that has been radically helpful in Integral Zen's new understanding of the world is the 4 quadrants.

The horizontal line divides the world into the individual and the collective. There is never one single individual without many individuals. The individual and the collective are not separate. There is no independent individual self, outside of collective groups of other selves.

The vertical line divides the world into an interior, and an exterior, thus, we arrive at 4 quadrants. The individual interior "I" space in the Upper Left Quadrant. The individual exterior, the "it" space in the Upper Right Quadrant. The collective interior, the "we space" or cultural realm in the Lower Left Quadrant, and the exterior collective social realm in the Lower Right Quadrant. The Four Quadrants can be used very powerfully as a typology of themselves. The founders of Integral Coaching Canada wrote a very interesting article on the quadrants as a typology.

I was invited to be part of a group that evaluated all the articles that were submitted to the *Journal of Integral Theory and Practice*. It was led by Ken Wilber himself; this group met for about a year and a half to two years. We spent every Friday afternoon together, and we reviewed this article explaining how the Four Quadrants could be used as a Typology,[3] submitted to the *Journal of Integral Theory and Practice*, by Integral Coaching Canada. Ken loved this article.

Some people are most interested in the upper left quadrant, in personal inner subjective experiences, feelings, thoughts, beliefs, values and emotional states. Others are more interested in the upper right quadrant in the objects of outer experience, such as: bodies, behaviors, emotional energy and reactivity. Then there are others who are more interested in the lower left quadrant in the collective cultural aspects of the inner realm, such as: the shared collective values, beliefs and collective moods. The "we" space of inner collective emotional realms of groups, cultures and whole peoples. And then some others that are more interested in the lower right quadrant. The actual social structures, the actual organizations, laws and systems, the outer manifestations of collective emotional fields and reactivity. The collective religious movements, organizations and the external formations such as: lynch mobs and fans of sports teams. Now, I've had many conversations, one-on-one with Ken about Carl Jung, and there's some aspects of Jungian psychology that he loves. He told me that he studied it all deeply and there's some aspects that he felt were problematic. Carl Jung's Typology, the 4 cognitive functions, is one of the aspects of Jung's depth psychology that Wilber told me that he deeply respected and found very useful.

The Quadrants as a Typology

	Interior	Exterior
	Most Interested in UL:	Most Interested in UR:
Individual	Inner Experience Mind Beliefs & Values Emotional States	Outer Experience Body & Behaviors Emotional Energy
	Most Interested in LL:	Most Interested in LR:
Collective	Collective Culture Shared Values & Beliefs Collective Moods & Emotional Realms	Social Structures Laws & Systems Manifestations of Collective Emotional Fields

Carl Jung published his book *Psychological Types* in 1921. In it, he laid out a very sophisticated Theory of Psychological Types that is incredibly useful in understanding another of Jung's unique contributions, The Process of Individuation, the process of becoming a whole healthy individual. During WWII, a popularized version was introduced as the Myers Briggs Type Indicator (MBTI) by Katharine Briggs and her daughter Isabel Briggs Myers. The MBTI became very popular. Like many original works that are popularized, certain liberties were taken that watered down the original ideas in a way that made

Jung's Four Cognitive Functions

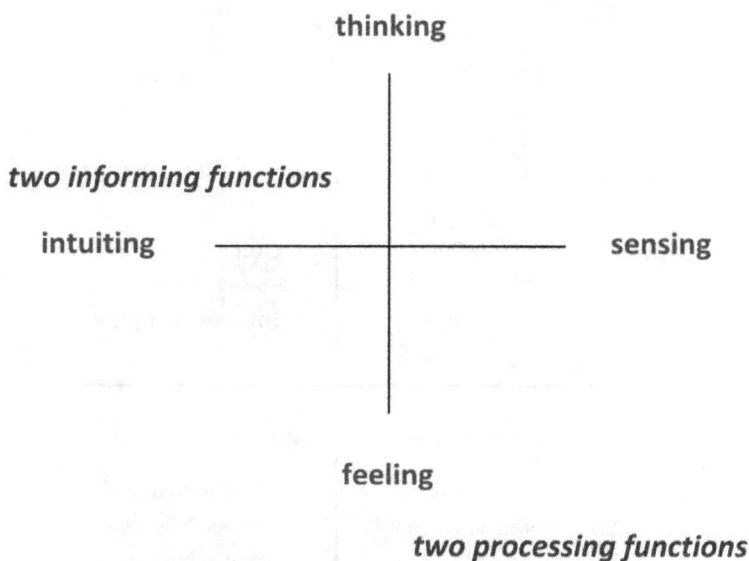

thinking

two informing functions

intuiting ———————————————— sensing

feeling

two processing functions

them more understandable but less valuable. From my perspective, they added something that was of questionable value and removed the most valuable and powerful components of Jung's Theory of Types which was the integration of the shadow into a more whole, healthy individual personality. Jung's Theory of Types involved a Herculean effort of examining many of the world's typological systems.

In his Theory, Jung proposes that there are essentially 4 cognitive functions, which human beings use to find their way in the world. There are two cognitive functions that inform us and two rational functions that we use to process that information and make decisions. The first informing function is sensation, or what is known in the modern world as the five senses. The second informing function is intuition, which Jung defines as direct knowing. The two cognitive functions that we use to process the information that we receive are the feeling and thinking functions. I would like to point out that both of these rational functions are dualistic. Thinking is dividing things into categories of good and bad, right and wrong, hot and cold, etc. The feeling function needs a little more explanation, especially in English. From my perspective in the context of Integral Zen, this is what we're really pointing to when we talk about emotional intelligence. For me, emotions are not intelligent, they are reactive. There is tremendous confusion about feelings and emotions in modern and postmodern Western Culture. The feeling function is intelligent, it is a rational function that we all use to process information and make decisions with. For example, I like to be safe. I don't like to be afraid. I "think" I will only go places where I "feel" safe and am not afraid. Emotions are reactive. For example: someone jumps out of the darkness and grabs me, and my reaction is fear. The actual intelligence that we attribute to emotions is actually what Jung is pointing to as the cognitive feeling function. Oh, I like this, I'm going to get more of this. Oh, I don't like that, I'm going to push that away. This is moving toward and moving away, which is a rational, intelligent function of cognition that we use fundamentally from almost the very beginning of our lives. (Buddhists might notice the similarities between Jung's feeling function and the first two poisons of attachment and aversion of the *five kleshas*.)

In the Myers Briggs Type Indicator, they left out one of the most important aspects of Jung's Theory of Types. They left out the dynamics of the dominant and inferior functions, which is extremely helpful for individuals to become conscious of their shadows. This is the first step on Jung's Process of Individuation, his process of becoming a healthy whole individual who becomes capable of living a productive, fruitful life.

The dominant function is the one that we trust the most, is the one that we learn to rely on as we grow up in the world. In Jung's Depth Psychology, the persona is the part of ourselves that we are conscious of, the mask we wear in relationships with others. Our persona naturally identifies with our dominant function. As the conscious persona begins to develop, it emerges along the same trajectory as the dominant function. For example, I am an intuitive type and my persona and whole ego structure has developed relying upon my intuition. This is what I learned to use and came to trust. This is how I have developed and found my way in the world. My second function is thinking, which means that I am informed by my intuitive function and process those intuitions with rational thinking.

The shadow on the other hand, is the part of ourselves that we don't know, the blind spot in our personality. It emerges along with the inferior function, the one that is opposite of the dominant function and in my case the dominant function is intuition and the inferior function sensation. This typology becomes an extremely useful tool as we begin the process of acquiring more complete self-knowledge, that includes the hidden shadow. As the self emerges and the ego begins to develop in relationship to the inner aspects of the psyche and outer aspects of the world. It gets even more important when considering deeper aspects of the psyche, the light and the dark aspects of the interdynamics within individual and collective relationships of personality and culture. This is really important and although we probably won't speak a lot about it here, it is foundational and has been used in creating the structure and content of this course.

Janel

So what Doshin just presented as we start exploring healing, it's important to keep in mind because whatever your dominant function is, this is where you're going to be much more aware of where you are healing. However what is actually happening, is it's happening in all four quadrants. Would you like to comment on tetra arising?

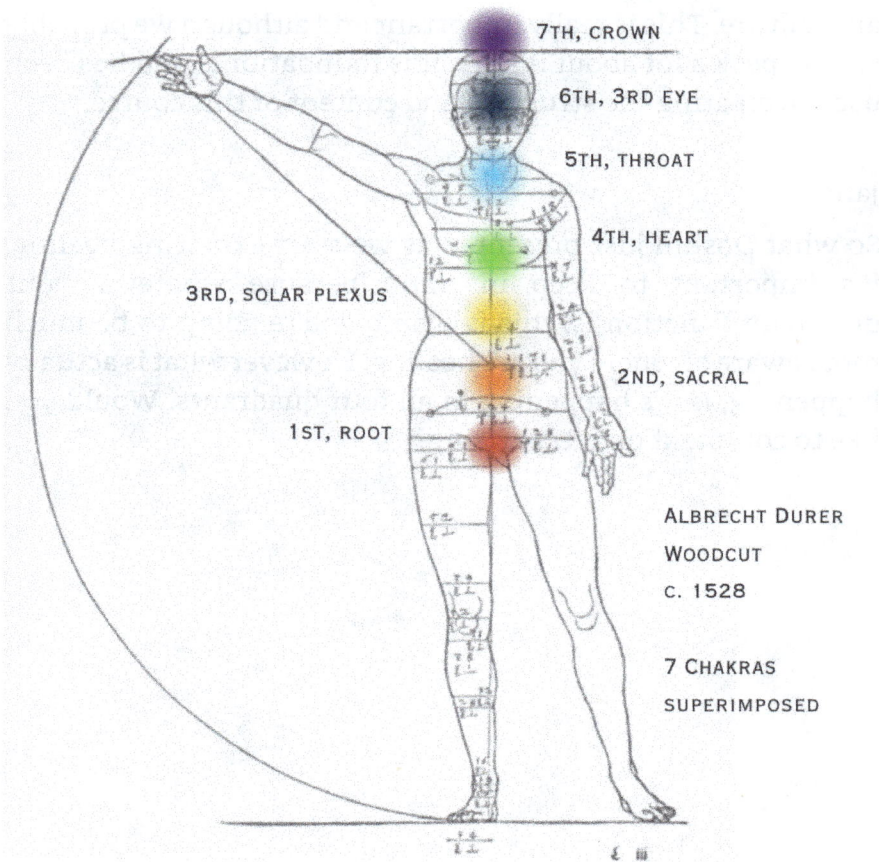

Figure of Woman Shown in Motion, Albrecht Durer, 1528. From Four Books of Human Proportion. Albertina, Vienna, Austria, image public domain, superimposed with text and color

Doshin

Yes, so both Wilber's *Four Quadrants* and Jung's *Theory of Types* are cognitive maps. They are conceptual tools that can be studied and used to help us understandand more skillfully interact with ourselves and the world in which we live and interact with others. Each alone is a powerful tool that can be used to heal and awaken. And when used together as we do in Integral Zen, their power and usefulness are exponentially increased. As for the Four Quadrants, it is helpful to keep in mind that if something arises in the lower left quadrant of the collective interior, the culture, it is also "tetra arising", meaning there's an aspect or impact of it simultaneously arising in all quadrants. Let's take for example dualistic thinking, the knowledge and assessment of whether something is right or wrong. This simultaneously arises in all quadrants. There's an individual aspect of it; there's a collective cultural aspect. There's an external object being experienced by an internal subject, and there's an aspect that resonates through the social structures. So, things are tetra arising in all quadrants, which makes it so helpful for us now. The scientific method emerged as a powerful tool that allowed us to conduct experiments, create hypotheses, test them, and evaluate the results in order to prove or disprove our hypotheses. That particular method is extremely effective in the upper right quadrant, the world of individual things. It is not so useful in the upper left quadrant of the world of our inner life, the religious and psychological aspects of our individual experiences, nor is that particular methodology useful in the lower left quadrant to understand the interdynamics between different cultures. So, understanding that everything is tetra arising, and seeing the relationship between what's arising in one quadrant and tracing it as it arises simultaneously in other quadrants, as it tetra arises in all quadrants, is an extremely powerful tool, and way of consciously interacting in the world.

Hopefully we will explore some examples of that in the exercises we're doing.

Janel

Yes thank you Doshin. As all of you come to know and understand better what your dominant function is, it's important to bring more attention to the opposite, which is your inferior function, what quadrant that might be, and really inquire. For example, what am I blind to? Where am I undeveloped? Because once you are paying attention, it will keep coming up again and again.

Doshin

Wilber says wherever you find one individual, you'll find many individuals; you'll never find one without many. That's just kind of a way of restating the third mark of existence of no self, nothing exists as an island unto itself. Everything is interrelated, interconnected, inter-penetrating with other things. There is not an individual that exists outside of a collective of individuals. You know, every deer has a herd. Every bee has a hive. Every goose has a gaggle. We don't exist as independent islands, so that's just kind of a loop back into basic Buddhist wisdom that I chuckle about. And apparently, Janel does too.

Janel

This map is important for when you start to recognize where you're needing karmic healing. The way the world is now with so much global change, a lot of people are really faced with a need for what we sometimes refer to as ancestral and karmic healing. It's much bigger than me, or you-for example, the second you may think "I'm healing…" it's actually much more than that.

I'm going to jump around a bit in terms of what we're looking at, remember you don't necessarily need to understand this, because I'm covering a big web which includes many traditions.

First of all, you may wonder, how are we going to use chakras for this course? Most people know the basic meaning, that the -origin of the word *chakra* comes from *wheel* or *cycle*. The first description was said to be an ancient Hindu teaching going back through millennia, a model that would become central to tantric spiritual traditions, including yoga. Most traditional systems used between three and six chakras, and the seven chakra system that has become popular, emerged relatively recently.[4] Also when we're using this, we're definitely not saying that there are only seven chakras. There are many chakras in the body, it is said even hundreds, but it's dynamic and varies with different systems, frameworks and the approach you are using.

Wilber begins to use chakras in *Sex, Ecology and Spirituality*, and explores the shadow dysfunctions in *The Religion of Tomorrow*. I know that ROT may seem like an intimidating book, but it works well as a reference, where you don't necessarily have to understand all of what he is presenting, and it contains a lot relative to what we're talking about. Doshin, is there anything you would like to comment on here?

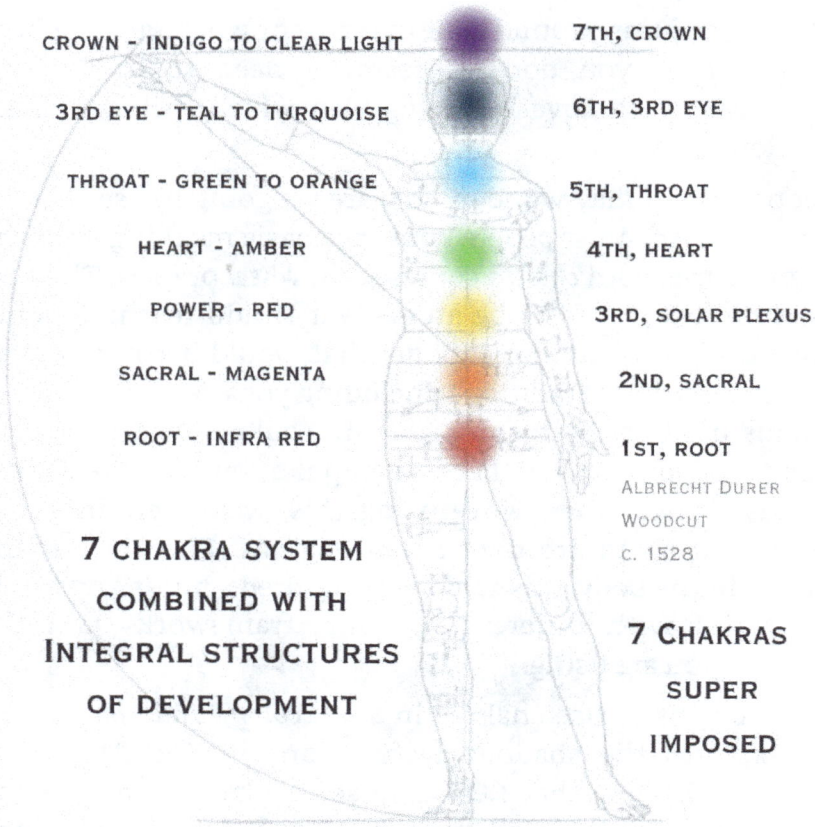

CROWN - INDIGO TO CLEAR LIGHT   7TH, CROWN

3RD EYE - TEAL TO TURQUOISE   6TH, 3RD EYE

THROAT - GREEN TO ORANGE   5TH, THROAT

HEART - AMBER   4TH, HEART

POWER - RED   3RD, SOLAR PLEXUS

SACRAL - MAGENTA   2ND, SACRAL

ROOT - INFRA RED   1ST, ROOT

ALBRECHT DURER
WOODCUT
C. 1528

7 CHAKRA SYSTEM
COMBINED WITH
INTEGRAL STRUCTURES
OF DEVELOPMENT

7 CHAKRAS
SUPER
IMPOSED

Doshin

Yes, in *Sex, Ecology and Spirituality* and in another paper Wilber published he outlines a way that he uses chakras that I want to mention; he's using chakras to describe ego development. For example: the root chakra is roughly equivalent to the infrared stage of ego development. The second chakra is synonymous with the magenta stage, the third chakra, the power chakra with the red stage of development.

The fourth chakra, the heart chakra with the amber stage. The fifth chakra, the throat chakra with both the orange and the green stages. The sixth with 2nd Tier and the seventh with 3rd Tier. So, we are using the chakras in a similar way, intermingling a lot of this chakra information, with developmental theory as Wilber uses it. I mention this here, and it'll become more evident as we move on. This is the way Janel and I have really started using this material as we are working with individuals, which you'll see reflected in the exercises. I have been personally blown away by how powerful this is with the people who we are both, simultaneously working with, and with myself as well, getting into the karma, the deep karma that I couldn't reach, without these lineage teachings and ancient healing methods.

Janel

In terms of physical location and area, each chakra has a gross location in the body that has physiological effects within the body, so with physical manifestations, as well as energetic qualities and impacts. Dr. Nida Chenagtsang says they function similar to hormones, for example the endocrine system is related to the gross chakras. Energies are subtle, and then causal is going to be less obvious or not visible to most people, with few likely to ever reach that stabilized level of state realization or understanding. So the chakras serve as body/mind energy centers, relating to the control and flow of vital life force energies, and energy channels. Further on we will also look at different traditions and frameworks. I'll get to a Chinese perspective later and go more in depth with the Tibetan frameworks.

From a more scientific materialist or matter view, the cardiovascular, lymphatic, and acupuncture meridian systems work similarly to the chakras. These correspond with brain, nervous, plexuses and acupuncture points; note that the channels and chakras are closely interrelated. Chakras interchange the physical and subtle, subtle and causal. Subtle energy can be transformed into physical life force energies. This is something that most of you probably won't understand yet but later on may become more clear.

Again how we're using the seven chakra system in part corresponds with the integral structures of development. We start with the first root chakra which corresponds to Integral infrared, this developmental period, initially is usually considered birth to six months, but now I actually expand this in that it's not only conception, it's even what happened before conception into the first six months (more on that later). Let's not forget then what a dramatic transition the baby faces when it is born out into the world. It goes from being limited within the mother's body, to a sudden stark experience of coming out, and separation without understanding what that is, is important to keep in mind, since it is how we first experience (up)rooting in the world, outside of our mother.

The second sacral chakra is generally referred to as physically located about four finger widths below the belly button and back into the spine;[5] it corresponds to Integral magenta period, so 6 to 18 months roughly- but remember, the developmental periods are going to vary individual to individual. I didn't mention before, the root is pre-pre-first person perspective. What that means is there's just no sense of a separated individual self for the baby. So, sacral is then the pre-first person perspective.

The third power chakra is located at the solar plexus, is at Integral red, so from about 18 months to 3 or 4 years old which is the beginning of first person perspective. That means the child declares, "I me mine", or attempts to, again this is dependent on each setting and individual.

The fourth heart chakra is in the center of the chest, it is Integral amber, that's the beginning of second person perspective and this is where the child is indoctrinated into whatever belief system they live in, of their family, culture, etc. *We are all indoctrinated into some belief system, culture and context.* This period is usually starting around ages 4-6 or 7, again this is debatable and will vary. Second person perspective means now there is not only I, but *I* can see *you*, as an object. The indoctrination usually happens at the age of five to six. These significant developmental markers are only able to happen when the child is developmentally ready. So trying to expect that children meet developmental stages too early is considered potentially harmful (for example forcing children to read too early); they will not have the capacity to do so, the timing has to be right. (This is the case for learning in general).

The fifth chakra at the throat–located at the throat–is Integral orange to green. So at about 7 or 8 years to late adolescence, early adulthood. This is where we have third and fourth person perspectives and at this point, not everyone living now, will reach these developmental levels, or levels of perspectives. Again it's going to depend on the individual, the culture, their development. Many individuals just stop developing. Remember likewise cultures have limits. Primitive (not meant to be pejorative–meaning undeveloped, preliterate, etc) cultures of which there are probably less than a handful left in the world now, isolated indigenous cultures, may still be at an infrared level of consciousness. We will cover this more in the next course.

The third eye sixth chakra, located slightly above the midpoint between the eyebrows, (corresponds to the start of the second tier) Integral teal, is known in many traditions as an important place for the dawning of transcendental wisdom and intuition, for connection with the archetypal realm of gods, deities, angels and devils. Most people aren't going to experience anything beyond a gross expression of this. If one is spiritually developed this is where one can experience siddhi powers, purified intuition, clairvoyance, etc..

The seventh crown chakra at the top of your head, corresponds to the start of the third tier, Integral indigo to clear light, (from the top of the head extending above the body). I also want to mention that there are relationships between the chakras, pairings and more, so the root is very connected to the heart and the crown, they are linked. The second chakra is connected to the throat. The power chakra is connected to the third eye. Also what it means when a chakra's energy is balanced, is that at that location, the individual is equally open, receiving energy, and sending out energy. That is a balanced, energized chakra. There are all kinds of energetic patterns for example blockages, energy leaning more Yin (feminine) or Yang (masculine), partial openings, strong blocks, and most problematic is when a chakra can be energetically dead, meaning shut down, no energy moving. If this remains long term, this is when we're most vulnerable to disease and sickness and problems.

I t is interesting as one starts to explore this you can see how the regions of the body are (inter)connected. For example the root is from the genitals below, down to the feet, we can see that people just can start out life with a lot of issues in this whole area of the body. Then over time you might notice that they are more vulnerable to health problems in these locations. Then depending on the framework that we're using, this can be expressed in many different ways such as Ayurvedic, an ancient Indian system, or a Tibetan view where negative emotions block your channels, so actually these are energy blocks in the chakras. So when the chakras are paired, if you have a dysfunction in one, the pair is often impacted. The lower three chakras are really the ground, so it's like each one is kind of building up on a foundation of the prior, and then the heart balances lower and upper chakras. It's really important for healing, to help ourselves discover what supports us, first at the first three areas and their corresponding themes, so we can potentially return back into some state of balance. Also if you overdevelop the upper chakras without healing the lower chakra issues, the dysfunction can have severe consequences, not just to the individual but to everyone they're connected to.

Again, we're just introducing the chakras now; in the next course we're going to explore the Integral Framework in more depth, and the first three chakras more in depth. Also in terms of a wider Buddhist cosmological context, it is helpful to remember the view- that we can't actually fix samsara. This is where our spiritual path is so important, and coming back to realize what it is that we can actually work with. What do we have control over, and what do we not? If you're stuck, addicted, and really don't want to let go of samsara, you are like a hamster in a spinning wheel...a poor, pitiful creature, which is not unlike many if not most of us.

Following our introduction course, with the more in-depth exploration of the chakras, we will explore the cultural context of what we were born into, and what our parents were born into. We will look at this broadly in the Western World, but not just the West, but beyond. For example if we were looking at the Victorian era to pre modern eras. At this time Western countries like England and America were undergoing really dramatic changes like industrialization, where industrial employ

Samsara, or "we are little hamsters running in a wheel"

-Dr. Nida

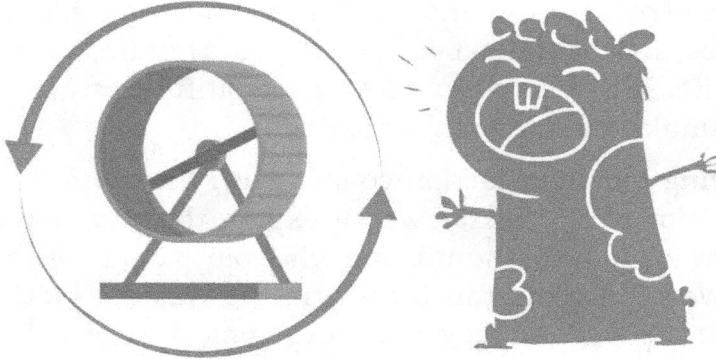

ment changed people's lives dramatically. There was increasing immigration, urbanization, changes in class and racial stratification, dramatic changes in science, and we can really look at the impact of science on culture and people's beliefs and families in the ways children were raised. Life really changed for mothers in the late 19th and early 20th centuries; mothers increasingly (in the US and the UK) lived in urban environments. Chores changed with time saving time, saving technologies, and health hazards of urban living are a few of the many of the many dramatic changes in the early 20th century really impacting how families lived.

Introducing The Root Chakra[6]

root, Sanskrit Muladhara

womb-six months, Integral Infrared
pre pre-first person perspective

- Location: Front, perineum, back, tailbone
- Essential functions: Survival, mother earth, nature, connection to ancestors and family karma
- Meridians: Urinary bladder, conception vessel, governing vessel, sushumna (the nadi or channel connecting root and crown chakras)
- Areas of body: Whole pelvic girdle, sacral and L5 vertebrae, hips, legs, thighs, hamstrings, adductors, knees, ankles and feet; bones
- Environment: environmental conditions from conception to six months
- Identity: Physical Identity with the body

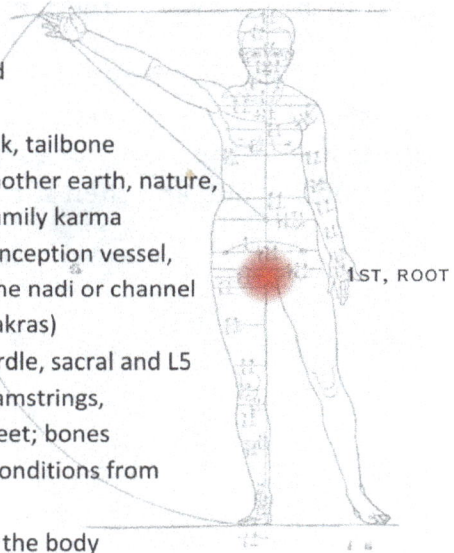

1ST, ROOT

ALBRECHT DURER
WOODCUT
C. 1528

CHAKRAS
SUPERIMPOSED

root chakra themes

Grounding and Rootedness - Safety – Security – Instinct and Instinctual Needs – Primal Sexuality – Body – Schedules – Rest – Nourishment – Earth – Mother

I'm going to talk a bit about the root chakra and then we're going to do our first exercise, which is a self-reflection and evaluation exercise. After that, we'll do a group exercise. Then we'll come back and we'll talk about self-work. There are lots of different things you can do to help support your root on your own. The root chakra is located around the perineum, and tailbone. The corresponding developmental parallel/period we're looking at includes the circumstances that led you into this world including conception and before, through six months. This is the six month framework that we are using in Integral Zen, and again there are differences between different developmental theorists, and it also varies with individuals. People are on their own timeline, so to speak.

So this is an Integral infrared pre-pre-first-person perspective. The essential theme is really just survival. This means the infant is just at the mercy of caretakers first. It's being in the womb, coming out, and then surviving your first six months.

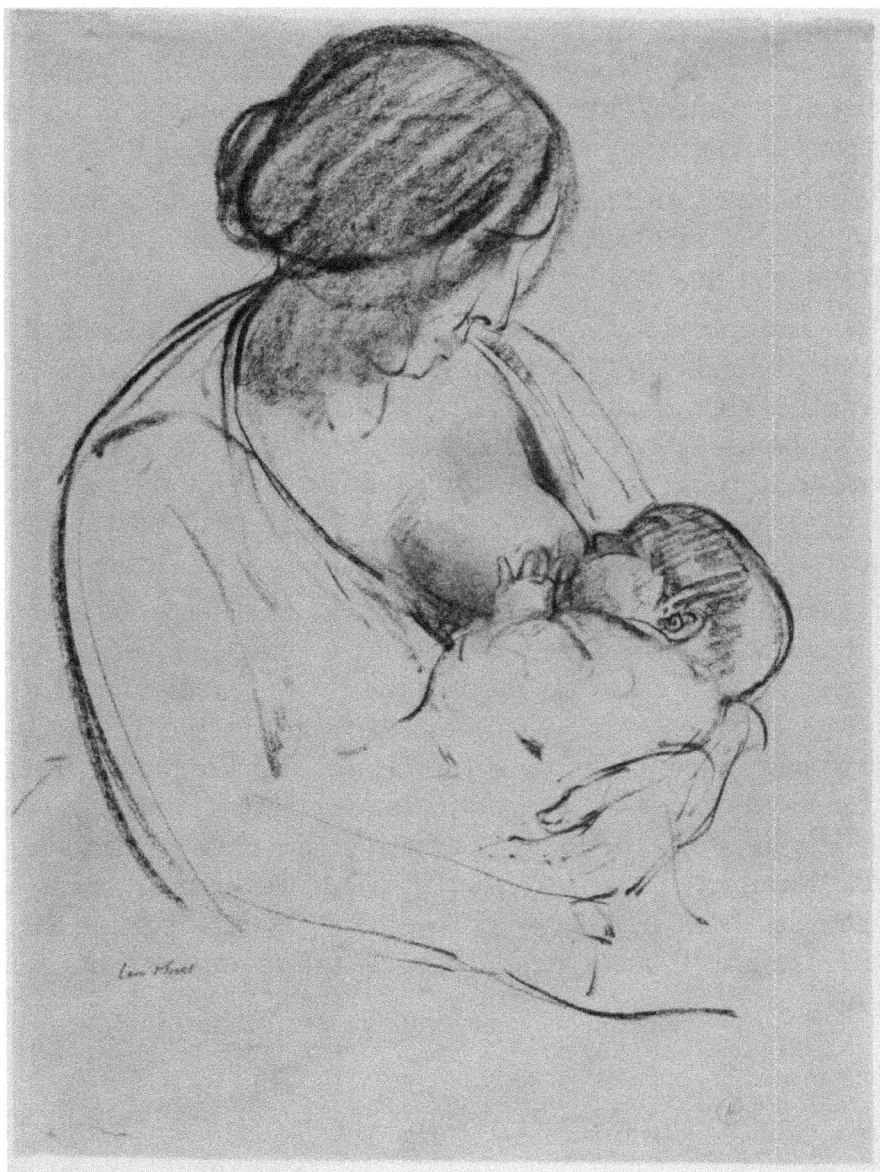

Leon Kroll, Mother and Child, 1904-1925. The Art Institute of Chicago. Creative Commons Zero (CC0)

It's often connected to the concept of mother Earth and

nature, and to ancestors and family karma. The urinary bladder, conception vessel, governing vessel, and *sushumna* channel connecting the base and crown chakras are meridians associated with this area of the body.

When I work with people and first do an evaluation, I ask what is your health history in different places in your body, or is there anything notable?

For example do you have pain that you can't necessarily connect to anything that you know of, in areas of your body? Another big question, do you notice more on your left or your right hand sides of the body? Because sides of the body make connections to our parents and their ancestry, although this will vary with cultural background in terms of matriarchal or patriarchal cultures.

Babies again are at the mercy of the mother and womb environment, completely dependent on her and sometimes others' care, the first six months. In Tibetan medicine there's a lot of information which describe very specific influences that can impact a being as they come into the world, from the circumstances at conception and on. For example in the Tibetan system, the foods the mother eats during pregnancy can impact the typology that the child inherits. There is a whole system, just like in Ayurveda in Tibetan medicine that helps to determine typology. We will explore some of that later on.

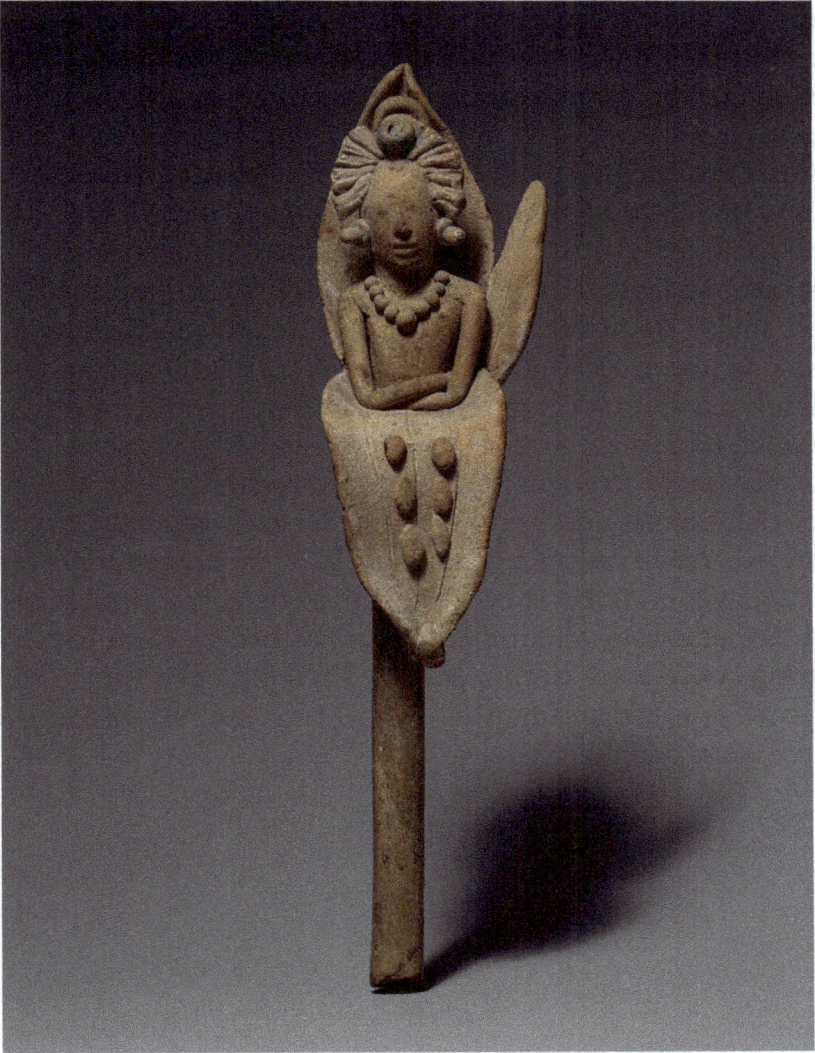

Whistle with the Maize God emerging from a flower, Maya artist(s), 600–900 CE, Mexico, Mesoamerica, Campeche, Jaina Island, Maya, The Michael C. Rockefeller Memorial Collection, Bequest of Nelson A. Rockefeller, 1979, The Metropolitan Museum of Art, New York, Public Domain

There are what I like to call root chakra themes. One is the baby just coming out into the world and learning to move its body, a very primitive level of body identity. The circumstances early in your life corresponding to this time can develop as particular themes in your life that are challenges. So if you were on what we might call shaky ground early on, extending to your family and ancestors, this will connect to themes including grounding and rootedness, and safety: safety is just a huge one; security and instinctual needs. The root corresponds to a primal sexuality, whereas when we get into the second chakra, it's a more sense and emotion based sexuality. We also mention how we relate to *schedules* here because if you look at your life, you look how you relate to these themes, you can often see the interplay, and patterns, of balance and imbalance, the seeds of which may have started not just early in your life, but in your family and ancestry. Nourishment is another big theme. How do we relate to food, how we relate to having enough food or not enough food, eating dysfunctions, overeating, or overly controlling how we eat. For example, all kinds of eating disorders seem to have a strong connection to this period. Then big basic (primordial) themes of earth and mother. In the next course we'll explore these more deeply.

Root Exercise 1

root exercise 1

Identify briefly

- significant family / ancestral karma before I was born
- unusual events or trauma in my life from in utero - six months
- was I a planned or unplanned pregnancy?
- was I the first born in my family?

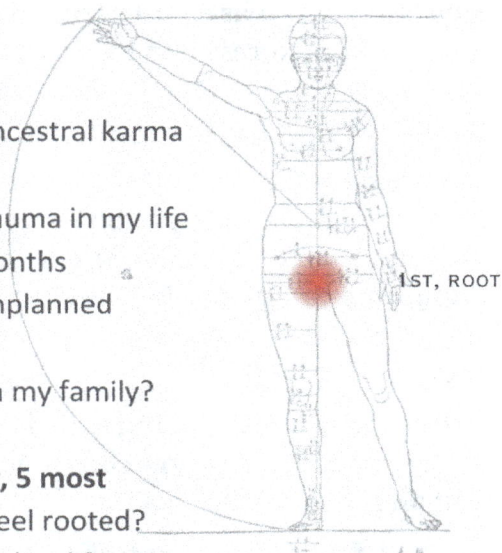

Answer scale 0-5, 0 least, 5 most

Presently in my life do I feel rooted?

Presently, do I feel generalized fear or anxiety?

Presently, do I feel generally safe?

Presently, do I feel generally grounded?

Presently, do I serve as a "ground" for others?

1ST, ROOT

ALBRECHT DURER

WOODCUT

C. 1528

CHAKRAS

SUPERIMPOSED

One of the things that I do when I'm working with people is first we really want to look at family history, and ancestral history. Many people don't know much about this. Important reflections such as was I born in the same country as my parents? Was my family uprooted (if not recently, then generations back?) All kinds of situations that people can identify in their family histories, appear to really impact our experience in the root chakra. Generations of war, for example.

In the present day, from the scientific materialist view, this can really be established increasingly using epigenetics. Epigenetic research first broke through by establishing a link between grandparents and grandchildren's health, in a study in Sweden. There was significant famine in Sweden in the 19th century[7], and so researchers were able to discover and map out the epigenetic connection between what the grandparents experienced with the grandchildren's health vulnerabilities.

If we look to the other Integral quadrants, aspects of life, these "karmic" impacts can be seen, everywhere (tetra arising in all quadrants). From a wider perspective of traditional healing, this can go far back in time. This includes all kinds of uprootedness, upheaval or dislocation, any kind of ancestral karma.

The first exercise we're going to do is, and this-you could spend years exploring this if you choose-we're just quickly going to reflect and make notes.

Questions for self exploration: Can you identify significant family ancestral karma before you were born? Do you see patterns, is there something you can identify? (The developmental period from the time you were in the womb to the first six months, but for your family, anything that preceded your life).

Also, in each chakra, we're going to review any unusual events, or trauma that occurred for you, your family or community or culture within each developmental period. Anything disruptive; many people often don't even really realize some of the events that could have impacted them. It requires some stepping back, really reflecting, did anything out of the ordinary happen?

Was a parent sick, or lost work, for example? I mean, there's all kinds of things that you might not have thought much about, but really impact a child. Again for example, if you're in the womb and something happens with your mother, it impacts you. A baby is floating and completely connected to its mother's body and nervous system. There is someone in our sangha whose mother was in medical school when they were in the womb. At a certain time every day, the mother would study. This person, in their 30s, would experience an altered state at this time each day, heightened awareness, tension, anxiety, exactly at this time. Finally in a conversation with their mother, she mentioned this study time. It's a fascinating connection, and not the only I have heard of.

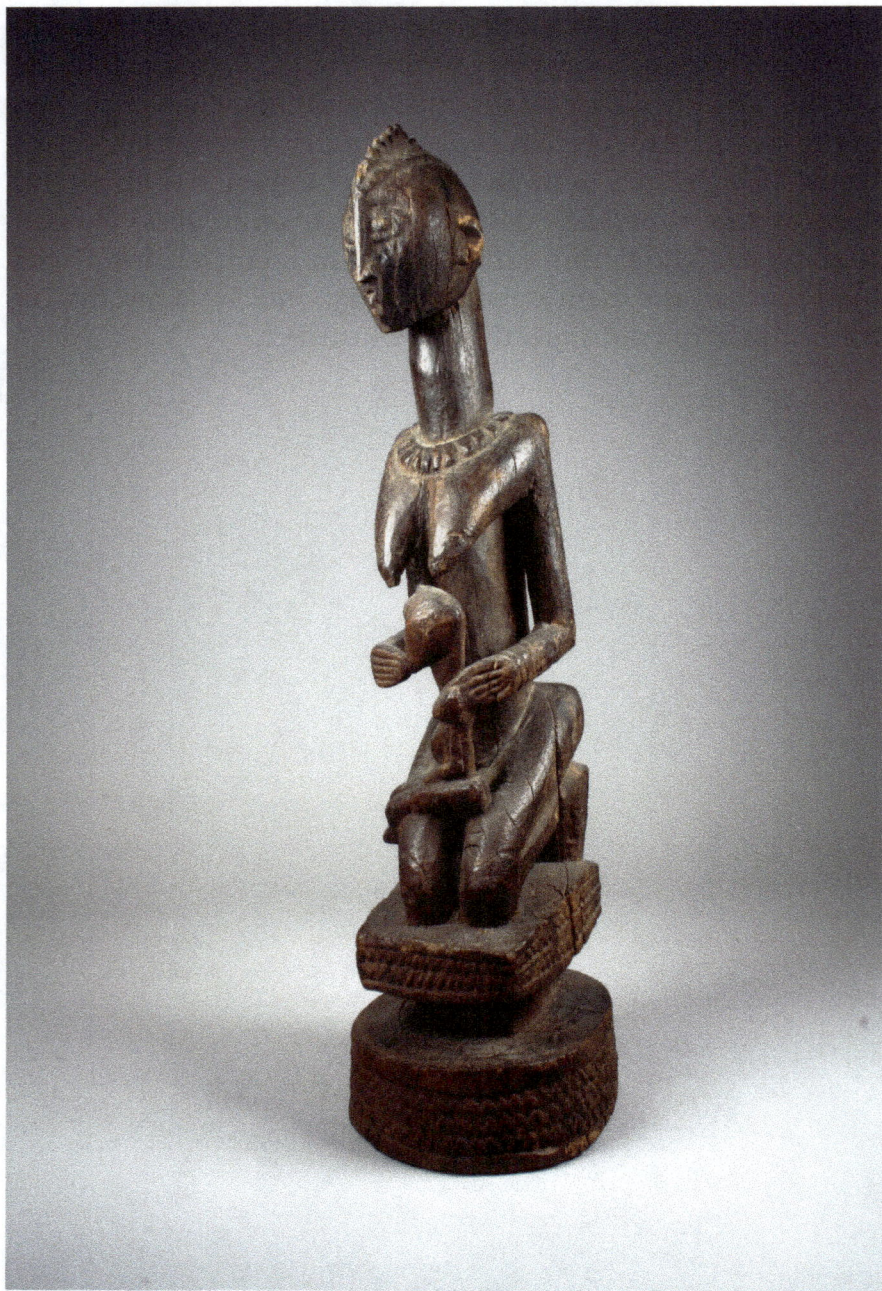

Mother and Child, 15th–19th century, Mali, Dogon peoples, Wood-Sculpture, Gift of John and Evelyn Kossak, The Kronos Collections, 1981, The Metropolitan Museum of Art, New York, Public Domain

Normally when I work with people I spread the process over a long period of time (for different reasons), and one of the important requests I ask of everyone I work with is to have some kind of meditation, or stillness, some reflective practice.

This is partly because of the need to develop the ability first to observe ourselves, but potentially and ultimately to "witness" ourselves, without reactivity, which requires many years or practice. In the meantime, practice builds up the capacity to be able to revisit, without great reactivity (meaning without getting very triggered, retraumatized, upset), so that we can even begin to look at our history, calmly.

Also I know a lot of you on this call but I don't know everyone. What we are talking about can be very triggering and so please know for yourself, that even one sentence I'm saying to you here, can incite all kinds of reactivity. So please know to take care of yourself; if you notice this, do what you need to do to take care, take a break, there is no urgency to this.

What we are reviewing in this course is not something anyone *must* do. We want to be in the right frame of mind and calm, open state to do these explorations. It's important to remember, there's no pressure around this at all. All of that said, we're going to take five minutes to just jot down whatever you want to. Identify any significant family ancestral karma before you before you were born. Unusual events or trauma in your life during this period, or potentially to a parent or parents, mother, father, siblings, other close family, anything you have knowledge of.

I'm sure many here are aware, in the past, and still in many places in the world, it has not been easy to give birth. One of my friends, her mother, had three miscarriages before she had her. So you know, this becomes relevant to how your mother may have related to her pregnancy with you. Also you don't have to tell anyone else, this is for you. Were you a planned or unplanned pregnancy? This is significant, because it reflects a mother or parents with different states of mind. If they're experiencing themselves as a solid family together, really wanting to have a child or all kinds of circumstances, versus not wanting to have a child, it's just different. Believe me, in doing this work with people, one encounters everything you can imagine. People are born into all kinds of scenarios.

Was I the first born in the family? There's also not enough research about how much the impact of siblings affects people in terms of their whole development and psychological growth. Observing people, it appears extremely impactful.

Next, answer on a scale zero to five (*zero meaning not at all, five meaning completely well*). Do you feel rooted now? What this is asking, is do I feel generalized fear or anxiety, as I go about in the world? This is what we can call in this context, *root insecurity*. One of the big signs of this is living in a state of fear as the kind of general way you live..and sometimes, if not often, people just don't even realize that this is going on, that this is their "normal." This is also connected to trauma, which we look at more in the next course. Presently, do I feel generally safe? The same kind of thing. We're considering more your state of how you go about your life, what is the experience of safety and security internally (or are you always looking externally, and have not yet tuned into the internal experience?)[8] This is not related to relative conditions–we're talking day-to-day, you go about things, you know, so there's not some tangible reason or situation (remember we are projecting mostly our internal experience onto our external circumstances, and not seeing that this originates within). Day-to-day presently do I feel generally grounded? The same thing. Another question is do I serve as a ground for others? The mature expression of these themes is that we've dealt with these themes and developed ourselves, and we now care and serve (or have done so in the past) as a ground for others. Often either we've healthily dealt with the themes and are acting as a ground for others, or we could also have bypassed our own development and healing and may be acting as a ground for others unconsciously to escape ourselves, in which often, this will just pass along the unhealed family karma, so that maybe the next generation will be able to work on it. That's just something to check in and reflect on.

Doshin

I'd like to say a few things about some of the correlations between different types of psychological work, such as: Freudian and Jungian theory, trauma work, different forms of trauma work and insecure attachment work. As we look at the same human experiences, we can understand them with many different theoretical maps and models from different perspectives. The particular emphasis on family karma and karma in general is where what we are presenting here is very unique and most valuable. Generalized safety is one the first attachment milestones. If the infant doesn't feel safe, it's unlikely that they will ever feel safe. Until the insecure attachment is, in an orange view "repaired," we will never feel safe. I personally think this view is a misnomer, because we're not machines, we are human beings or "holons." We can't just be repaired like a car, we must heal and we must heal on multiple levels. So whatever your background is, whatever your orientation is, whatever you've explored, just understand that these things all correlate together and we're presenting a framework here that is integrating many perspectives both modern and ancient. We are providing a more integral context where everything can be examined, experienced, felt, understood and integrated. Many different perspectives and views are being presented. I think this is really important to keep pointing out.

root

solo or group exercise
Identify briefly, rootedness

- *where was I born, was I raised there or other places?*
- *where is my ancestral rooting, in one or several places?*
- *was my family displaced, why?*
- *do I feel rooted where I am now?*
- *where have I felt most rooted, can I describe why?*
- *is there somewhere I have wanted to live that I haven't? what is it that draws me there?*

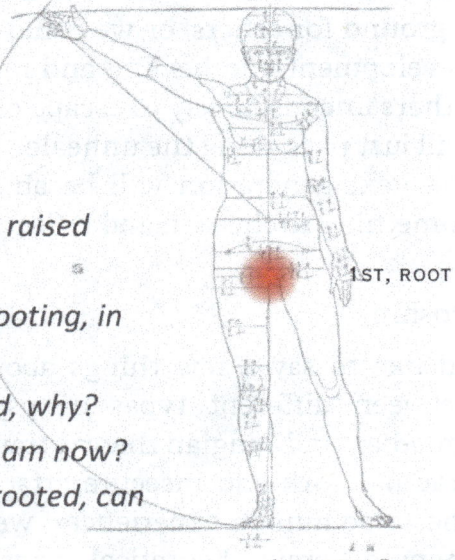

1ST, ROOT

ALBRECHT DURER
WOODCUT
C. 1528

CHAKRAS
SUPERIMPOSED

Janel

I suggest people keep all your notes because you can build on what you discover. The more we do, the more you may suddenly have insights, and also the root is very much going to connect to the heart. How you relate to groups is going to go back to the ground of the root.

Let's explore some more root questions now, looking at where you were born. Were you raised there or other

root - on your own

- connect with the earth, gardening, bare feet or sitting, laying on the ground, time outdoors in silence
- attention to less processed, nutritious food
- allowing enough time for work, rest, sleep in a fairly scheduled routine
- hot / cold baths especially natural springs, or using epson salts, swimming in a pond, lake, ocean
- time with animals, pets
- take a half hour or more to pick up trash at a park or a beach
- shamatha, chi gong, tai chi, internal martial arts, all of these should be traditional versus new age
- Nejang Tibetan Yoga, lineaged schools of Yoga

places after that? Where is your ancestral root originating from, in one or several places? Was your family displaced? This includes a few generations ago, displaced by war, moving to different countries, all kinds of situations. Do you feel rooted where you are now? Where have you felt most rooted? For some people you may actually be asking this for the first time. Can you inquire as to why that is? You may not know. Is there somewhere you've always wanted to live that you haven't? If so, what is it that draws you there?

Let's look at the *homework*. In doing this, I mean healing or whatever we want to call all of this work we're exploring. There's stuff that you can do immediately, for example one of the things to ground yourself quickly, is to jump in very cold water and then take a hot shower to immediately ground yourself. There are methods for immediately grounding yourself, then there are short term things, and then there are long term things, different categories of work we can do.

For attachment issues, this may be life long work, so getting in the right mind about what is reasonable to expect going forward is a good idea, and we will look at attachment more over time. Watch your internal agenda maker throughout all of this. You can't speed up healing, like grief, it's on its own clock.

Connecting with the Earth, for example gardening, *literally* grounding is getting your feet in the dirt. As human animals/ beings, we live amidst and are composed of all the elements. Getting outdoors, also being in silence, being near water is just important, any kind of water, but natural water settings are best. Hot and cold baths, natural springs are very healing. Using Epsom salts, swimming in ponds, lakes, the ocean, or just going near the ocean. Food which from the Tibetan view, is medicine, can also be poison. Paying attention to less processed, nutritious food makes a huge difference for health. This is a whole branch of health care in Tibetan medicine. We will talk about it more in time, but just slowing down to make your own food, including local foods if you are able to, organic foods, this is very good for your root. Allowing enough time for work, rest, and sleep in a fairly scheduled routine is also important. From the Sowa Rigpa Tibetan view, we consider an 8-8-8 schedule, which means 8 hours of rest, 8 hours of work, 8 hours that you do what you choose with your time. This is a model for balance and just using that and considering how you're actually using your time can be very helpful. As you start to do this more and you start to realize, oh, I'm not grounded, getting back to that will help.

Time with animals and pets is very helpful for the root and other chakras; simply being with an animal is very healing. Time to pick up trash at a park or beach or clean your house. How do you feel when you just clean things up? But again, that can also be looked at in a framework of balance. If you're obsessed with cleaning, cleaning all day long, that can be a root imbalance. Meantime, going out publicly picking up trash can be a great grounding exercise. We will explore more traditions of working with subtle energy, so shamatha meditation is a particularly grounding meditation, and Qigong, Tai Chi, internal martial arts. I emphasize, all of these are better done traditionally versus new age, which means connecting with a lineage, and there are reasons for that. Also, Nejang Tibetan yoga, I'll share more information about that.

Nejang is a form of yoga that's very simple for people to do, it helps balance the three internal mental poisons (desire, anger, ignorance) in your body. It's been used in Tibet for a thousand years. It's balancing for your root and then I would encourage lineage schools of yoga because of the healing power and transmission power of a living lineage.

What we mean when we say *lineage*, is that what is transmitted has a timeless legacy, a power of people practicing and interconnected, through the ages. This also points to how whenever you study with someone, you want to inquire, to whom or what do they bow down to? Do they bow down to something greater than themselves? Whatever that may be, we take on that karma too. If they don't bow to something greater than themselves, then to whom are they bowing down to? They may be bowing down to something and you're bowing down to it too, that neither of you know. (Their ego?) I would assume you want to know what that is?

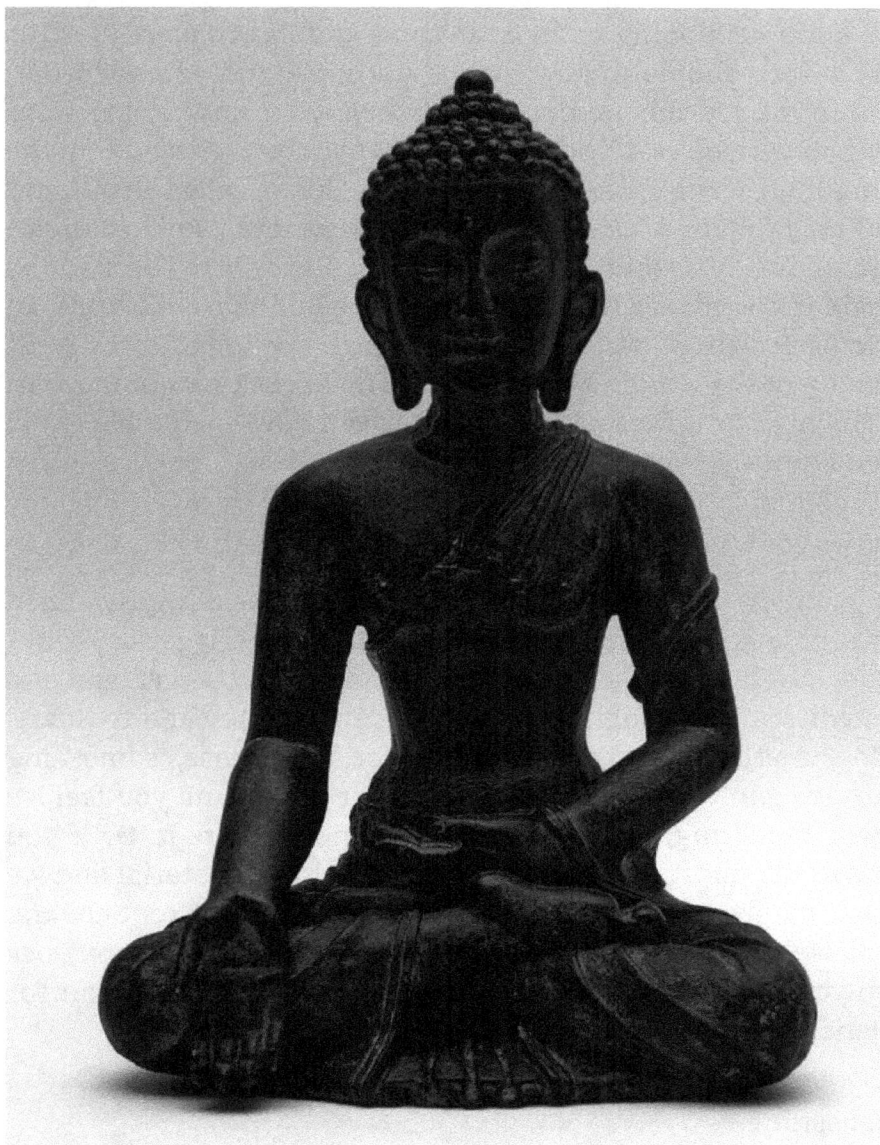

Mudra of the Fulfilling of the Vow

Buddha, Varada Mudra, Photo credit: nomo/michael hoefner, http://www.zwo5.de, CC BY 3.0 via Wikimedia Commons

We are also going to look at some different *mudras*.[9] This is a very simple mudra; it's your right hand extended out, so if you try this mudra, just observe your body going from whatever you're doing initially to what changes by doing the mudra, there's an energetic change. This is called the *Mudra of the fulfilling of the Vow*, Senganin (Japanese), Shih-yuan-yin (Chinese), Varamudra, varadamudra (Sanskrit). The Buddha said if one makes this mudra then the Buddhas will fulfill all vows. It's about dana, or charity, which is giving for the well-being of the world. We will explore different types of mudras. The history is fascinating and they can have incredible ritual and healing power.

Doshin

So earlier we let you all connect, and then we abruptly ended the connection. Isn't that exquisite? Did that trigger anybody? No, no, let me back, me! Don't end it now, don't end the meditation by ringing the bell! So, now's the time to share. If something happened, an insight that arose, something exciting in your interaction with your group, and you feel it's worth sharing, now would be the time to share it. Or if you have any questions, since we covered a lot of material and we just barely scratched the surface today. The first root chakra. Oh well, we could spend lifetimes digging in the dirt here. Does anyone have anything you'd like to share or a question for Janel, or myself? Go ahead.

Question

Hi, for our purposes in this course, what is the working definition of a chakra?

Doshin

I think in the context of this course, working definitions are going to be a little difficult to pin down because we're not examining it specifically with upper right quadrant language and tools. We're looking at all four quadrants. We're looking at all four cognitive functions, so we're really concerned with how things interrelate and interpenetrate, and the inter dynamics of things that lead to health and awakening. So precise left brain, upper right quadrant, conceptual definitions are not going to be helpful. This is Zen. I think the important thing is to open the heart and listen with curiosity to learn how the chakras are viewed and used in the ancient traditions, and how they relate to the modern explorations of ego development. We will examine many different traditions. Many wars have been fought over the question: what the hell is a chakra and why is that important? Yes, blood has been spilled and shed over this question. We are looking at many traditions and many different perspectives of this that go back thousands of years and then we're integrating it with what is the most recent understanding of developmental theory, always keeping in mind that developmental theorists don't seem to agree on very much either. They're all arguing about what ego development is and what is important and what is not important. To pin down a precise definition is really not only difficult, it's a waste of time if we are trying to expand the context of learning. I would suggest that you just take it in and if it's useful to you, use it and if it's not useful to you, let it go, and find something that is useful to you. That's what this is about. Finding something that is useful that you've never considered before. Because I'm telling you what we've done in the past hasn't worked very well for most of us. And that's what this is all about, awakening and healing. Yes, how's that?

Questioner

I mean, part of me just does not like the fact that if someone asked me what's a chakra I have to honestly say I don't know.

Doshin

Beautiful answer. That's a Zen answer.

Questioner

That's good, I mean I'd I'd say that.

Doshin

Ask me exactly what a chakra is?

Question

What is a chakra?

Doshin

I have no idea. There's so many perspectives. It's this wondrous thing that has captivated human imaginations for thousands of years that has created opportunities for such healing and opened the door to such awakening. How's that for an answer?

Questioner

Yeah, I can take that. That's good.

Doshin

Good.

Questioner

Thank you.

Doshin

You're most welcome. Great question.

Also, any insights in your own self reflection? Stir up anything for anyone?

Question

When you asked us to rate 1 to 5, I noticed that I was trying to see around the quadrants. For example, this answer around if I feel fear or anxiety and I notice the different conditions, I feel different ways for example.

Janel

Oh, that's great.

Questioner

I feel very comfortable in, I'll say upper left and then, there is the lower right. Like I don't know how to say, my English is not quite good. So these two I feel very comfortable and the other two, I feel a bit uncomfortable.

Janel

That's so good. I mean, that's so informative for you. This is wow, you're taking it to a new level.

Questioner

And then when you said that you, you just mentioned that root chakra is related to the heart and how you relate to groups. Then this made a click for me. Because I'm very comfortable in my self-awareness and the way I step into the world. This shows up. The other ones, either behaviour or related groups, is where the fear and securities come from. It's just something that I notice.

Janel

Yes, that's exactly what we're looking for. Perfect.

Question

Yes. Thank you. It was very interesting to me to listen to these root chakra problems. Because I could connect very easily to the family history of my wife, and observing some of her behaviors that match almost exactly what she was. Like spending time with animals, internal martial arts. Then looking into her family history, coming and being displaced, the grandmother from Hong Kong. Escaping the war and then being born in a place that is full of immigrants and then in Canada and then her father forcing her to take on the French culture, and not being able to root into either one of them. Yes, you know, she wanted to cohabit at the same time with the father's family as I was taking her away from that and trying to plant her into this culture. This translates into the issues that you describe in the questions, "I always feel insecure". So my question is. What is the value and the healing power of observing this?

Just sitting with it? Maybe a lot of people here are conscious of this. Maybe basically just now through examining these questions, is there a practice? It seems to me that one thing you could do with this information is sit with it. And then contemplate your life history and then that in itself could have a healing effect.

Janel

Absolutely.

Questioner

And then my question is that if that doesn't work, then what? Are there other things? Crystals, reiki, maybe some shamanic ritual? That could, you know, heal that root chakra?

Janel

So yes, this is where an Integral perspective is really helpful, and it's also individual. This is the start of a real internal exploration for people and so, first if we recognize that we want to heal, we need to discover what, and how can we heal? What directions are going to work for us? For some people, internal martial arts or yoga are somatic approaches that can be very healing. For another person you may know, you may be aware that you have attachment problems, so you may need an attachment specialist for certain attachment issues. There are many factors. For example, simply sitting with, what is? This is where Zen and a spiritual practice is so important, because let's say we are bringing all this content up; alright, I see this pattern is in play in my life, in my family, then we just sit in silence. Just sitting with it. One of the things I first say to people is just acceptance: *things are as they are, and can be no different.* Acknowledging this, making space, not resisting the way things are. Normally, we may not notice that we're often internally fighting against the experiences we have had, and are having. We may suddenly notice that we are living in a constant state of resistance. If it was the past, we may be constantly resisting, unconsciously thinking, why was it that? I didn't want it to be that way.

This is the first part: acceptance. This was, this is, my life. This is it. Sitting with this is so important. Then if you can, as Doshin does in working with people, you could always try a process like *Big Mind, Mondo Zen* or his *Touching the True Face* Koan process, or you may have a spiritual practice, which aside from other benefits, gives you a chance to rest, *in the perfection.* To step away from the relative. However, it's important to note that there's a threshold, so with certain kinds of attachment problems, and with trauma, we may have to attend to what is happening to us, more immediately, or urgently.

Also in this process, we're also getting to know ourselves,

which can include getting to know our traumas. Say something is triggered, related to a trauma. So getting to know how we actually deal with stressors. This can be the beginning of a process of really deeply getting to know yourself, then learning and exploring how to actually care for yourself, also how and when you may benefit from reaching out to others. Also remembering, some aspects of healing are going to take a long time. Doshin, would you like to bring in some Zen perspective on this?

Doshin

Well, to me there is no separation between this and that or healing and awakening. We live in a time that is incredible; we have access to so much information. We have access to so much knowledge and we have access to so many different presentations of teachings, it's overwhelming. How can we possibly sort it all out? What do we use to tell which is the direction we should go, and which is the direction we should avoid? A simple question. Well, let's see if I need a brain surgeon. I'm gonna find one that graduated from a good medical school and has lots of experience. I'm not gonna settle for one that just declares that he's a brain surgeon. So how do we tell? How do we separate the skilled from the unskilled? How do we evaluate who's good and who's a charlatan? Isn't that an interesting question? How do we find the best source of healing help? In this time where everything is out there and nobody seems to know who's good and who's bad, across the board.

Ken Wilber's suggestion, which is something we will go into in these courses in much more detail, is the way you tell, is by using *Kosmic Addressing*. This is a methodology that Wilber invented that I learned directly from him, in a group that evaluated articles submitted to the *Journal of Integral Theory and Practice*. This is a method that can be used to evaluate everything. I'm constantly using this method to evaluate myself and to evaluate every student I work with, every healer I engage with and every teacher I encounter. What we want to do is use the 5 AQAL maps: the Four Quadrants, Levels (Structures), Lines of Intelligence, States and Types (typologies). In terms of what we are doing in this course, we are giving special attention to the levels (the structures) of human development, which we are correlating to the chakras. We are also keeping in mind the State Vantage Points of awakening: gross, subtle, causal, nondual, and non-dual suchness. Then the lines of intelligence, and the types. Using all five of these Integral categories to evaluate where someone is the foundation of *Kosmic Addressing*, at least at this introductory level.

We want to inquire, what is a person's center of gravity? What chakra is really active or alive for them, and what chakras are asleep, stuck or have not yet been activated? We consider the states of the gross, subtle and causal realm. This is a methodology that we can learn to use now even though it will likely take generations for this to develop and be useful to a whole culture. It will most likely take a long, long time to develop an integral science that's capable of doing this. But you can get a felt sense of how to use this Kosmic Addressing out of this course. We can at least know that it's possible to evaluate ourselves and everything else in these new powerful ways. For example, who am I going to go to if I break a bone in my leg? Who am I going to go to if I have arthritis? Who am I going to go to see if I have an overwhelming karmic experience, or I'm suddenly overwhelmed by my family karma. You know, one of the questions I ask, and I always get the same answer. I say. Raise your hand if you have messed up family karma? Come on, be honest. All the hands in the audience go up. Who am I going to go to see to help me heal with my screwed up family karma? Do they give a PhD for that at Harvard? Do they teach this at Oxford?

Janel

Someone will be selling it soon, a "certification."

Doshin

So I am going to lay this out now right in the beginning, because it's a really important question. And this is where we go. On the one hand, we go to ancient lineage teachings that have generations and generations of teachers and wisdom behind them. And on the other hand, we go to modern experts in the field that have deep non-biased scientific studies to back them up. And consider how different it is in each quadrant. What is the truth test in the upper right quadrant? The scientific method works beautifully. What is the truth test in the upper left quadrant? Well, I have to just believe what you say, because I can't really see into your direct experience. So the truth test is Truthfulness. What about the lower left quadrant? This is where energetic congruence is important. Where the compatibility of cultural values becomes important. And the lower right quadrant? This is where the external collective organizational structures are significant, and the structural functional fit is a significant factor. There's a different truth test for each quadrant. And in Integral Zen we bring Jung's theory of types that brings the four cognitive functions into awareness where they can be consciously examined as well. With these powerful tools we can begin to investigate our individual and collective preferences and prejudices and the impact of three poisons of greed, hatred and ignorance on our lives both individually and collectively. There's just so much juicy stuff to explore. Is that helpful? Probably not yet. It will take a while. Be patient.

Questioner

Yes, of course, definitely it is helpful, and interesting. Some of these questions that you've posed, I have the feeling that they haven't been answered yet.

Doshin

They haven't even been asked, let alone answered.

We've had these conversations before about what would be the equivalent of the scientific method for the other quadrants and what IS a useful method in the other quadrants that asks for truth? That's just one question we could spend a long time examining.

Question

Then if I may ask what you say in terms of recognizing who to go to? In the past. I think we had this conversation, but the way I found you for example, was not through any knowledge of Kosmic Addressing because I didn't even know about Integral theory, but it was an intuition in terms of being in the face of something that felt truthful and authentic, and I just went with that. The right thing, probably even more efficient than trying to find what your Kosmic Address was.

Doshin

And we call that *gut knowing* and *gut wrenching*. It is the gut wrenching that drives you searching, and the gut knowing that leads you to finding.

Questioner

Yeah, and something I really like about you is the fact that you said something along the lines of, well, you don't have to stay here. If you find it useful, just stay the moment. If you don't find it useful, then go find something that is useful that works for you. Which I mean it's great. Then you also pointed out something very important, that we should take a little bit of time in identifying whether the teacher that you are with has an agenda.

Doshin

Yes, that is most important.

Questioner

And be careful, be careful of this. When it's not present, or at least not so not so strongly present, then it's probably a good sign.

Doshin

This is a really simple criteria that I look for when I'm looking for a teacher or a healer actually. I want to know, are they awake enough to see the one right thing to do in every set of circumstances? Are they awake and healthy enough to know when to do that one right thing and how to do it? And then, are they doing it for the right reason?

Questioner

At the right moment.

Doshin

At the right moment in the right way. Yes, but the right reason is where the agenda comes in. You know, I'm delighted that everybody's here, but I'd be delighted if nobody was here. It doesn't really matter to me. Now I care deeply about the people that are here and want to help them in any way that I can. But if nobody was here, I'd be just as happy. It would not disturb me if no one came. I don't care if you like me or if you don't like me. I don't care if you stay or if you go, if this is great for you, if it's working for you, great! Stay as long as you like. If it's not working, go find something that does work for you. With age, I have let go of so many of my agendas that I have had in the past.

Janel

Doshin, we have one minute left.

Doshin

Ok then, thank you. That's a polite way to say: Enough Doshin. Okay, I hear you.

Janel

So for next week, continue exploring with the questions we presented. I would try to tune into the themes and look at how you see and experience these themes in your life? For example, schedules, do I need a schedule all the time or do I prefer being spontaneous? Really start to reflect and just look, look around the theme of safety, security, food. One other thing is with the root, dissociation from what is being experienced in the body can also be a sign of root dysfunction. So hypochondria is a good example. It's like a fear of what's going on in the body. Something interesting to explore, so thank you everyone for coming. Even though he says he doesn't care. We deeply appreciate it, and it's really wonderful to see all of you.

Doshin

I care deeply for all of you, but it's none of my business if you stay or go.

Deepest gratitude thank you so much.

Janel

Thank you. See you next week.

CHAPTER 2, THE SACRAL CHAKRA

Doshin

Here we go. So, let's jump right in. Healing and awakening. With a focus today on healing.

Week two, the second chakra, the sacral chakra. Healing first requires knowing yourself. Knowing what needs to be healed, and preparing yourself for healing. To know ourselves, we have to explore the whole of the human psyche. Now that's very different in today's age than it was in the past. I want to just put this in context. The human psyche is often characterized symbolically in dreams as a house. The house often has basements, and in the basements, we find the hidden aspects of ourselves that we can't see. Then if we drill down beneath the sub-personalities and the shadows, we'll find the preverbal traumas. The disowned sub-personalities emerge from these preverbal traumatic experiences that create dysfunctions, and from the insecure attachment issues that they leave buried in us. Trauma therapy and attachment work are other ways to begin exploring at least some of the same material that we are exploring using the chakras.

**Healing Requires
Knowing Thyself**

**Explore all of the
Human Psyche**

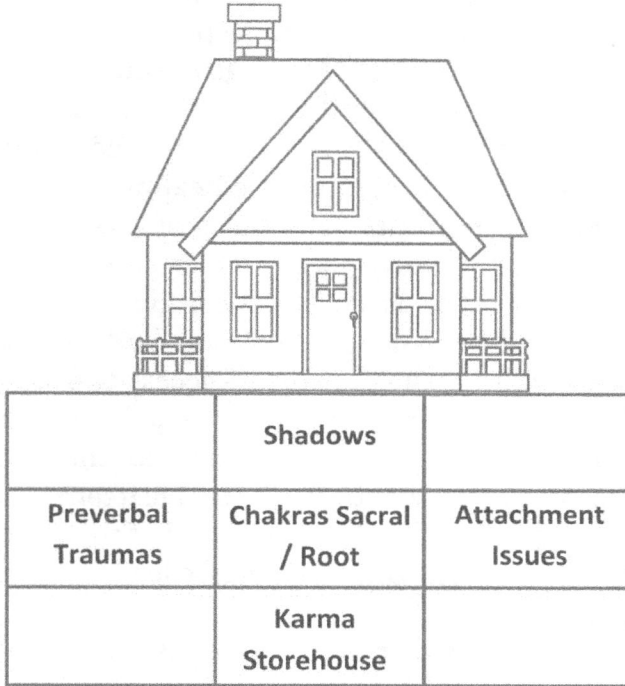

	Shadows	
Preverbal Traumas	Chakras Sacral / Root	Attachment Issues
	Karma Storehouse	

Today we're looking at the sacral chakra, last week was the root chakra. In my experience this is very similar to exploring the insecure attachment issues. Attachment therapists usually talk about "attachment repair," but this modern metaphor seems out of place because human beings are not machines that can be repaired. From an Integral perspective, that is a very orange mechanistic view, but that is a false view, because we are living organisms. We are "individual holons," living beings. So rather than being repaired, we have to heal. This is the one thing that I've found on my personal path that led me into Shadow work in the first place. After many years of seeing and then integrating split off shadows, I started doing trauma work because I realized that just working on the shadows was not enough. Then I realized that working on the traumas was not enough. That led me into attachment, exploring insecure attachment therapies. I realized that wasn't enough, and that led me back to the Depth Psychology of Carl Jung, and the ancient lineage teachings of traditional Eastern Wisdom Traditions, especially Zen. It wasn't until I discovered Wilber's Integral theory that I was able to build a framework that could hold all this including the healing methodologies and the chakras. I found that this was a way of dealing with the deeper territory of my own psyche and the collective archetypal aspects of the psyches of those I was working with. By this time I had become a Zen Master and had practiced meditation enough that I was able to access the storehouse, which is what I understood Jung to be pointing to as the collective unconscious. This finally created the conditions where the karma itself could begin to resolve itself. I wanted to present this context before we jump into all of this. So take this and do with it what you will. Janel, please lead us further into the territory.

Janel

So we're going to pick up again and look a bit more into different chakra systems, and then start introducing different energetic, subtle energy systems from the East. Again, this isn't necessarily going to make sense. Hopefully by the end of this course the framework of healing will seem more interconnected and make some kind of "sense". If you're confused, just go with the flow.

Hindu yogic traditions are the model for how we are working with the chakras. The Upanishads of Hinduism called them "psycho-spiritual vortices", or "physiological psychic centers". Medieval Hindu and Buddhism empha

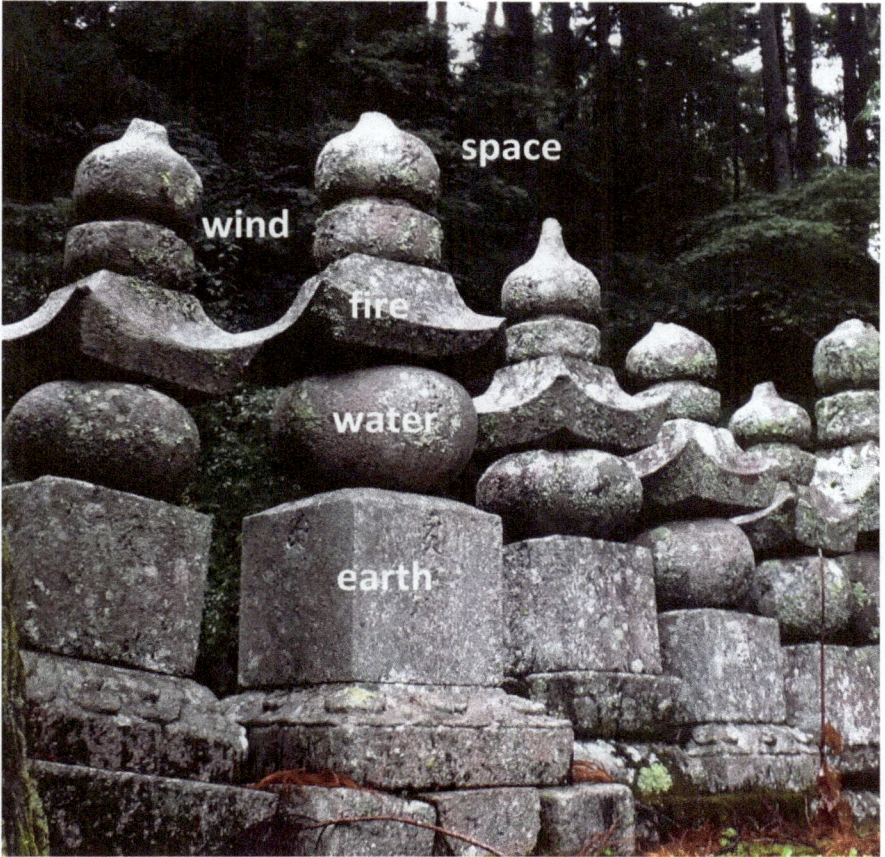

sized how the chakras related to prana or Vayu life energy along with Nadi energetic channels. Tantric practitioners aspired to master the chakras by awakening and energizing them,

Tibetan Sowa Rigpa chakras and elements

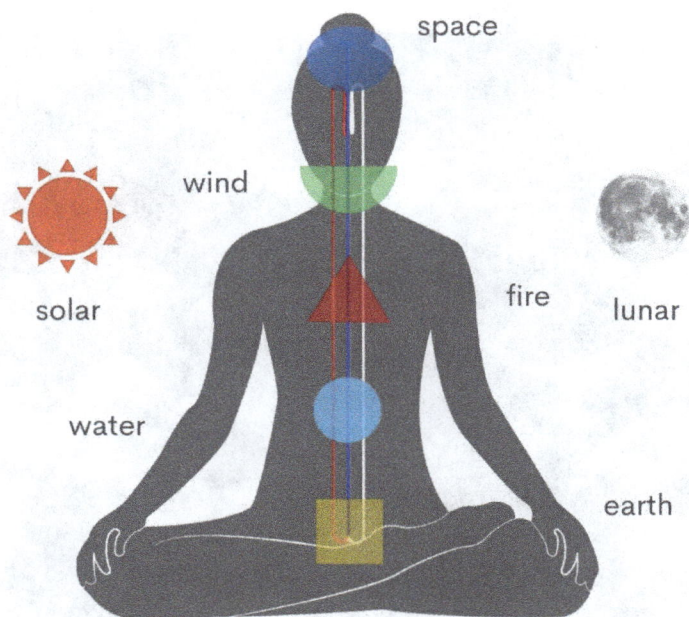

using breath techniques, with the guidance of teachers. I may have mentioned before that in some of the lineages I study in, with breathing techniques, it's very clear when a teacher approves a student to teach others; in lineages this doesn't tend to be ambiguous. Once a student has mastered a technique, and the teacher decides they are ready to teach, they may tell them to start teaching. So I really recommend if you're learning any kind of lineage breathing technique that you just be sure that the person you're learning from has been given the "ok" as a teacher by their teacher. That doesn't mean they have some kind of certificate, but usually there's been a clear instruction, versus someone who chooses to teach without that.

So I find this quite interesting; in Japan, Vajrayana Buddhism is called *Shingon* and it does not seem to be as well known in the West as Tibetan Vajrayana traditions are. The forms in the photo are called "stupas". One will see these all over Japan, at temples and in cemeteries, funerary stupas. What's so fascinating is this formation represents the five elements, and is the same "stack" as in the tradition of Tibetan Buddhist lineage I study in, it's a five chakra system, with the same order and symbolism. It's not always represented this way in the Hindu tradition, but it often is. So this is one way of representing the elements in the body: at the bottom is earth, then water, fire, wind and space on top. So while it's the same as the Tibetan lineage I study in (Yuthok Nyingthig/Sowa Rigpa). It's not universal in all different lineages, so some of them will have 6 chakras, and I've seen less, but 5 seems to be more common. So in the Tibetan Medicine Buddha lineage, we work with five chakras, the same as in Japan.

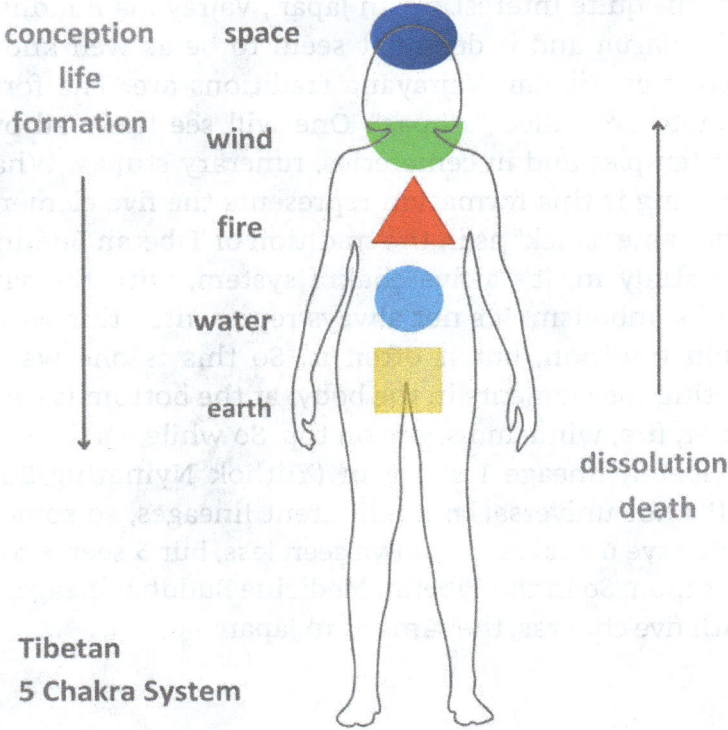

conception   space
life
formation   wind

fire

water

earth

dissolution
death

Tibetan
5 Chakra System

This continues to be interesting as this is tied to our energetic body. At conception solar and lunar (feminine and masculine) essences come together, Sowa Rigpa teaches that the solar essence comes from the mother, and the lunar essence comes from the father. From the lunar essence, the male brings the elements of earth and water, and the solar brings wind and fire, joining at conception. Back to the elements, the lower part of the body is associated with earth, then it goes, water, fire, wind and these form the five chakra (Tibetan) pattern during our life.

At death, we experience a *dissolution* of the elements, which begins from the bottom. First earth, then second water, third fire, fourth wind, last is space. Again in Tibetan Buddhism, this process is laid out in considerable detail.[10] The process of death is described, where you can even start to see signs of the earth element starting to dissolve as long as six months before death, there are a number of signs as each element is dissolving. There are obvious signs (external, internal) and subtle internal, so called *secret* signs. Part of death preparation, to prepare for your, and others' death, is to learn what all these signs are. One can contemplatively practice one's own experience of dissolution of the elements. Then there are practices to prepare for the bardos, (leaving room for flexibility, it is said to vary on an individual basis). It's really fascinating to see this whole cycle and circle, through conception, birth, life and death, and rebirth.

I will say it again, there are many variations of chakra systems. Kabbalah for example, which I know nothing about, lays out a scheme of ten emanations and attributes of God, said to be equivalent to a chakra system.

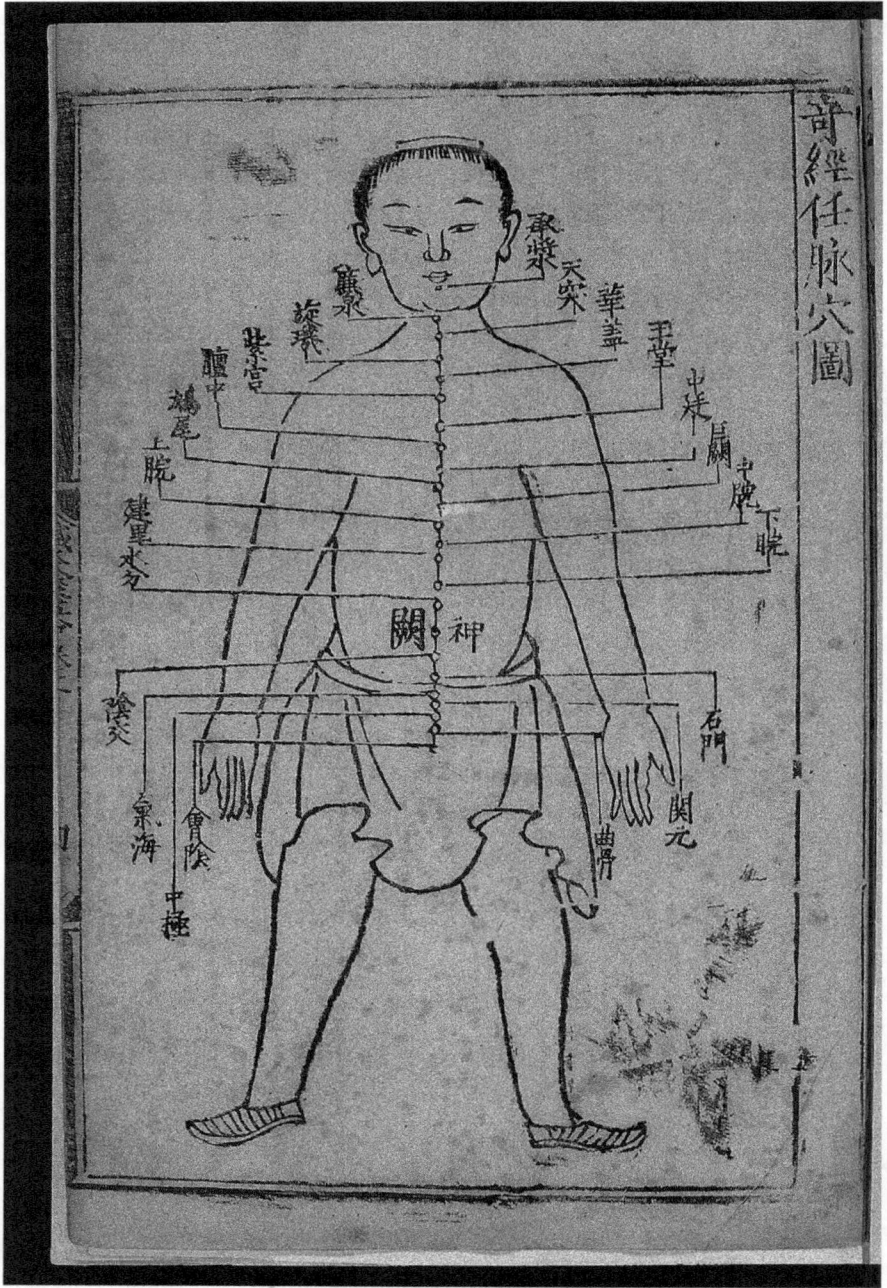

Acupuncture chart, renmai (the Director, Woodcut illustration from an edition of 1537 (16th year of the Jiajing reign period of the Ming dynasty). The Director Vessel (renmai)

In Chinese traditions, even though you have five elements, it's not the same. About 3000 years ago, during the Chao Ch'in dynasties, practitioners of medical arts and Shamans turned to Taoism. Life energy called Qi is worked with as potentially unlimited. The more you look into some of these ancient systems, the depth of complication can be astonishing, especially with numbers. All this cosmology comes down into the human body. For example the Meridian system works within 12 hours of a day, 12 meridians, every two hours changing where the energy flow is going in the body, connected with different organs; acupuncture works within this map.

Taoism doesn't use chakras, but three Qi roots, there are three dantian in the body, so there's the upper, the middle and the lower. They're different from chakras but have similar functions and effects.

In India, where the principal medical tradition is Ayurveda, there is an ancient system of *Marma* points, still worked with today. In the Siddha tradition in South Asia, many practitioners were masters of Ayurveda, including Nagarjuna.[11] A lot of information was exchanged between Southern India and China, the Middle East. Even the apostle of Jesus, St. Thomas came to India.

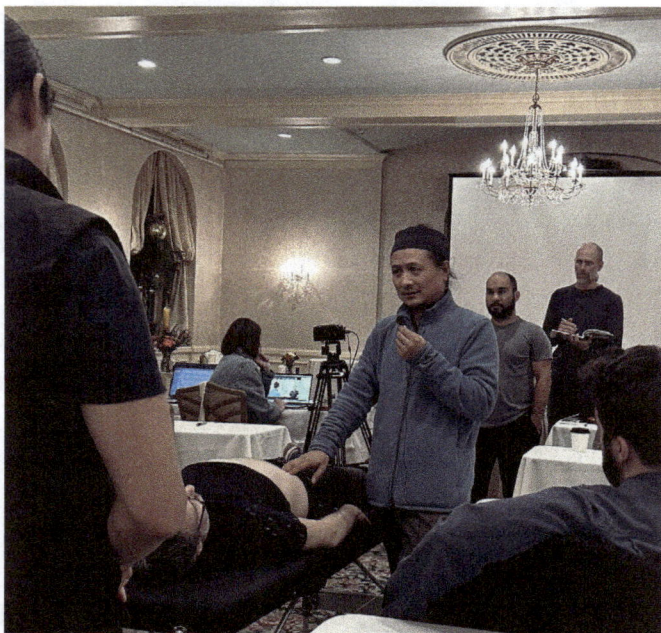

Dr. Nida teaching Tibetan Medical points, December 2024, photo by Janel

Marma points are vital points that can be worked within many different ways; the points can have positive and negative effects on health. If you get injured in one of these points and it is not attended to, the energies–unhealthy energies-- can seep out to other locations in the body. Also within the whole system there are points which provide antidotes to injuries, and all kinds of ways of working with them. This is intertwined with yogic tantric traditions. There's a gross, subtle causal body presentation, and generally a six chakra system is used. Again remember that there are many, many more chakras in the body, but most systems narrow down discussion to the essential ones.

Sowa Rigpa, three channels in the subtle body

central channel, blue, wind humor
(wind, loong), rooster, craving,
attachment, desire

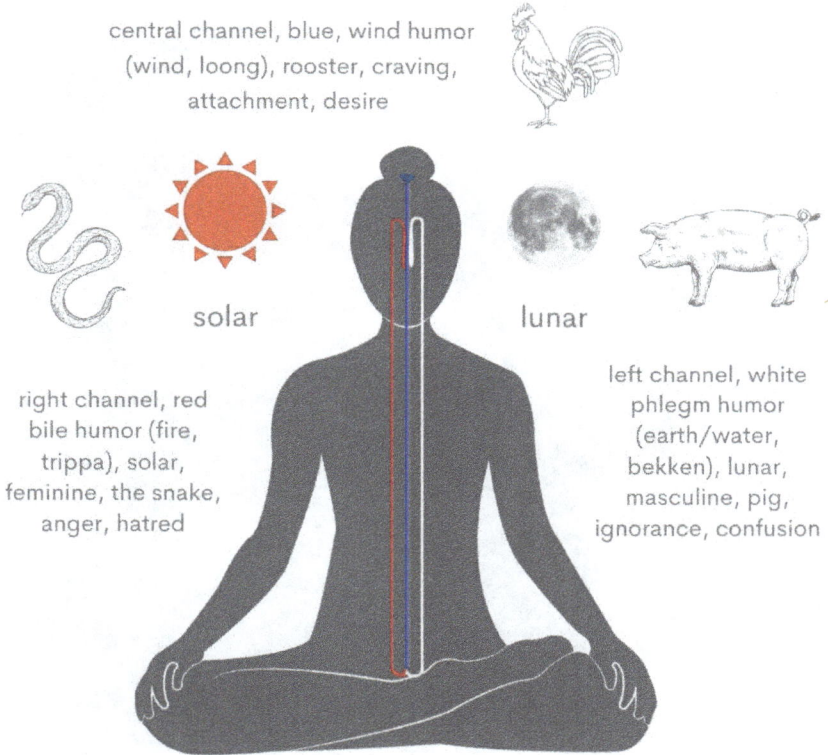

solar   lunar

right channel, red
bile humor (fire,
trippa), solar,
feminine, the snake,
anger, hatred

left channel, white
phlegm humor
(earth/water,
bekken), lunar,
masculine, pig,
ignorance, confusion

Some of these points can be used to cause grave harm to people. It's a very interesting system. What is exciting is Bodhidharma[12] came from this Marma region where it is said the first martial art was practiced, which was called Kalahari. It is believed that Bodhidharma brought this ancient martial art to Shaolin Temple. Also of note is there are 108 Marma points, a significant number in Buddhism. In the early martial arts a main strategy was attacking the points so as to easily defeat an opponent. Again, they're vital energy locations, from the passing from the hair and the head down to the soles of the feet, circulating like a field or net, all over the body. Every single hair is a marma, approximately 300,000 hairs.[13]

Dharmakaya, Sambhogakaya, Nirmanakaya

Doshin

Traditionally in Buddhism there are three "bodies" of the Buddha. There is the *Dharmakaya*, which is the Absolute or truth body of the Buddha, what is realized and embodied upon awakening or attaining enlightenment. The *Sambhogakaya* is the bliss or energetic body of the Buddha. Then the physical body of the Buddha is the *Nirmanakaya*. This traditionally is the Mahayana Buddhist view.

Now this is really interesting if we look at it in the context of an Integral Framework. If we consciously place the *Trikaya* inside the four quadrants, which is what we all experience and we articulate this in a graphic form, we can start to think about it in a new way. The Nirmanakiya, Sambhogakaya, and Dharmakaya. These three bodies of the Buddha are all viewed as being in the upper right quadrant, the individual exterior quadrant. If we go into the upper left quadrant of our individual internal experience, what are experienced as bodies in the upper right quadrant are experienced as states of mind. So here in the upper left quadrant, we have a gross state of mind, subtle state of mind, and a causal state of mind, which in Zen is a mind empty of self and all its impurities of greed, hatred and ignorance or delusion.

Gross - Subtle - Causal
in the Four Quadrants

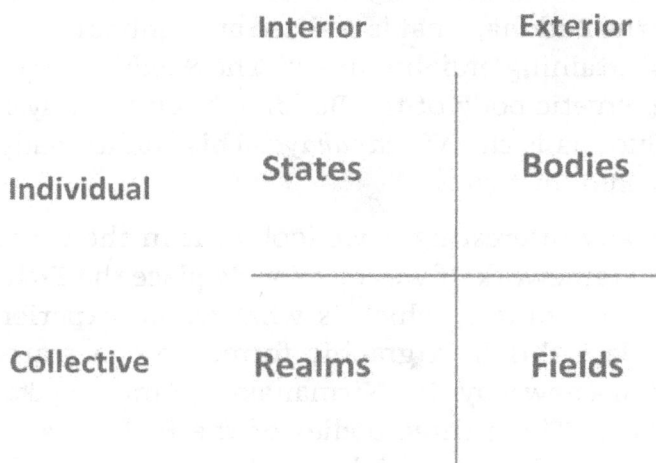

	Interior	Exterior
Individual	States	Bodies
Collective	Realms	Fields

In Vajrayana Buddhism, this causal state of mind is usually viewed as "very, very subtle," almost empty, but not quite. This is a very interesting difference between Zen Vajrayana Buddhism. Wilber calls Zen *Essential Buddhism,* going right to the essence, to the heart of things, and he calls Vajrayana Tibetan Buddhism, *Complete Buddhism.* In Vajrayana, there is a whole pantheon of very, very subtle states, energy bodies, wrathful and benevolent deities, and there are practices to become one with each of them. And if we go into the internal collective realm, the lower left quadrant, the cultural realm, we can experience a gross realm, a subtle realm, and a causal realm.

If we move into the lower right quadrant, the external collective, then we can look at these realms as fields: we have a collective gross field, of physical manifestation, we have a collective subtle field of subtle energetic manifestation, and we have a causal field. We can view the causal field either in the Tibetan view as "very subtle," or the Zen view as "empty." This is very helpful if we want to understand ourselves, and this quadrant view of the gross subtle and causal body states, realms and fields ivery powerful tool to aid our understanding. There are

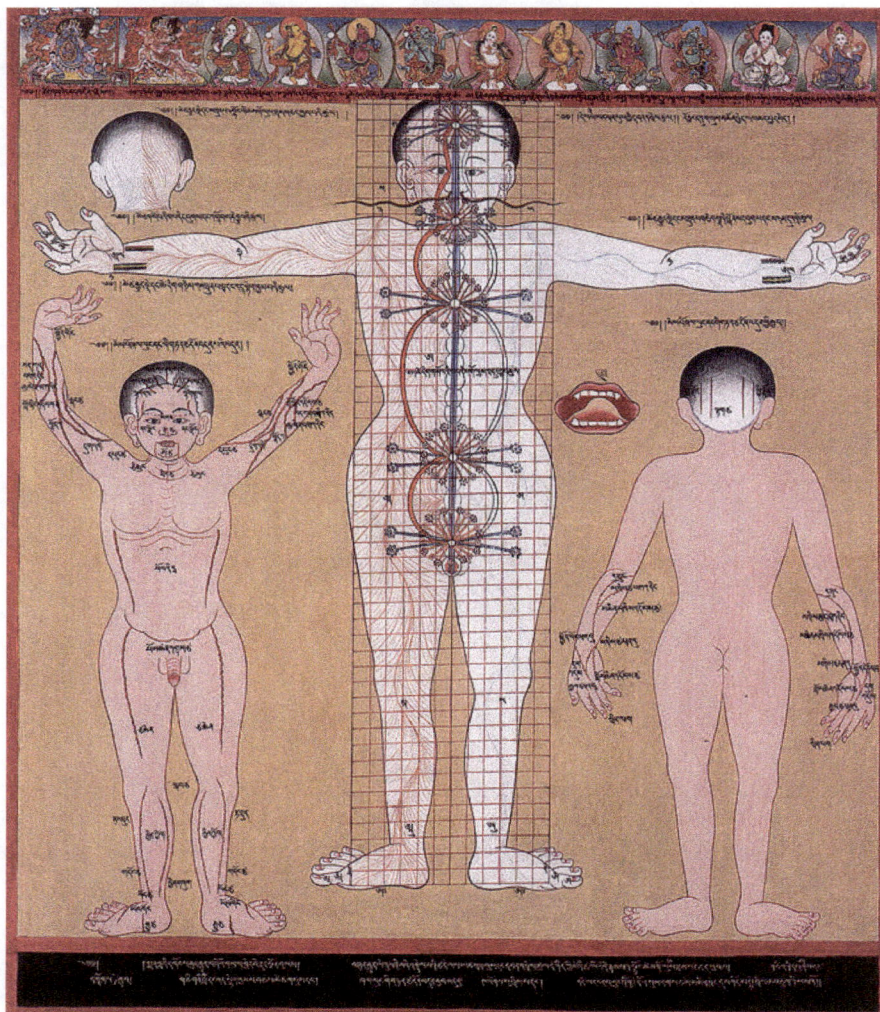

Tibetan Medicine Chart of the chakras and channels. The Blue Beryl medical charts were designed and commissioned by Desi Sanggye Gyatso in the late 17th century. This file is licensed under the Creative Commons Attribution 2.0 Generic license

many things we can do with this. When I saw Wilber present this, he had the upper right, the upper left and the lower right quadrants described as *bodies, states and fields* respectively, but he hadn't described the lower left, which I found quite interesting. So in a private conversation with him, I showed him what I have outlined here and explained it and he said, yes, that that makes perfect sense.

Janel

Thank you. In Vajrayana we have a Vajra body, a subtle energy body, made of subtle luminous energy. Within this energy body these are the three main energy channels that you can work with which I will introduce now and we will talk more about later. This is similar to practices where one visualizes oneself as a Buddha body, within a process of retraining perception, to redefine and purify the basis of all our gross conditioning and karmic manifestations. However, for the more simple practices that I share on retreats, we first envision ourselves, the shape of our body like a crystal or clear, light, and empty. Then we envision the three channels. It is a way, one of my teachers describes it as a way of going "in the back door" for purification. Also this is connected to how our consciousness is operating. Along with this we bring awareness of the empty nature of things, envisioning this clear channel view is a significant part of subtle energetic practices worked with in phases.

Doshin

Yes I mean this really relates to what I was saying about essential Buddhism (Zen) and complete Buddhism (Tibetan.) If I'm on a Zen path then the front door is emptiness; and this would be a side door or perhaps a front porch if I'm on a Vajrayana path. Working with emptiness would be more of a beginning. And I see these two things as extremely complimentary because you can start with one path, and then flicker between them, in a way that they can complement rather than conflict with one another.

Janel

Thank you Doshin. The Sowa Rigpa/Tibetan Medicine, the Medicine Buddha tradition is one of a number of Medicine Buddha lineages. Within this comprehensive system, it is said there are 72,000 channels in your subtle energy body. There's a five chakra system that I mentioned before, which is comparable to the endocrine system in Western Biomedicine. In Sowa Rigpa chakras and

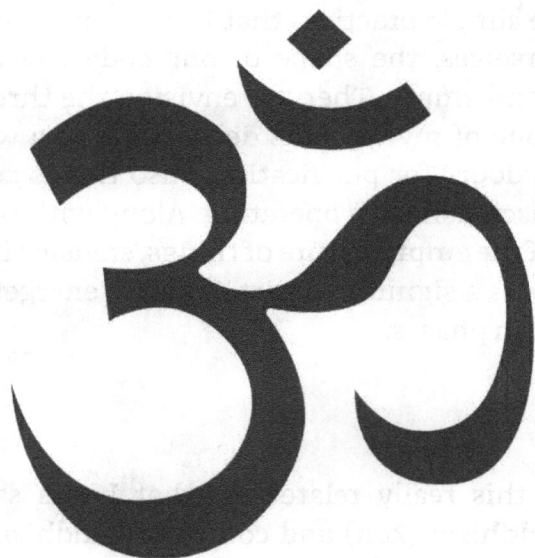

ॐ

OM

channels connect to sound, color, and energies which relate to the innermost functions of the body. It is said that knots in the channels are caused by negative emotions. This is really interesting to consider, to compare, if we look at our day to day experience, we might notice an experience of feeling *stuck or blocked*. But again this is from this view from this subtle energy, that's how it's described.

In terms of human conception, from this framework, we have vital essences, which are white and red, in the subtle energy body that join at conception, called *tigle.* There is a white male lunar essence, when we are formed, that eventually is located at the top of at the crown. The white lunar masculine essence is associated with bliss and emptiness. Red feminine essence is associated with bliss and creativity. A red feminine solar fire essence is located at the base of the central channel, four finger points below the navel below and back. The white essence channel is on the left side, and the right channel relates to the red essence. At conception they come together, then at birth they separate, and at death, they rejoin. These essences are referred to in different subtle systems. In Hatha yoga, this is very essential and central to the practice of Tibetan Tummo, an internal fire practice. Chinese Taoism works with their own variations.

I'm going to start referring to mantras soon and we start with the seed syllable OM (OM is a mantra *containing all mantras*). Within Tibetan Buddhism and Tibetan mantra healing arts, seed syllables are described as the *original sounds of the universe.* Mantra literally means *mind protection* (Sanskrit "man" means mind, "tra" means protection). This use of "mind", means mind, heart, body. It's mind, as in mind-only Yogacara Buddhism. As "seed syllables," these sounds in the universe connect to specific locations in our body. When we voice the sound of one of these seed syllables, it creates a vibration that opens locations in the channels in our energy body, so therefore these are used for healing and awakening.

Mantras are one of the most powerful healing arts and have been used for centuries by Tibetan Tantric practitioners, mantra healing forms a significant branch of Sowa Rigpa/Tibetan Medicine and has been widely used by Tibetan doctors, healers and yogis (ngakpas) for restoring health, pacifying negative energies, increasing the strength of therapies, herbal and medicinal substances, as well as for prevention of further disorders. The tradition has been passed down in continuous transmission and lineage over centuries. Mantras have been collected through the ages by masters and sages, and revealed as treasure revelations, in sacred texts.[14]

What I wish to convey is, it's not just speech, it actually is the vibration, and so as we do practices, one can chant mantras silently, but for some things actually making the vibration sound with your voice is needed for opening channels (from what I've been taught, this isn't always the case, sometimes doing it silently is better). I have also been taught that the shapes of the seed syllables replicate the actual shapes of the channels in the body.

An important point about energy in Tibetan medicine; I mentioned there's a system of vital energy points where seed syllables are connected to locations in the body. The points are connected to what is called *La* energy, in Tibetan Medicine, one's vital life force energy. Each of these locations and our energies are connected to phases of the moon, along with a healing seed syllable sound (and shape of the seed syllable). We have a number of different types of life force energies within this context. One of the most critical vital life force energies, you can recharge from both the sun, (sunshine) and moon (moonlight) which is most available during a full moon. Going out and *moon-bathing* can charge us up, which can actually be too much for people! It's well known what happens on full moons to people and animals, so this intense life force energy is related. This is related to the meaning of the term, *lunatic*.[15]

This life force energy is a key to vitality and what is said to be the predetermined, general length of your life, your gross physical form, life on this earth. Since I mentioned there are a number of different life force energies, some can be recharged or boosted, so to speak, while one is limited (and individually determined coming in with karma, at conception). So when a human is initially conceived and then when you're born, you have a unique karma that also relates to this life force energy, and length of life, that has a limit on it. The way it's been taught to me is it's not so much necessarily a life-will-end-on-this-day kind of situation, but a range of time (although Tibetan doctors can check your life force pulses, when they examine you). Impending death will show particular signs in the body, so basically, we can say that while you can do a certain amount of things to support your life energies, one of those energies will be limited, predetermined according to karma.

The Second, Sacral Chakra

sacral, Sanskrit Svadhisthana

six-eighteen months, Integral Magenta
pre-first person perspective

- Location: Front, two finger widths below the navel; back between L4 and L3
- Essential functions: Sexuality, emotions, movement, energy of movement, the energy of life vitally expressed, Magic and Ritual
- Meridians: Kidney, solar and lunar channels / nadis
- Areas of body: Lower back, kidneys, adrenal glands, sex organs, bladder
- Development: Beginning to receive enormous amounts of information through the five senses, and process it, with feelings and emotions.

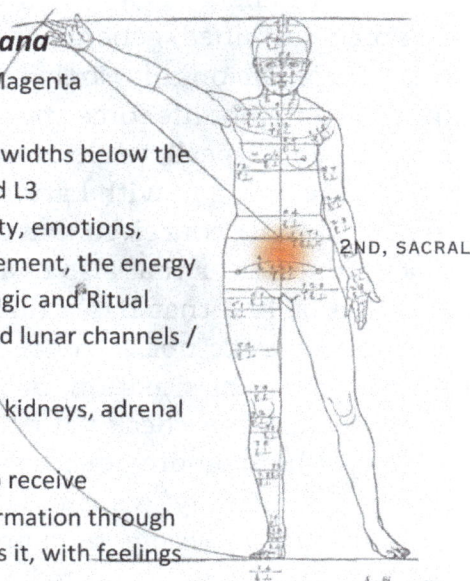

2ND, SACRAL

ALBRECHT DURER
WOODCUT
C. 1528

CHAKRAS
SUPERIMPOSED

Sacral themes

Emotions & Feelings (liking and disliking) - Childlike Innocence and Creativity – Sensuality – Sexuality – Play – Nurturance – Tenderness and Attunement – Compassionate Touch – Magic

Okay here we are at the second chakra; there's a lot to look at. This corresponds to 6 to 18 months (roughly) of development. In integral structures it is pre-first person perspective, so again, how to describe that, first note that the first two chakras/developmental periods, the child's awareness is not yet separated from their caretakers and environment. The child has *not* come into a first person perspective where it will declare "I, me and mine", not yet. So what that means is that the environment, the caretakers, the emotional atmosphere, everything going around the child is *really, really* impactful. In some sense we can say the child is a sponge to what it is surrounded by.

Six to eighteen months in the general developmental view is when the child really is just coming into their sense awareness, sense development and emotional

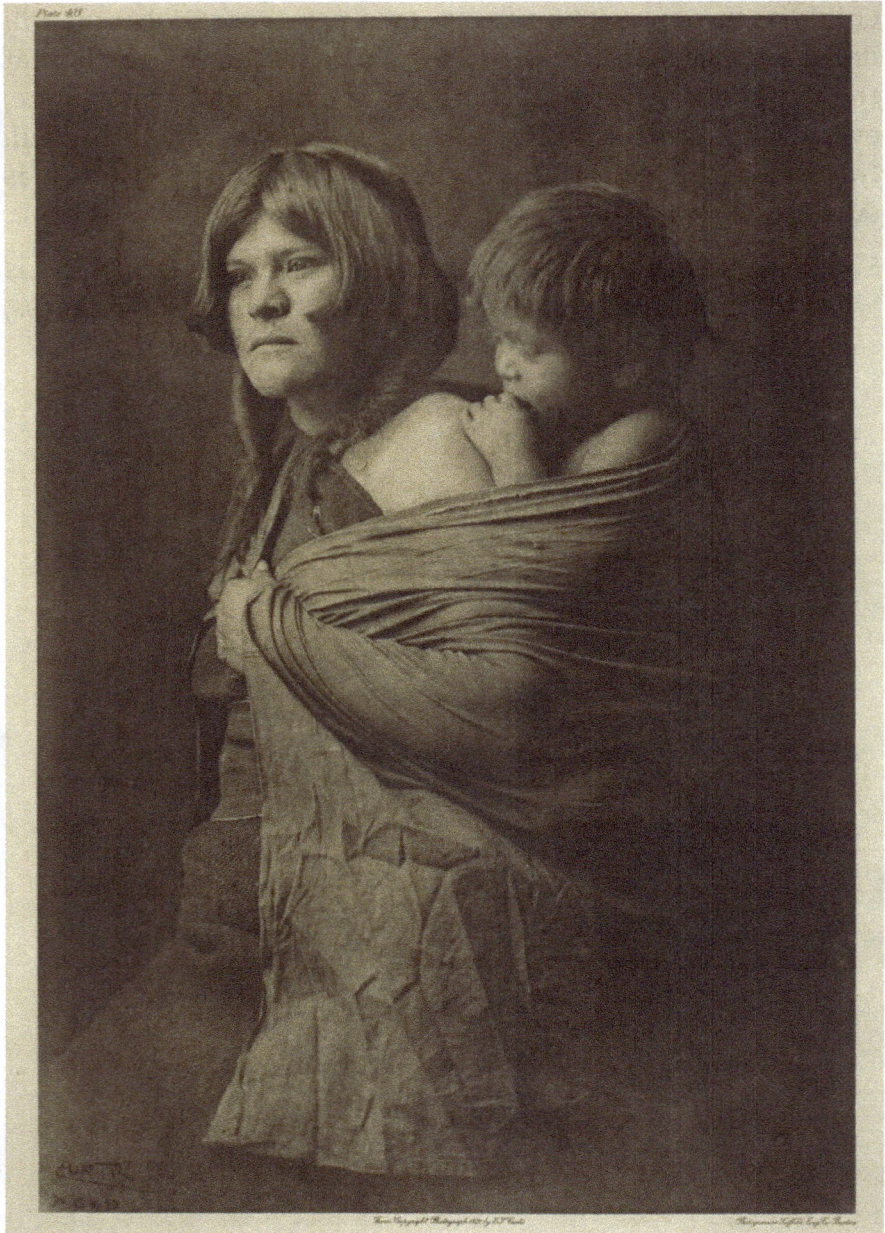

Edward S. Curtis, A Hopi Mother, 1921. The Art Institute of Chicago. This information, which is available on the object page for each work, is also made available under Creative Commons Zero (CC0). Additional data about artworks in the collection is available using our public API

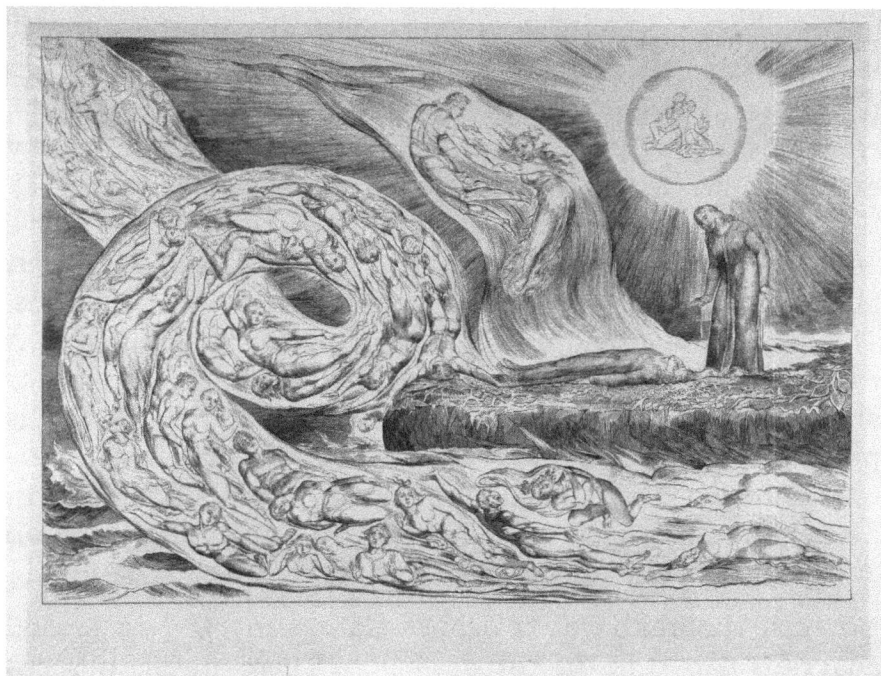

Circle of the Lustful: Paolo and Francesca, Series/Portfolio: Dante's Inferno, Canto V, William Blake, British, London, ca. 1825–27, Rogers Fund, 1917, Metropolitan Museum of Art, New York, Public Domain

development.[16] This means the child is developmentally ready for this, which also means, before this, the child does not yet have the capacity. This is important to remember through all developmental levels. You cannot force a capacity onto a being that lacks what is necessary to engage with that capacity. This is one of the biggest factors of understanding integral structural levels- partly why people are frustrated with each other so much, they expect other people to have capacities, where they may not have, and then judge, penalize, assume they should be, in ways that they simply cannot.

In the body, the location is central in the body, below the belly button maybe three to four inches around the spine.[17] Some life themes that this area impacts, is first awareness of the senses, and emotions. The seeds of sensuality, sexuality, emotions, movement, the energy of movement, life, vitally expressed magic and the experience of magic and later ritual. During this developmental period we are beginning to receive enormous amounts of information through the five senses, and learning to process them with feelings and emotions. This is also the development of starting *liking and disliking*. A theme that carries throughout life also is childlike innocence and creativity. Play is a big theme, nurturance, which is pretty obvious, tenderness and attunement, compassionate touch, and again magic. The health of one's root chakra developmental period is really going to impact the situation and set the ground for the second chakra.

Now also chakras have a "pairing" relationship, and the second chakra is paired to the throat chakra. There are many seeds that are planted in the second chakra for dysfunction that may blossom in all kinds of ways, from gross sense based addictions and obsessions. If they connect to the throat, the fixations of obsessions can become ideological, which we'll explore later. This is where *hungry ghosts* are born. So a hungry ghost in Buddhism lives in a realm where it has a really long neck and really long arms, and it's just endlessly desirous, and not able to satisfy thirst or hunger.

There are other types of longings people can experience. An experience of never being satisfied, roaming around; never fulfilled.

To describe it simply, basically we each have needs as an infant and child, as a baby to be responded to and met in the most basic ways for survival, protected, fed, responded to,but emotionally (loved) as well. Response via affect, joy, and the mirroring of emotions are actually critical for human development. In terms of receiving care it's not severely restricted to mother and father, or nuclear family, other caretakers can step in, *as long as there is consistency*. If there is a lack of consistency or minimal interaction, this generally leads to significant attachment problems. For example, in integral magenta level cultures, it is common for a mother to bundle and attach a young child to her body as she goes about her day. This is actually ideal for their development in so many ways, one of which being that she's right there. She can just sense the baby and take them everywhere, which is very healthy for necessary bonding. Again since the baby doesn't experience itself as separate yet, it is very aware of mother primarily as the ground of safety and protection, assuming the mother has a stabilized level of balance[18] to offer to the child, since this isn't always the case.

But you know in the Western world the style of mothering and parenting of children at this age goes through so much change historically, in the next course we're going to explore this more in depth. From the late 19th century to now, for example, American culture just goes through so much change with science and economic change, which greatly impacted families and child rearing. Class situations changed as society saw more advancement and prosperity, as women started working more, people's lives also changed greatly with technology.

All of these factors impact children, families and the second chakra. This is a really important area for emotional health and well-being, and almost everybody I talk to, did not get their needs and nurturance fully met, I mean very few would be met in an ideal way, and in the Western world this is especially the case. I see a lot of imbalance and dysfunction.

Doshin

Yes I think this is something that we will explore in much more depth in the next course. Exploring your own life, your own history in the early chakra development is such a rich exploration, and it can be a bit disturbing because we have to look at things that we aren't accustomed to looking at and often do not want to look at. We have to look at things that Western psychology doesn't necessarily have tools yet to work with and integrate some of these aspects of our psyches. I would point to being possessed by demons as an example. Just because we believe that demons don't exist, doesn't mean we can't be possessed by them or by some mysterious force that science has not yet acknowledged, because it cannot be found in the upper right quadrant. So, let's keep open minds and hearts as we are filling in the gaps and the connecting dots between what we don't yet understand. Individual and collective psychology, which Western psychology is just barely beginning to look into is still in its infancy. We have a lot we can learn from ancient lineage teachings and noble wisdom.

For example: some of the work the psychologist and author Jonathan Haidt[19] is looking at and exploring morality, this is where we've just barely begun to scratch the surface of our explorations into the lower collective quadrants. This is what I'm really most interested in exploring and finding methods to heal and awaken in the areas where we have to dig very deep. We'll have more to say about this pretty soon but right now I just want to mention sexuality, spirituality, magic and emotionality–Jung borrowed a term from Kant and he was looking at noumena and phenomena. Phenomena would be objects in the world that exist in the right hand quadrants. Jung was more interested in what Kant referred to as the *pneuma*: these are the objects that have this feeling of sacredness, that he called numinosity. So it's this feeling of sacredness of numinosity, arising in the sacral chakra that we find naturally in cultures that are pre-scientific, before there's been a separation between inner and outer, between mind and soul, or ego and nature. It is a very different experience growing up in a culture like this, than in post-scientific culture. This is an area where I really get excited and have been working for many years. I am just foreshadowing here, planting seeds for things to come.

When we really look at emotions with Integral Zen tools, we begin to see that emotions are something that in the modern and postmodern West, we don't

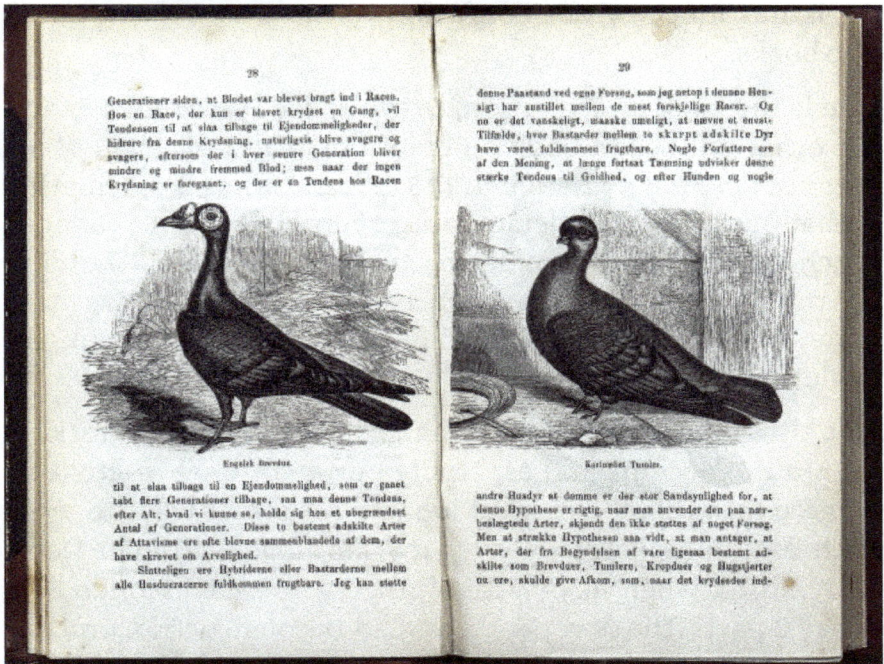

Danish translation, Origin of the Species. These illustrations were inserted in the section in which Darwin discusses the differences in domestic pigeons. Shown are the Engelsk Brevdue (English Carrier) and Kortnæbet Tumler (Short-faced English Tumbler). The illustrations originally appeared in Darwin's Variation of animals and plants under domestication published by Orange Judd & Co., New York, in 1868.

adequately understand. Lisa Barrett[20] is a neuroscientist who has spent her life studying emotions. She spent twenty years trying to duplicate an experiment that linked facial expressions to universal emotions, and she was not able to duplicate this experiment, which led her into really questioning our whole understanding of emotions. In her book *How Emotions are Made* she describes how she failed to duplicate the results of this experience long considered to be the gold standard of the scientific views on emotions.

The way she literally deconstructs our understanding of emotions is brilliant. She really articulates this and she attributes much of our confusion to Darwin. Darwin wrote two books.

One is the book on Evolution, *Origin of the Species (1859)* and the other one was a book on emotions, *The Expression of the Emotions in Man and Animals (1872)*, and what is fascinating is that our current understanding of emotion hasn't changed much since then. There seems to be a picture of Darwin's on the altar of Western Science. So, in the West we have taken Darwin's work as gospel in both our understanding of evolution and emotions.

It is time to find better ways of understanding and working with our emotions and especially our emotional reactivity. I was led into this territory of looking for better ways to work with emotions karmically by my Zen teacher JunPo Denis Kelly Roshi, when he created a process he called Mondo Zen. It has 2 parts, the first part is an Ego Deconstruction process, which is a method of using modern koans to lead someone with language to or close to a direct fleeting experience of "awakened mind." The second aspect of Mondo Zen is what Junpo called an Emotional Koan. This led me into a journey of finding new ways of more deeply understanding what emotions really are and how to work with them from a perspective of liberation, looking out from "awakened mind," rather than from the prison of emotional addictions. I've been doing this work full time for the last twenty years. It has been quite a journey and my experiences have led me into a deep exploration of what emotions are and how they can be used as medicine and tools of awakening. I have combined my understanding of Jung and Wilber with Zen Practice and Junpo's emotional koans and I'm working with all of this in an Integral Zen Framework.

So an integral way of working with emotions inspired by Jung, Wilber and JunPo is what I have been passionately working with for the last twenty years. If we look at the quadrants, the chakras exist in individual human beings. In holons, they're linking the inner and the outer worlds. Right down the middle, if we move into the

Chakras and Emotions
Upper Left & Right Quadrants

Chakras

Inside   **Outside**

Emotional Feelings   Emotional Decisions

Emotional States   Emotional Reactive Energies

upper left quadrant of the individual interior, we have

emotional states. These emotional states are like all states that exist in the left hand quadrants. In the right quadrants, we have bodies, behaviors, and energies. These exist in the external, right quadrants. So we use what Jung called the *feeling function,* an example of which would be the liking and disliking without language or labels. We all have the capacity to discriminate between what we like and what we dislike. This feeling function emerges in the second chakra, where we're trying to figure out what we need to move toward and what we need to move away from or be afraid of. We need to discriminate between what we want to eat and what might want to eat us! We begin to make decisions–we like certain things and we remember what we like. We dislike other things, and we remember what we dislike. We begin using this feeling function clearly defined by Jung, in order to make decisions in the second chakra, the magenta stage of ego development. The objects that we feel we like and dislike take on an emotional charge to them.

Corresponding to our emotional states in the upper left quadrants, we have emotional reactive energies in the upper right quadrant. For example, when you walk into a room and you have a sensitivity which is really a "felt sense." We can be sensitive to the exterior manifestation of emotional anger, let's say, I can walk in a room and if anyone is angry, I intuit it, I can just smell it and I'm highly sensitive to looking for the emotional energy, the emotional reactivity which accompanies anger. This gets into a whole exploration of a much better way of understanding emotions that is extremely useful in understanding things like "why can't we just all get along?" What is the cause of war? Why do we have these culture wars that we don't seem to be able to understand anymore than natural disasters? To really begin to understand this, we need something that is not readily available in any social holon. We need an Integral Framework that provides a deeper understanding of emotions and the nature of religious phenomena, as well as our relationship to all of this. This begins with a deeper experiential understanding of the lower left quadrant, what Jung would call the *collective unconscious*, and what Mahayana Buddhism calls the storehouse or the *alaya vijnana*.[21] Then for the lower right quadrant, which we can begin to understand more clearly with systems theory. We need an Integral Framework, a whole new way of looking at the universe within and without. The universe behind the eyes and between the ears as well as the vast external universe, that extends endlessly or seemingly endlessly, into the heavens. So that's enough, for now.

Janel

Attachment includes patterning that is established in the early chakras/early development periods, which includes the style of nurturance as well as lack of nurturance; patterns of relating and affection. These patterns run deep within us, and if you look at babies, how they learn, babies learn so quickly by watching and modeling behavior. There have been all kinds of studies where you put babies in a room, and then someone starts behaving, doing some kind of movement or something, and babies and young children just completely mimic them, picking up the same behavior so quickly. Watching the mimicry of a very young child is actually shocking, especially when we consider how unconscious so many people are in caring for children.

Therefore basically these early patterns of relating become deeply established. When we do this work with more depth, we can really start to identify, and lay out patterns that we lived, that we experienced and experience, that we internalized, so that we can start to make them conscious in the present. Then once you start doing this, you can begin to connect all of this to your own relationships past and present. This can lead to a lot of discovery, as well as sober realization, when you start to see patterns that you just didn't see before.

There's just so much here that impacts us and how we live our lives, consciously and unconsciously. The first exercise we're going to do is going to be a reflective exercise. Again, you can start to take notes and work as much or as little as you want. If this is overwhelming, then please take care of yourself. There's nobody here saying you *have to* go through looking at all these chakras, or do these exercises. People put so much pressure on themselves in general in contemporary life. (Unconscious, internalized "should" and "shouldn't-ing.") If something triggers you, just take care. You may *not* be ready for this.

Sacral Exercise 2

sacral exercise 2

Identify briefly

- was my family able to provide me with loving, patient and attentive nurturance at this time (6-18 months) or if not, what got in the way?
- unusual events or trauma in my life from 6-18 months

Answer scale 0-5, 0 least, 5 most

Presently in my life do I feel nurtured?

Presently am I nurturing or supportive to others?

When do I feel playful?

Do I feel emotionally attended to?

Do I feel emotionally attending?

Do I feel emotionally nourished?

Where do I experience magic, now or in the past?

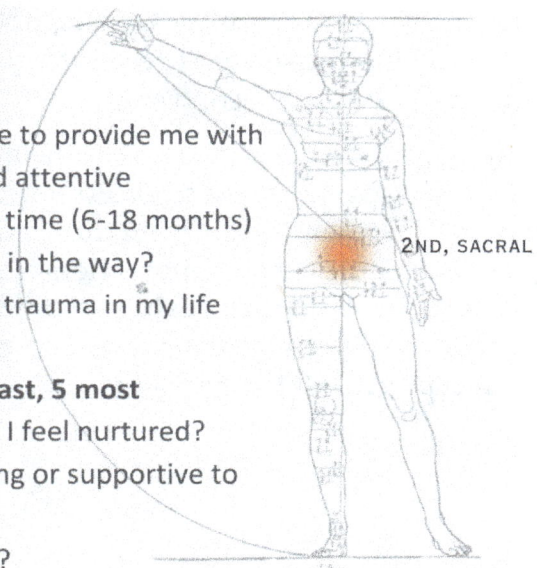

2ND, SACRAL

ALBRECHT DURER

WOODCUT

C. 1528

CHAKRAS

SUPERIMPOSED

First exercise. Was my family able to provide me with loving, patient and attentive nurturance during this developmental period, from 6 to 18 months? If you suspect or know they did not, then what got in the way? Were there unusual events or trauma in my life (or family) from 6 to 18 months? Again, every time there's some kind of disruptive element in a developmental period, this impacts us, and it's going to impact us in an individual way different from everyone else. Recognize that it can take some *sleuthing* to see how it did, and how it's manifested, or manifesting, or how we're just undeveloped in some aspects, and how we may benefit in developing ourselves. These two questions here are really fundamental to the second chakra.

Next, you can answer on a scale of zero to five (*zero is not at all, five is completely*). Presently in my life do I feel nurtured? Presently, am I nurturing or supportive to others (pets included)? (Supporting others is a mature expression of this, and that's if we're healthy in doing this to ourselves, we are then available to nurture and support others). Next, when do I feel playful? If the answer is

sacral

solo or group exercise
Identify briefly, attention seeking

- *Can I identify some areas of my life, even if quite subtle, where I am seeking and or craving attention, validation, etc., that may be out of balance?*
- *Looking at this, can I identify where I have early needs that have never been met?*
- *examples: behaving, acting out, pursuing goals for the purpose of receiving external validation or attention*

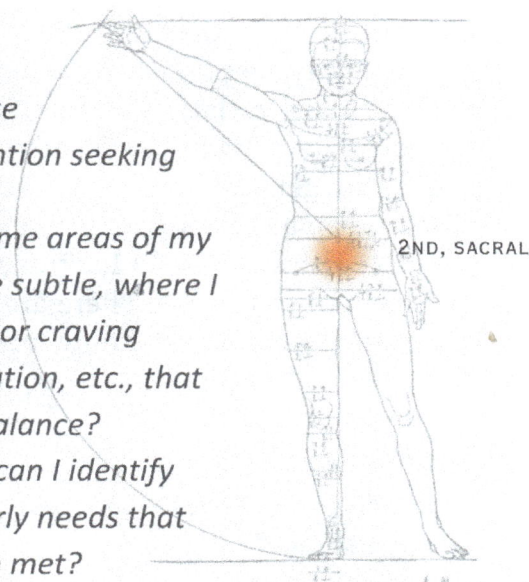

2ND, SACRAL

ALBRECHT DURER
WOODCUT
C. 1528

CHAKRAS
SUPERIMPOSED

never, that's some good information for you, for example. Do I presently feel emotionally attended to, relationally or internally, am I able to do this for myself? Do I experience emotional connection and attachment? Am I emotionally nourished? Where do I experience magic, now or in the past?

One of the various ways we can see imbalance (of many different ways) in second chakra themes, is *attention seeking* behavior. Can we identify some area or areas of our lives, even if it's quite subtle, where I am–or this can be in the past– driven to seeking and or craving, attention validation, etc., to a degree that may be out of balance?

Looking a little more deeply at this, can I identify where I may have had early needs that were never met? It's interesting because of so many variations of this, from the very gross level of acting out, like a young child might physically disrupt an environment to get attention (or withdraw too), adults do this too. Where people are seeking visual response, as in, people will just you know, actually look at you, you "turn heads". Gross sense manifestations. There are more nuanced degrees of course, some people you know, very sophisticated people have

sacral chakra - on your own

- *arrange time with children, doing playful, interactive activities*
- *make a special effort to be more nuturing to others, in a sincere way, get curious and see what happens*
- *try new bodywork, massage, craniosacral therapy*
- *start paying attention when you are triggered- there may be something you are not doing for yourself*
- *find something to do where you're moving your hips, dance with others or alone. Put on your favorite music and sing, and looking foolish can be healing.*
- *traditional Chinese or Tibetan sound therapy, or simply listen to music that moves you, aroma therapy, sense based therapies*
- *find someone young at heart and go to an amusement park, play games*
- *if you had a ritual practice you enjoyed in your life, try it again, or find a new one to practice*

their own ways, like wanting attention for all kinds of things and and the more sophisticated they are, the more subtle it may be. This is just an opportunity to look at yourself and really feel into some type of behavior or pursuit or, I mean, you know, I guess why don't I use one of my own examples. Also it's not necessarily purely like you're only looking for attention, so it can be merged with other things. So I love to paint (painting and drawings etc) but for a number of years I think I really wanted a certain kind of external validation as an artist (which eventually subsided.) This is some area where I think some of these early needs that were not met just kind of came out in that way. That's one example, but there's almost infinite variations we can imagine. Just explore this as you wish.

So what I referred to as homework, which is not really homework, but things that you can do on your own that relate to the second chakra and healing. Some examples, arranging time with children doing playful interactive activities. Making a special effort to be more nurturing to others in a sincere way, being curious and seeing what happens. Trying new bodywork, massage, craniosacral therapy. Paying attention to when you are triggered now in some of the specific ways connected to second chakra stage developmental needs. The mirror of triggers like this can indicate there is something that you're not doing for yourself. In Integral Zen we have been focused on shadow a lot related to this. Noticing the difference as well of minor triggering, and intense triggering, which will be more related to the category of trauma.[22]

Try to bring particular attention to the area of the body connected to the second chakra. Find something to do where you're moving your hips or just moving this area of the body because when you do move this area of the body, if there are energetic blockages, you can be stiff and awkward, which is not a huge problem, but an indication that you will benefit from moving, so dancing with others or alone put on music you like that makes you want to move. We can consider this a sense based therapy, anything that can engage our senses can contribute to healing the second chakra, or getting second chakra energies flowing. Looking foolish can be healing!

Other options include all kinds of sound therapy, traditional Indian, Chinese and Tibetan sound therapies can be very powerful. Listening to music and also aromatherapy, another sense therapy. Finding someone young at heart and going to an amusement park playing games, these are all great options to reconnect with our second chakra innocence. Especially playing. Can you be playful, and being playful is not like "I'm taking a course to achieve this;", we're talking about play for the sake of play.

Next if you had a ritual practice you've enjoyed in your life, try it again. Or if you want to find a new practice or just are curious about this, explore it. I often ask people because most people are not going to have memories from this time of their life because we don't tend to have memories before language. Occasionally some people do. But I often ask people, when you were young, were there any kind of rituals that were magical to you, singing things with your family, community, anything that really you remember that opened up a sense of *magic* for you, and sometimes it's really good to reconnect with that because remember, when you through integral orange indoctrination (rationalism), a period of your life where you're embracing science and reason, part of that is going to include, a rejection and even decimation of all that was magical to you, all that was mysterious. It generally in the Western world, is a rejection (not transcend and include as Wilber says, but transcend and negate, creating an aversion and causing people to hit a spiritual ceiling, which Doshin will discuss later). So part of this healing is wanting to reconnect with that, something that children just innately experience.

Self-Healing Practice For The First Two Chakras

self-healing practice for the first two chakras
message to heart-mind-body

- *place your left hand on your back at your root and sacral areas, your right hand on your heart*
- *visualize yourself as a baby*
- *tell yourself with no wavering, with complete, loving determination:*

"I was, and I am loveable, I deserved, and am deserving of love"

also you can repeat this traditional Tibetan healing mantra for the heart:
"A A Tsitta Sukha Sam Sam"

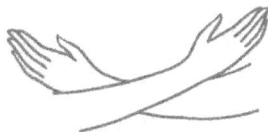

Next is a healing practice for the first two chakras to do on your own. Now you might look at this and just quickly dismiss it because it's so simple, but *here's the thing*. This is a message from yourself to your heart-mind-body that the body may not have necessarily received in the past. Your heart-mind-body may have not heard clear, confident, loving support all of its early life, and in fact, it may have taken in some real negative messages and experiences that are still in your body. This is good to do before you go to sleep. Place your left hand on your back at your root and sacral areas, your right hand and your heart, and visualize yourself as a baby and I think it's better not to visualize your own family. Instead, you're just a baby. This is really important and Doshin pointed out, this is the third chakra part to tell yourself this is a healing action with no wavering. Complete loving determination, saying to yourself, "I was, and I am, lovable. I deserved and am deserving of love." So this is actually you telling your body, giving your body permission, declaring the right to heal. This is, you know, mind, body, heart healing.

Heart Healing Mantra

Also I have a healing mantra from Sowa Rigpa:

"AH AH SITA SUKA SAM-SAM"

and you can repeat this as much as you want. The sounds are vibrations which heal the heart. Do this self-healing practice as often as you like.

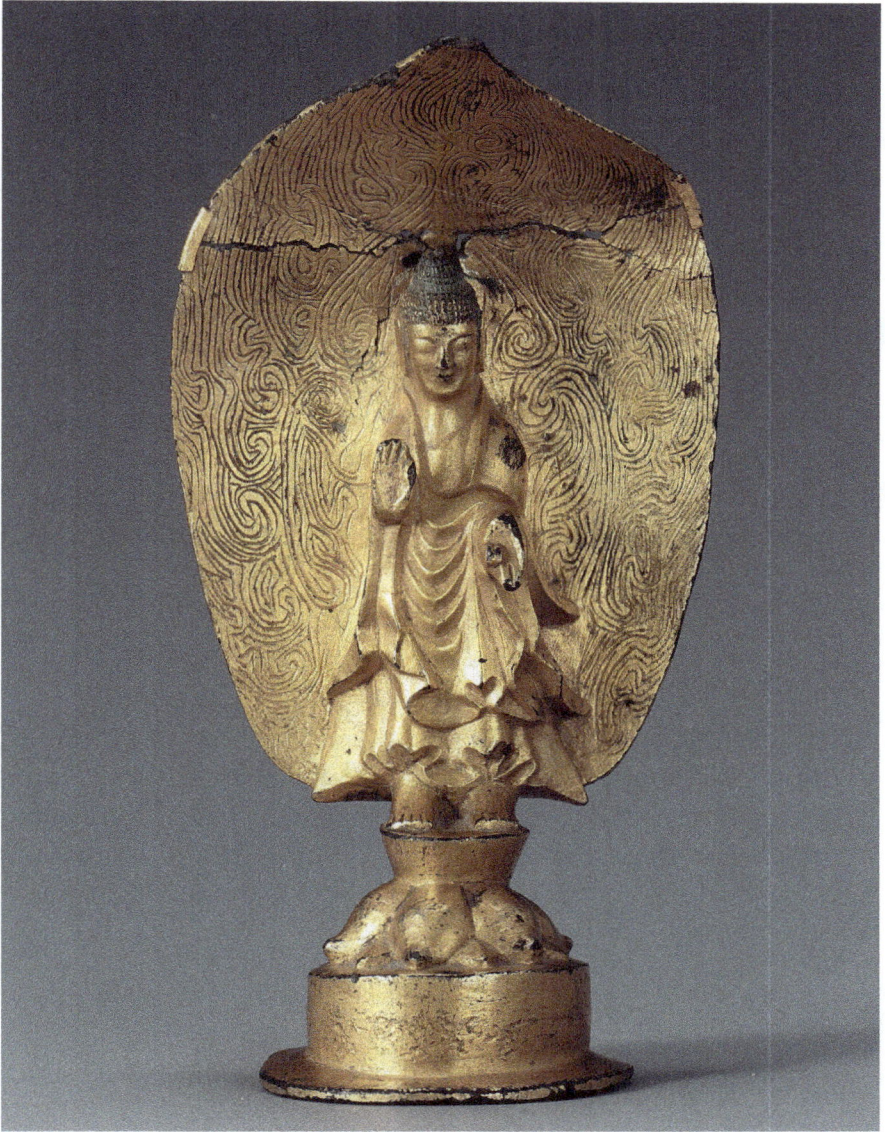

Mudra which Grants the Absence of Fear

Abhayamudra. Gilt-bronze Standing Buddha with Inscription of "the Seventh Yeonga Year," National Treasure of Republic of Korea No. 119 By National Museum of Korea (National Museum of Korea), KOGL Type 1, https://commons.wikimedia.org/w/index.php?curid=83991015.

Next is one of my favorite mudras, called the *Mudra which grants the absence of fear:* Semui-in (Japanese), Shih-wu-wei-yin (Chinese), and Abhayamudra (Sanskrit). This mudra has the power of giving tranquillity and absence of fear to all. When you do it, pay attention to the energetic difference between doing it, and not doing it.

This mudra comes from the legend of the malevolent Devadatta, who wanted to hurt the Buddha, and caused an elephant to become drunk. The elephant was about to trample the Buddha, and it is said that Shakyamuni raised his right hand with his fingers closed together, and this gesture not only stopped the elephant in his tracks, but completely subdued him.

Doshin

Are there any questions? You know, we covered an immense amount of material in a way that puts this material in an Integral Framework. You don't get to do this very often in my experience with people. So let's open it up. If there are any real questions where there's something you'd really like to know.

Question

Yes, at the risk of seeking attention. I was intrigued by your reference to the sense of the sacred emerging with the second chakra. I think that's what she said and it makes sense to me intuitively, but I can't quite understand it. A thought that emerged later, you know, age 6, 7, 8, whatever, when the child starts to learn the amber structure of whatever their parents hold sacred, can you say more about this?

Doshin

Yes, this is very important, and almost never seen. What emerges at 5, 6, 7 years old, is a 2nd person perspective. We then have the capacity to be indoctrinated into a social holon, a socio-cultural system that has its own moral values and ideological beliefs. So in terms of the second chakra question, the capacity for the sacred begins for the individual in the second chakra, the magenta stage of development, but the individual does not yet have even a 1st person perspective. the capacity to be indoctrinated into a collective social holon doesn't emerge until the fourth chakra, the amber stage of development. The interdynamics of what happens at the second chakra is, the second chakra is energized, so that a felt sense of sacredness begins to be felt in the individual's personal experience. The sense of self at magenta is pre-egoic. The ego doesn't begin to fully form until the third chakra, the red stage of development as the 1st person perspective comes online. The 2nd person perspective emerges with the fourth chakra at the amber stage of development around 5, 6, and 7 years old.[23]

At six months old, that second chakra starts energizing. Along with this, the emotional body, magic, the capacity of rational feeling, and the sense of sacredness all start coming alive. As the emotional/spiritual body comes online, the very emotions and magic that are emerging, are ignored and rejected by our collective scientific, materialistic, modern cultural belief system. All emotions including the sense of the sacred are rejected as irrational. This all comes online and is then indoctrinated out of us when we're born into an orange (technical integral term) or a green (technical integral term) culture. But these irrational human traits still remain in us, a part of us. Just because our modern culture tries to indoctrinate it out of us doesn't mean it's not there. One of the things that we're really doing in Integral Zen by dealing with awakening and healing is re-energizing that feeling of numinosity of sacredness. It's such a critical part of healing. You can't see, heal or liberate the deeper karma without religious practices. There is nothing in Western psychology that I have found that will touch the deeper healing which allows the karma to liberate itself. That we only find in religious practices. So that has to be re-awakened, seen and integrated into your life. Is that helpful at all to you?

Question

Yes. Yes it is, I was taking notes.

Doshin

This is something that we're really going to explore in a lot more depth, and it's something that we really get into in the next healing retreat that we're doing, a retreat/workshop. There will be a lot of deep healing work going on along with the awakening practices.

Janel

Yes, and just to spark your intrigue, we all have conscious or unconscious "altars" of things we worship, so to speak, and there are things on our altars, and even if we think, *I'm rational*, that means something is on your altar and *you don't know what it is*. So a lot of times, what I notice, one of the things that ends up on the (orange) scientific materialists' altar is sex. So for them, that's where the magic goes- into sexuality– or lack thereof. I mean, when I say sex, that means that it can be like obsession about sex, sexual dysfunction, like all kinds of possibilities. It's like we think we're really rational, but that means a lot of this is going into shadow. So we're going to explore that more going forward.

Question

My granddaughter has a developmental disease, she's seven years old, but I think she is maybe in between the first and the second chakras developmentally. Could you say something? Is it possible to look at her in this way?

Doshin

Yes, it is. If we're going to evaluate someone, we're using a measuring rod to evaluate them so it's complicated in this complicated world where we have so many different measuring rods, right? We have the orange psychological measuring rod, we have the green psychological measuring rod, we have the traditional religious measuring rod.

To really get a complete picture we need a new method of measuring. This is where the Integral Framework is absolutely priceless, especially when you combine it with someone who has meditated enough, that they have really cultivated a stable causal state of unbiased witnessing mind, a causal vantage point. This enables them to actually see more clearly; the third eye is opened and they are seeing *what is*. They are looking into the metaphorical *perfect round mirror* and they're really seeing, they're actually witnessing *what is*.

This is where Ken Wilber's *Kosmic Addressing* is priceless and going to become more priceless as we keep arguing over what is the right measuring rod? We have to understand what structural level of development an individual is at, for example. Your granddaughter is at a certain structural level of development and you know we have to look at that really non-judgmentally and with great compassion. Then we have to understand what is the level of consciousness of the environment, the social holon that she's interacting with? Then we have to look at the lines of intelligence. We have to look at the center of gravity of her overall ego development. Then we have to look at how developed she is emotionally. Is her emotional line of development at the magenta level? Or is it at a different level of development? Then we can look at her cognitive line of development, and her spiritual line of development? These are some of the yardsticks that we use when we're assessing Kosmic Addresses, when we're applying the AQAL framework to help evaluate anything. All quadrants, all levels of consciousness, all lines of intelligence, all states of consciousness and all types. What state has she stabilized in? We all begin in gross, and that's probably where she is. Then typologies are really important to help us understand ourselves and each other in new useful ways. When I first started studying Wilber, he only talked about one type: masculine and feminine. That's a really fundamental one, which is really important, but today we're adding and expanding the masculine and feminine to include light and dark. The Taoist yin and yang, balanced, unbalanced and then we're extending that. Today, we use the five element typology that has been around as a useful tool for thousands of years. It has been used for both healing and awakening long before they were differentiated as two separate processes in modern times. With an Integral Framework they can be re-united. There's an incredible amount of knowledge about the five elements that's been accumulated and passed on in oral traditions, and written down only recently. There's so much that might be useful in an extremely personal and practical way to help your granddaughter. Does that make sense to you?

Question

This is a way I can look at her, yes, with different things. But my question was especially about chakras because we are learning about chakras now, and, if so, my question in effect is, is it useful to use the knowledge about the chakras to look at her and see what she's doing?

Doshin

Okay, so you're listening to just the chakra part. I'm teaching everything that I described. You're only taking in what you're able to hear, and that's perfect. It is all any of us can do. So if there's something in what I'm saying that's useful to you, then use it. If it's confusing to you, then just let it go. Take what's useful and apply it. People will hear whatever they're capable of hearing, you know it. It's really difficult to find someone that understands how to use Kosmic Addressing. I only know of one person that I would trust using Kosmic Addressing, and that's Wilber himself. And I happen to have been given the great gift of participating every week in a group that used Kosmic Addressing in a very practical way. It changed the way I look at everything. So take in whatever you can and if you find something that's useful in the chakras or anywhere that helps you treat your granddaughter more kindly with greater compassion and greater clarity, then use it. I hope that's helpful. And if you have more questions about that, you know where to find me. You know we've been down this path, for many moons.

Question

Thank you, Janel, and thank you, Doshin. So I think probably like a lot of people here, it's just darkness when I'm thinking about prior to 18 months, just outside of my conscious recall. So what's your advice in trying to approach those questions ? You know so I'm looking back at, did I get, was I provided with loving, patient and attentive nurturance? Because I've got a sense of feeling, to say no. You know, I also feel that's my, that's me, rationalising post hoc. Then adding up what my part from my experiences more recently and then sort of projecting it back. I have to do some detective work, don't I?

Janel

Yes, so when I'm working with people, you know, there's a few things. We have information, and we can gather information from what we know historically from our family, but then we also can look, you know, assuming the people are still around, they may not be. To some degree you have to be like a sleuth. Hopefully if you--I mean some people didn't know their parents really, so then that's going to be really hard to do, but if you still have people around, then sure they've changed over time, but there are signs of how they interact with other people now that will give you information about the past. Really, you can take a look, and it may not have been *that different* when you were small, look how they relate to other people. I mean, if you have a mother that every time you talk to her, she only talks about herself, and you know, never asks you questions, never inquires. Then she *probably* wasn't hugely different when she was your mother as a young child. (She most likely was less mature, a general assumption one can make).

So we put together, and what I say when I start the root, I say, just based on what you know, and what you surmise, paint a picture of what your life might have been like at a particular time. What you *imagine* it was like, and even though we don't know for certain, we can't go back in time. The more we reflect, the more we look at different specifics, different perspectives (I guide people one on one), we can come up with something, some sense of how life probably was. (Sometimes we might have baby photos, for example, and we can look at these more closely, there's often a lot of information there we may have overlooked). Just as well, if we can't, sometimes that's a sign too. For example if awareness and memory is extremely blocked, then that's something we're starting with. Doshin would you like to talk about this at all?

Doshin

Yes, I would like to say a few things. Just the way you phrased your question, I think for you personally and for some other people, this might be useful, but not for everybody. Because we're all different. If instead of trying to understand it with your thinking-mind, if you just cultivate a deep curiosity without the need to understand it, just set your intention to exploring it and not needing to understand it, it will be much more helpful for you. How does that feel to you?

Question

Yeah, I think that makes sense, I just remembered when we were doing state shadows and you said something like the difference between I don't know and not knowing.

Doshin

Yes.

Question

Is that the same thing you're talking about?

Doshin

Yes, exactly. So cultivate a curiosity and then follow the curiosity into the journey of self discovery. If your parents are around, you can always ask them or you have older brothers and sisters, ask them. I'll never forget I was fifty years old and

I'd done a whole bunch of psychological work, therapy, shadow work, and all of a sudden I started digging into this first and second chakra territory that I had not explored before. And my mother was there and I asked her if there was anything that happened to me when I was an infant that might have had anything to do with this huge amount of anger that I've had to deal with all my life? And she says, "Oh yes, there was this one little thing." That one thing exploded into a complete exploration that made so much sense. It explained why I've been angry since I was born. At least, that is the way it feels, I was angry because something happened to me when I was infant, and had I not asked her that question, I may never have known. That opened the door to being able to heal this angry little infant that is still struggling for his life, and the three year old who is still throwing a temper tantrum. So get really curious, and let that curiosity lead you. This is an exploration, not an exercise in intellectual understanding.

Questioner

OK. Thank you.

Question

You mentioned the Japanese element system, and you said when death is coming on, the Earth base chakra starts to dissolve. Would you say some more about that, please?

Janel

There's so much to say about that. The dissolution of the five elements is basic to look at, it is a basic part of practice in Vajrayana to prepare for death and the bardos. One can review the signs of the dissolution of the earth element, for example, with the earth element dissolving, bones become weak, and break more easily. There are known, identifiable signs, like teeth breaking and falling out. There are stages, there are gross signs, subtle signs (also called external, internal and hidden) secret signs. The secret signs are the signs experienced by the person in the process of dying. This is partly the benefit of doing such a practice to prepare for death so one is familiarized with how it generally is said to proceed. So it's there if people want to study them. Also for people who work in hospice or if you are caring for people who are close to death, people can find this very, very useful. It's out there if you want to know. I'll give you references if that's useful to you.

Question

Hi, a simple question, but first I just want to appreciate you know, Janel and just for what you're presenting, and I mean it's tremendous. Then, of course, just such clear transmission, you know. Deep mind and heart, mind and things just coming through very clearly and a lot of gratitude; appreciate that.

A mere question just kind of kept coming to me, how I work with children and special needs children, I just kind of kept thinking about some of the healing practices for the chakras that Janel has been laying out and you know how interesting that could be to to look at those chakras in the, in the, in the context of your granddaughter we talked about, for example, you need to go to the hot springs or whatever, that kind of thing so. And then on that mantra, the *Sita,* I don't have it written in front of me, but is there a cadence to that? Could you just say it, verbalize it?

Janel

Sure, you can hear recordings of it online by this wonderful Tibetan teacher that has her singing. (Drukmo Gyal) So yes, I'm going to look and see if I can find that and I'll make it available.

Question

Mine is more of an observation in myself that I thought was relevant to the group that might have a question attached to it, but I'm also a painter and one of the things that I was thinking about was in the healthiest of ways, when you're making expressive art, there's a certain sort of wonderfulness you can lose yourself in. You paint for six hours and you know the world disappears and it's just you and this focus on this painting. But then there's something that happens when you have a show, and you have a work up on the wall and people come and you know if people really get the work. It's this amazing, to think I'm thinking of a spiritual term, *transmission*, that happens when somebody that's viewing the art gets the intention of the work. But there's this really fine razor blade edge right between having that because I mean it's very energizing, you know, when you feel like oh, everybody understands what I'm doing here, this is great. That sort of need for that external validation? I'm wondering about. Like there's a healthy piece, and then there's the, you know, not. Then I feel like, as I say, like this razor blade edge between the two and I wonder if there's a way to refine your discernment about that. You know what I mean?

Janel

I would say this is a dynamic situation of gross subtle causal state shifts. Flux and fixation and objectification and subject object stuff is going on every moment. Wherever you're at in your creation process, and suddenly you fixate. From being lost in the process and flow no separation then suddenly one can become self conscious or thinking, evaluating, seeing it as other, imagining others seeing it etc.. This is oh, this! Then other people are involved with their projections. It's so dynamic and I think if we're creative people, whatever we're doing is just evolving moment to moment. As our relationship to creation is evolving, and, Doshin, would you like to say something about that?

Doshin

You're the artist.

Janel

I haven't been painting much lately. I'll just say that, in part of it, is how we relate to it.

Doshin

Well, yes, someone just commented on how artistic the slides were, you know. Guess who created the presentation? Isn't it beautiful? The slides in the presentation are exquisite. You know, once the artist is there, it never goes away...until the body dissolves.

Janel

Thank you, I am humbled. As for the creation, I would say that even though I'm not painting lately, it is true we are creating this program now. What I miss with painting is it feels so healing. That's what I notice. Mixing colors, choosing colors and maybe that's part of the *play* aspect, you know that can vary like when it starts out as play, and then it can also quickly become an agenda. *I need to fix this!* I mean you can see all kinds of things happening. It's a great mirror, I guess, like everything.

Questioner

I think when you know the world really does disappear and you hear other artists talk about this as well, it feels like there's this thing that's happening where you are just the channel. You're not doing it, you're not making the choices. It's something else.

Janel

Yes I experience this too, and I especially experience it when I do artworks of animals, and it was almost as if this animal's being would come through me and the process would happen on its own, and then I'd stand there after, saying, oh, what was that?

Question

Yes, I heard what the other speaker said and I just wanted to say that eventually with age, there is a line that disappears and you don't care anymore, if you have been evaluated or not, it's just there and that's one thing I wanted to say, if to give hope that one day just doesn't matter anymore.

Doshin

Thank you. All of these things are so appropriate for the second chakra. The magenta development in the individual, the longing to be an artist. You know, at the gross level there's a need, and at the subtle level there's a different need. There is even a deeper need at the causal level, a need to liberate. In the gross realm we may want to become an artist to make money and succeed. In the subtle realm, we want to have a meaningful livelihood. We may find it very meaningful to be an artist. We may even have a hungry ghost that's starving to have others see us as being meaningful. In the causal realm, we have purified or emptied out our self, and its need for success and meaning. I always kind of jokingly say, I just don't give a shit whether you like me or don't like me. Of course this isn't completely true, but there is considerable truth to that. What's more true is I care deeply. But I really don't give a shit whether somebody likes me or not anymore. The most important thing is liberation from self, from suffering.

Questioner

So you're talking about, meaning making, the last show that I was in was called imploding meaning. I think it's relatable to that.

Doshin

Well, you described your creativity. In your creative process you described attaining something where there was no you, no self. That is actually a causal state. The meaningfulness longing for meaning is not causal.

Questioner

Right.

Doshin

It's a subtle state, and when it includes a feeling of sacredness, a feeling of numinosity to it, then it's what the Tibetans would call a high subtle state. There is a very thin line between the word causal as it's used in Tibetans Buddhism and it's used in Zen Buddhism. It is not just black and white, there are many shades and densities of blackness and whiteness in all this.

Janel

We're a little over time, thank you all.

CHAPTER 3, THE SOLAR PLEXUS, POWER CHAKRA

Doshin

Wonderful, so here we are, week three. Have you ever heard anyone scratch their head and ask, why can't we all just get along? Have you ever wondered why it is that we fail to understand why we all can't just get along? What would it take to understand this? What do we each need to do to understand and clearly see why it is that we all can't just get along? Well, that is an even more interesting question.

In order to be healthy human beings, we need to heal. In order to fully heal, we must awaken. In order to fully awaken, we must also heal. It's so simple, for us to all get along we must heal and awaken. It's so simple.

I'm going to remind you every time we start one of these sessions, remember: this is an experiential course. It's not a class. It is not our plan to teach you a specific set of knowledge. In the first place, there is no agenda. We have an intention to present an experience and we use the chakras in the context of an Integral Framework to do this. We are presenting a broad overview of many ancient healing lineage teachings that have been around for thousands of years. We are focusing on both healing and awakening. This is a very different approach. We are integrating ancient wisdom with modern knowledge.

Prior to the emergence of the W.E.I.R.D.est people in the world (Western Educated, Industrialized, Rich, and Democratic), Europe was coming out of the Middle Ages which lasted from about the 5th to the 15th century. Then, about the time the printing press was invented and Protestantism emerged, the Modern Age began. The age of Reason, the Industrial Age and the Age of Science all followed. It was here, in this Modern Age that things were radically split apart. God died, and the modern rational ego assumed the throne and place on the altar. With empirical science, everything that wasn't measurable and everything that wasn't rational, was ignored and negated. This included anything religious or spiritual. Human reasoning ruled and the human spirit died. An unhealthy form of self-centered egoic reasoning was born and the paths and practices of spiritual healing were lost. The ancient methods and practices of spiritual healing and awakening were ignored. So, please let go of any agenda to learn anything and instead, set your intention on trusting that you will take in something that will be fresh and helpful to you. Just let the rest go. Let the experience be healing and get curious about what is out of balance within you and outside of you.

I think it will be helpful to say a few words about what an Integral Framework is. I'll keep it as brief and as comprehensive as it needs to be. The Integral Framework is a more user-friendly version of Wilber's Integral Theory. It is usually presented as AQAL, which is short for: All Quadrants, All Levels, All States, All Lines and All Types. These are 5 cognitive models and methods of looking at the universe. These are integral tools, which form the foundation of an

Integral Framework–a new way of looking at the universe.

Last week and in the beginning, we started covering a little bit of the four quadrants. So to review: if you draw a vertical line right down the middle of the page, and a horizontal line across the bottom, the middle of the page, what you have is everything on the right of the vertical line is outside, and everything to the left of the vertical line is inside. Everything above the horizontal line is individual, and everything below the horizontal line is collective. This gives us a complete picture of the four quadrants of our experience, and this is a new and profound tool that can help us understand ourselves, each other and the whole universe in which we live. It's a foundational beginning to understanding why we can't all just get along. (Notice the overlap between the inner and outer quadrants with Jung's Theory of Types of Introversion and Extraversion.)

Now, in addition to the Quadrants, which is the first piece of the Integral Framework. The second piece is All Levels of conscious development. We are roughly using the ancient teachings of the chakras along with the modern knowledge of the levels of ego development or self-development. Janel has a little deeper and broader understanding of the chakras, so she's going a little deeper than I'm going into them. I will link ego development with the chakras as Wilber does in his book: *The Religion of Tomorrow.* I'm simplifying the chakras and using them as a metaphor to describe the levels of ego development. I am doing this with a deep understanding of Jung's Theory of Types that I have been studying and using for the last 50 years.

The karma of everything that has ever been enters the individual being at conception.[24] Beginning with the first chakra is this karma, starting at conception and continuing through the development in the womb, birth and the first six months of life. That's the infrared color or level of development in the Integral Framework. The second chakra is roughly equivalent to the magenta level of the ego development from 6 months to around 18 months of age. There is not a solid sense of self until the third chakra, the power chakra is energized. This 3rd chakra corresponds to the red level of development where the self first emerges with a first person perspective, a solid ego. When the perspective of *me* becomes firm, then suddenly *everything is mine*.

In the fourth chakra, the second person perspective emerges. This is where the individual me, finally has the capacity to be indoctrinated into a collective cultural set of rules, roles and values. All the things that the individual "I" should and shouldn't do according to the rules. This is the period of life beginning at approximately five or six years old and continuing to about puberty when the third person perspective begins clumsily to emerge (this will vary in different individuals, circumstances and cultures). Then, sometime after the third person perspective takes root, it is possible if the culture is advanced enough for the fourth person perspective to begin to emerge. The third person perspective is roughly equivalent to the orange stage of ego development and the fourth person perspective to the green stage, the stage of development that Integral Theory describes as postmodern.

In Integral Theory, the fifth person perspective begins to emerge at 2nd Tier teal and turquoise levels of development. This can be equated roughly to the sixth chakra, and the transpersonal aspects of ego development. Here the opening of the third eye becomes possible in peak states of gross, subtle and causal experiences. The crown chakra can be equated roughly with the 3rd tier structures. The sixth chakra is equated with the 2nd tier in our Integral Framework and the seventh chakra, the crown chakra is roughly equated to 3rd Tier levels of development where we naturally become more concerned with liberation. So that's two of the pieces of AQAL, the quadrants and levels.

The third piece is the lines of intelligence, and their corresponding level of ego development. To what degree have the individual lines of intelligence developed through the structural colors? Examples of some lines of intelligence would be: cognitive intelligence, emotional intelligence, spiritual intelligence, moral intelligence, culinary intelligence, kinesthetic intelligence. All of these separate lines of intelligence develop through the levels just like the center of gravity of an individual does. So it's possible to have a level of cognitive intelligence that has developed to 2nd Tier, teal, and also have a much less developed level of spiritual intelligence that is stuck in the red or even magenta level of ego development. These lines of intelligence are not all at the same level of ego development.

The fourth piece of AQAL is the states of consciousness. Last week I described the states of consciousness that we find in the upper left quadrant of the four quadrants. In the upper right quadrant we find the gross, subtle and causal bodies of consciousness. In the lower left quadrant we find the collective gross, subtle, and causal realms of consciousness. Finally, in the lower right quadrant, we find the corresponding collective gross, subtle and causal fields of consciousness organized into external systems.

The fifth piece of our AQAL framework is types. Human beings have used typological maps to better understand ourselves, others and the world around us for thousands of years. For example yin and yang, the four or five elements and astrological types. These tools have been used for thousands of years and have been an integral part of all of these healing lineages we are presenting here. The five elements are an incredible typology for working with healing and awakening. It is an incredibly powerful and useful typology. Janel is going to go into more depth with this.

So in addition to these five AQAL models, Wilber's Integral Framework includes his integral understanding of shadows, described in *The Religion of Tomorrow* where he outlines in meticulous detail, his integral understanding of shadows, which he describes as addictions and allergies in both states and stages of consciousness, as well as what drives them. It also includes an understanding of split-off sub-personalities that seem to have a life of their own. They seem to be fully operational without our consent or knowledge in our blind spots where we can't see them. Then some more really sophisticated tools are Kosmic Addressing, Integral Semiotics and an Integral Framework that includes subtle energy. So now that I put you to sleep with too much integral babble, Janel, it's your turn to wake them up.

Janel

Oh goodness, I was just noticing, that even though I've heard this so many times, that I was getting overwhelmed. But thank you for providing all of that necessary context. So from this point until the end of the class, we will be looking at Buddhist frameworks for health.

We'll get into the very basics of Sowa Rigpa and the Tibetan Medicine Buddha lineage I study within, and then at the end we're going to start to touch on Zen and Chan lineages.

Again, I will be jumping around here. First looking at this excerpt from *The Essence of the 8 Branches of Medicine*, considered a core text in Ayurveda and Tibetan medicine from the great master Vagbhata.[25]

> "Homage to that original Doctor who eliminated without
> any residue the diseases such as desire/attachment,
> which are spread throughout the being, creating anxiety,
> confusion, and restlessness/dissatisfaction."

ASHTANGA-HRIDAYA SAMHITA SU. 1.1[26]

This points to the interconnectedness between the traditions, the parallels with major Buddhist thought. Next session we will really start getting into *the three poisons* in their relationship to health and pathology in the medicine Buddha lineage.

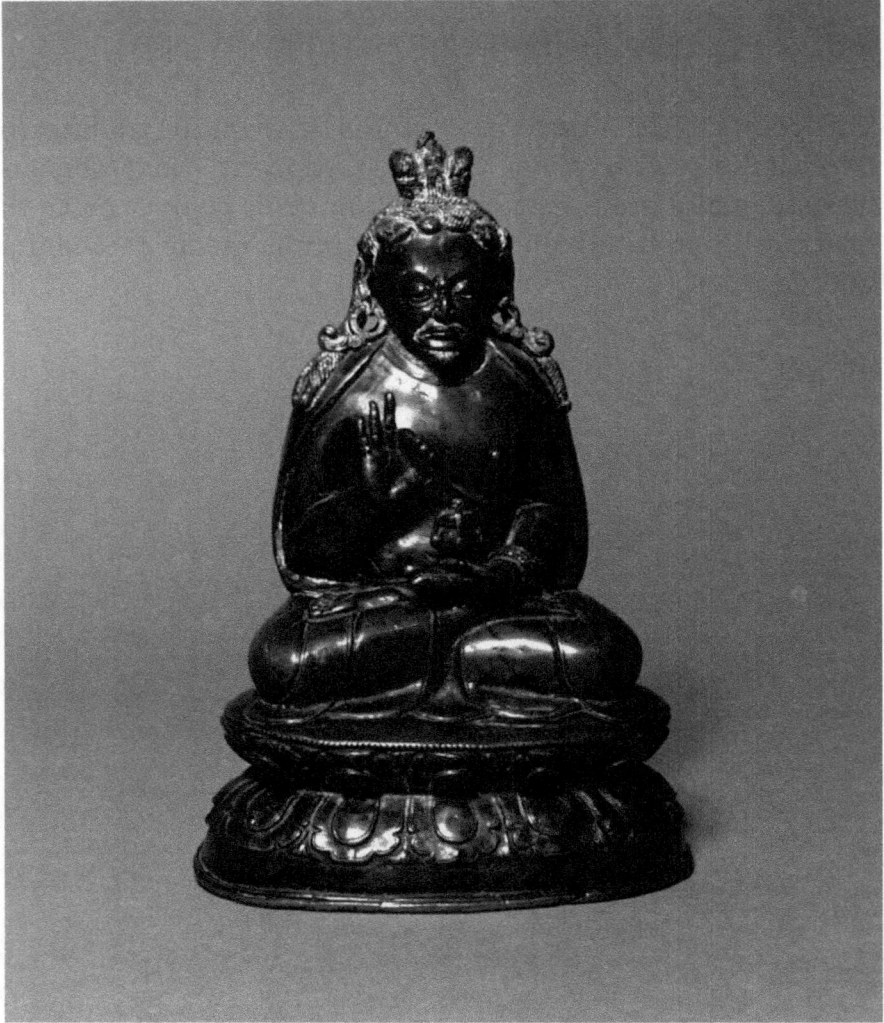

Yuthok Yönten Gonpo (1127-1203) or Tangtong Gyalpo (1385-1464), Eastern Tibet, 16c
Sculpture, Public Domain, LACMA, www.lacma.org

The main teacher in the Medicine Buddha, Sowa Rigpa
tradition I study with, Dr. Nida Chenagtsang, says this is one of
his favorite quotes:

> *"I myself am my own master/lord/protector. There is no*

one else I can look to be my (own) master (for me)"[27]

The Buddha

And then more recently, His Holiness the Dalai Lama

"Without your own effort, it is impossible for blessings to come."[28]

His Holiness the Dalai Lama

So this is a reminder, it's up to you, just as it is up to all of us.

Throughout time there were many Medicine Buddhas, they are not limited to the Eastern world. All great medical figures can be considered Medicine Buddhas.

Shakyamuni Buddha had a doctor named Jivaka, and there is a story often told, where Jivaka takes his students through the forest. As he walks with them, there are lots of footprints, broken branches, and so Jivaka questions the students, asking what do you suppose happened here? Jivaka's students don't really say much. They see some big footprints, and make some simple observations, and then Jivaka tells them:

"those are footprints of an elephant, not male, but female. She is blind of the right eye, and about to bring forth young (pregnant) today. The woman is too blind, also blind of the right eye; she will bear a son today."[29]

The students are naturally astonished, and want more of an explanation.

> *Jivaka says, "being brought up in a royal family, one knows that footprints of male elephants are round, whereas those of female elephants are oblong."*

Then he explains that if you look carefully you can see she had eaten grass only from the left side of the road. Next, she was pressing hardest towards the right side, which suggested that the calf would be a male. Then last, he explains that the woman riding the elephant was blind in her right eye, and that she picked flowers that grew on the left side upon descending, so that the heels of her feet made deeper than usual impressions, and her backward lean suggested that she was pregnant. So this

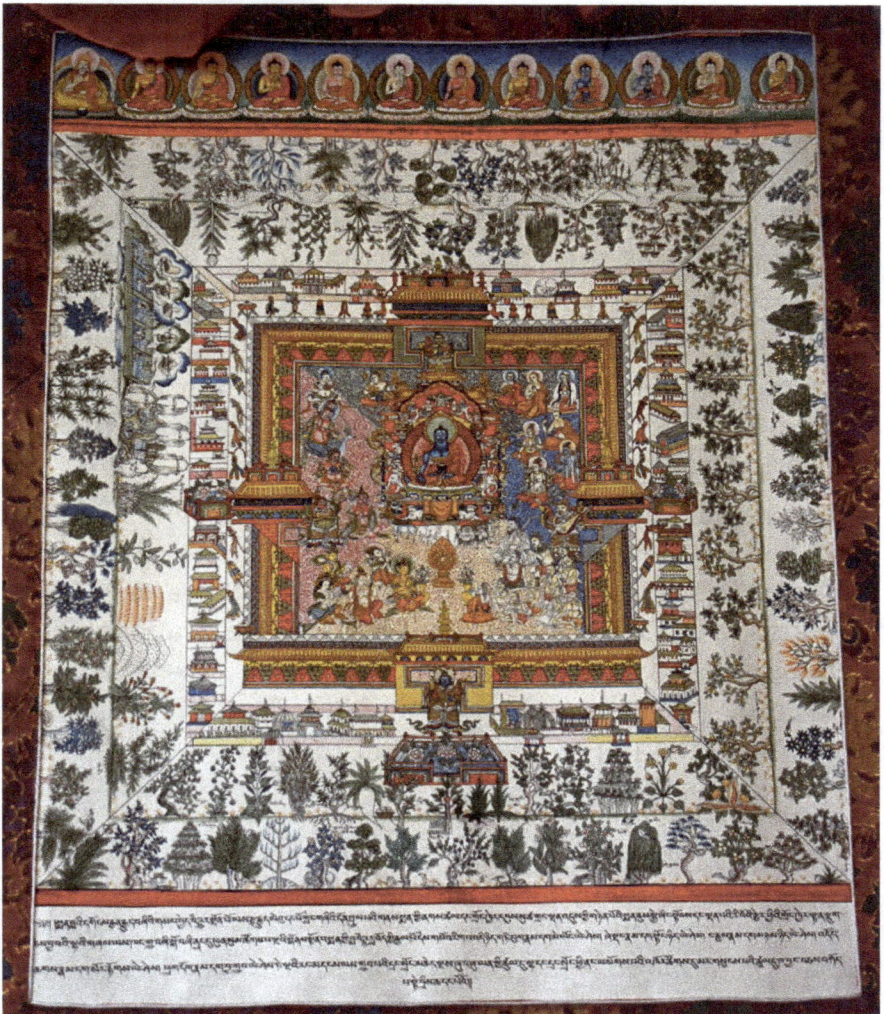

The blue Medicine Buddha, Bhaisajyaguru, sits center in the first of the medical thangkas. This placement illustrates his vital importance to the practice and study of Tibetan Medicine. This painting consists of a walled 'City of Irresistible Beauty' where a host of deities reside alongside the Medicine Buddha. The city itself is square with four gates opening up in each of the cardinal directions. Outside the palace's walls lie four mountains where medicinal plants grow and animals roam.

Growing in the Snow Mountain to the north of the city are white and red sandalwood, camphor, arecanut palm, chiretta along with many other plants and trees. Although it is not clearly visible in this photograph, the moon is located in the center of the top row of the north mountain. The east, south and west mountains each contain different plants corresponding to their climate. The figure in the top left of this painting is the Fifth Dalai Lama (1617-1682) who was responsible for communicating the teaching of Tibetan story reveals the incredible interconnected awareness with the natural world that the Buddha's doctor had.

The Medicine Buddha in Tibetan is called *Sange Menla*. The tradition of *Sowa Rigpa* can be translated as "healing science", or "nourishment of awareness." A big emphasis of this tradition is based on the interdependence between human health and nature.

It is said that the *fruits* of Sowa Rigpa are longevity, freedom from disease, Dharma, wealth, happiness. Something you may notice is missing, and that is awakening. Sowa Rigpa was intended to be taught to everyone and anyone of any religious or non religious background. In other words, it separates the awakening path from the healing path. There is a spiritual path connected to Sowa Rigpa, (Yuthok Nyinthig[30]) but it is separate from the healing path.

There are many *mandalas* used in the Medicine Buddha lineage. In Sanskrit a mandala means *mind circling* or *mind spiral*. A mandala is geometric, usually a circular design, a kind of map, of the universe, representing a pattern of forces that make up external/internal "reality" in pure form. Each mandala is a symbol of the perfect balance of all 5 elements.

Yuthok Yonten Gonpo, the elder (708-833)[31] is recognized as the father of Traditional Tibetan Medicine (TTM). The head of the Sowa Rigpa lineage which has continued to the present day, he was said to have lived to 125 years, and recognized as having achieved *rainbow body*, spiritual realization of body speech and mind.[32]

There are two main schools within Sowa Rigpa, known as Southern and northern schools since the 14-15th centuries. The lineage I practice in is the Zur School, the Southern School. I mentioned before the Root text, the Root Tantra, which is considered Buddhist scripture, composed of four tantras. There are four sections, one is called the Root Explanatory tantra, then oral instructions, and the subsequent tantras. I have the Root Tantra here which I believe was only first translated into English in 1995.[33]

Within this the medical tradition is part of the Root Tantra, and I mentioned there's a spiritual tradition connected to this, a Vajrayana tradition, Yuthok Nyinthig Anutara Yoga tantra. These teachings were transmitted through various Indian Masters, to Padmasambhava (also known as the second Buddha), Vairocana, Yuthok the Elder in the Eighth century, then to the historically notable Tibetan King Trisong Detsen who actually hid the teachings, revealed later in the Eleventh century as a treasure revelation, *terma*, eventually to Yuthok the younger, (1126-1201) the Root Guru of the tradition that continues today.

Many different Buddhist schools use Medicine Buddha teachings throughout Asia, but I have mostly studied Tibetan schools. Part of the teaching starts with this *mandala* of

Tanaduk, which can translate to *enchanted garden* and it's believed this represents the Himalayas.

How this is described, is a central garden, with a palace with five precious substances, stones and jewels, that have the power to cure what are classified as the 404 diseases. Arising from disorders from the three humors, the three typologies (which we're going to start to introduce today), those are derived from the five elements. These numbers are complex and interconnected.

Within the Sowa Rigpa tradition a round of mala counts to 101, (usually it is 108.) 101 relates to classification of illness/disease. Disorders can be classified by differing methods related to location in the body, type and typology, environmental factors, etc.. [34]

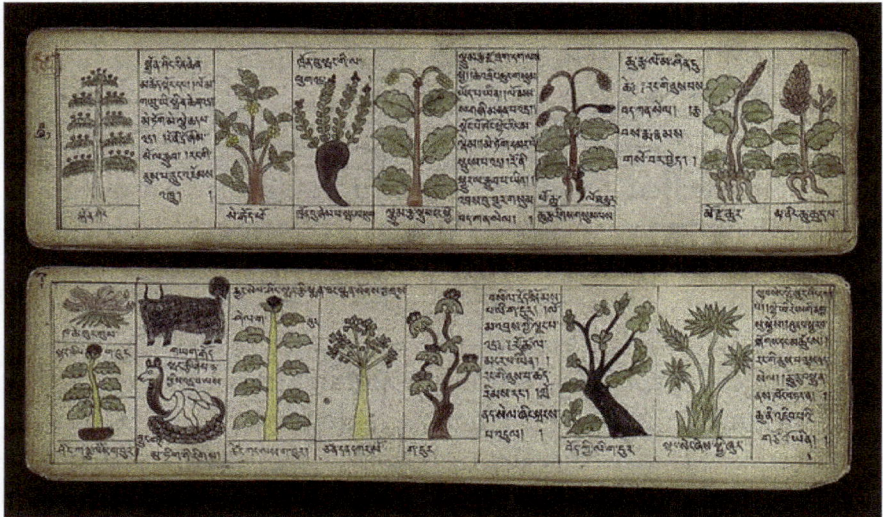

L0038345 Illustrations of Tibetan materia medica, Credit: Wellcome Library, London. Wellcome Images images@wellcome.ac.uk http://wellcomeimages.org Illustrations of Tibetan materia medica, plant and animal, used in the production of medicine. This anonymous manuscript is written in the 'Trungpa' ('khrungs dpe) genre of Tibetan medical literature. Entitled, 'Sman bla'i dgongs rgyan rgud bzhi'i nang gi 'khrungs dpe re zhig', it deals with various material medica, plant and animal, used in the production of medicine. Copyrighted work available under Creative Commons Attribution only licence CC BY 4.0 http://creativecommons.org/licenses/by/4.0//

404 Disease Classifications

The main classifications are:

101 disorders strongly influenced by action/karma from previous lifetimes

101 disorders of the current lifetime, having causes in the early part of life and manifesting later

101 disorders related to "spirits" or "provocations"

101 superficial disorders, categorized because they can be resolved by following dietary changes, lifestyle changes, without medication or other therapies [35]

G etting back to Tanakuk Garden, within this garden, in each of the cardinal directions, everything which grows and is available there can pacify disturbances of heat and cold, and rectify all of the barriers that interfere with good health.

In the middle of the mandala sits a palace with what are called the 5 precious substances, including precious stones and jewels, which have the power to cure what are known as the 404 diseases, which arise from disorders of the three typologies, or humors.

Southern garden has the power of the sun, including precious metals and medicinal substances which heal cold disorders

Northern garden called "the Snow Capped Mountain", contains lunar qualities, plants with medicinal qualities to heal heat disorders, fever

Eastern garden has fragrant mountains, which cure many disorders and diseases, also bones, body, channels and ligaments, skin, hollow, sense organs and vital organs

Western garden is the Garlanded Mountains with the six Good substances, nutmeg, clove, saffron, bamboo pith, black cardamom, and green cardamom. These pacify many diseases, along with other substances[36]

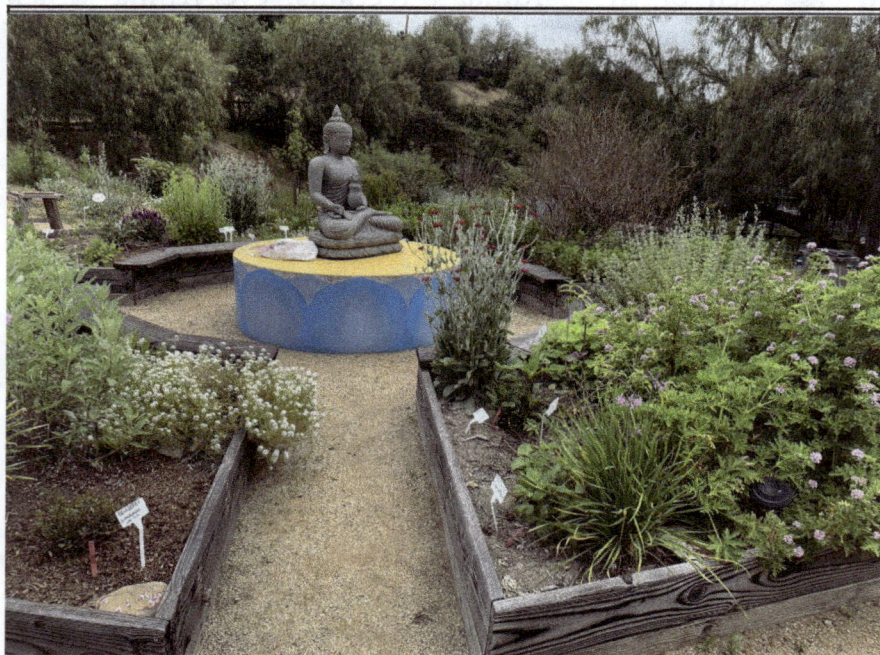

Tanakuk Medicine Herbal Garden at Pureland Farms, Topanga, California, photo by Janel

We even know all of these substances, in these drawings, this is what we work with and use in Sowa Rigpa. Many of these substances also grew in other places as well. There's many parallels in Europe, especially with early Greek medicine. There were interrelationships with Greek medicine in Persia and different locations. There's a remarkable book called *Physica*[37] by Hildegard von Bingen who was an Abbess in the 11th to 12th century, a famous Saint, Mystic and healer. You can read her instructions for healing, alchemy and herbs, and there are many parallels with Tibetan medicine and subjects I am mentioning here.

Getting back to the Tanakuk Gardens, the framework for medicinal healing in Sowa Rigpa, starts with the Southern gardens, which are related to the sun within;

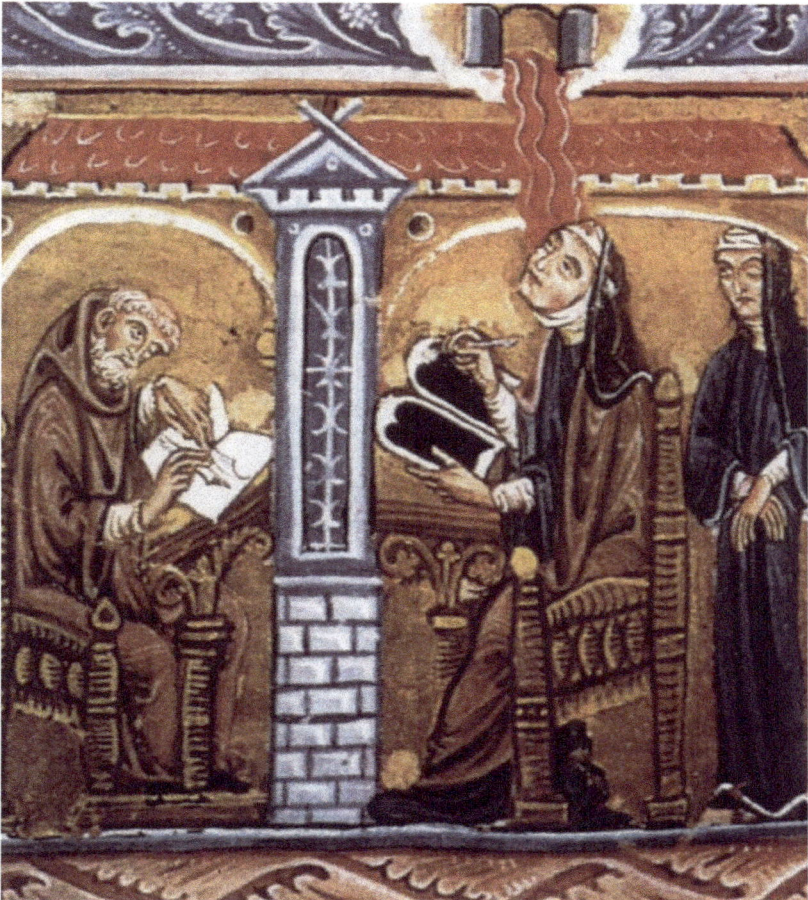

this is where we find the medicinal substances to heal cold disorders. The Northern gardens are imbued with lunar qualities, with plants to heal heat disorders. The Eastern gardens contain substances that cure many disorders, the bones, body channels, ligaments. In the Western gardens are the *Six Good Substances* which you may be familiar with: nutmeg, clove, saffron, bamboo pith, black cardamom and green cardamom. These are powerful healing materials that have been used for since before the emergence of our species.[38] This is a whole mandala that we can actually use. Not only does it have actual technical/gross information, it is also a mandala to practice from, and to determine all kinds of healing techniques.

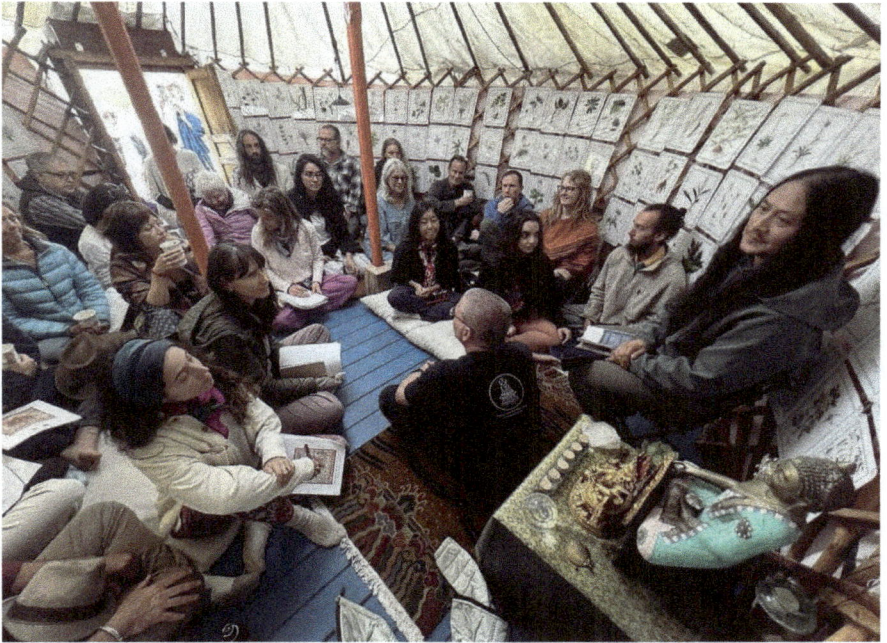

Pureland Farms, Tibetan Medicinal Herbal study with Dr. Nida Chenagtsang and Dr. Ed Coughlin, 2024, Sowa Ripga photo

Last session we introduced a mantra. Mantra means *mind protection*. Remember also, the highest form of mantra is silence. This is the short medicine Buddha mantra which has powerful healing properties, and can be used by anyone, and done for others.

Tibetan Medicine Buddha Mantra (Bhaisajyaguru Mantra)

TADYATHA OM BEKANDZE BEKANDZE MAHA BEKANDZE

RADZA SAYMUDGATE SOHA

English translation: Homage to the Three Jewels!

Homage to the blessed, thus-gone, worthy, completely perfect Medicine Buddha![39]

One can find many recordings online and various translations. So Doshin, would you like to talk a little bit about the five elements here?

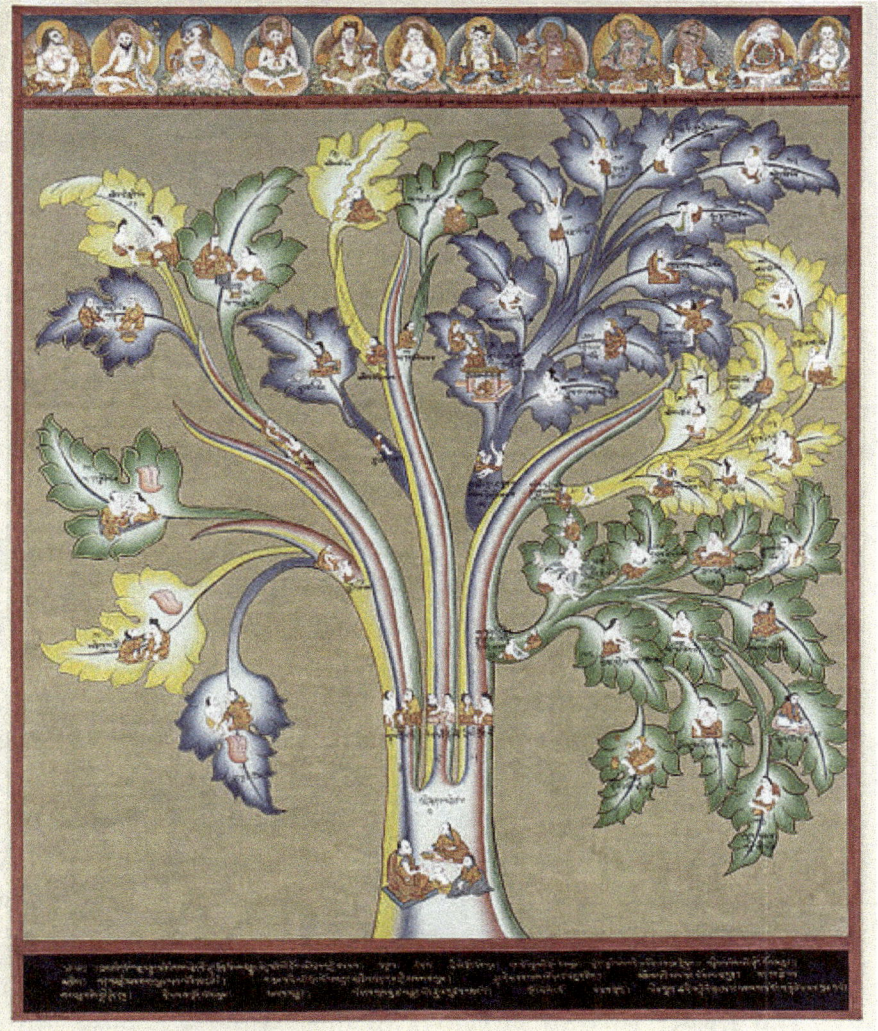

The Blue Beryl - tree of diagnosis plate, Date between 1687 and 1703, This work is in the public domain in the United States because it was published (or registered with the U.S. Copyright Office) before January 1, 1930. Photo Credit: Brian Bald, AMNH Division of Anthropology, © 2008 American Museum of Natural History, Division of Anthropology, NYC

Doshin

I just wanted to reiterate how important and how ancient and deep this five element typology is. There has been so much experimentation, so much studying, so much knowledge and wisdom accumulated over thousands of years, first in oral traditions, passed on from teacher to student, often secretly, that has contributed to the healing that we have now, even in the West. Where do you think these drug companies go to find the miracle drugs? They go into the ancient teachings, and then they experiment from there, but they are building on the ancient foundations of traditional teachings. Scientists don't usually talk about this because it's not rational and it's difficult to measure. And it's certainly not fashionable. You don't get any articles published in scientific journals by doing studies in alchemy in any of the hard sciences.

What excites us about this is when you get sick if there's no cure available to you, you will start turning to the wisdom traditions. That is what often happens to Zen Masters when they contract Zen disease. In Zen practice, we take a shortcut. We learn to be disciplined and follow instructions religiously. And then we focus on meditation practices, which bypass the subtle realms and the high subtle Deity realms. And then, we often get sick! There are not many practices in Zen that facilitate healing, even this Zen disease. There are some secret teachings about healing that were passed on orally, but there's no healing lineage directly in Zen.

When Hakuin, an 18th century Zen Master got sick, he went into the forest to find a Taoist healer, and he begged him to help him find a cure, to help him heal, which the Taoist did. Then Hakuin began to introduce some of these healing practices secretly, and a few publicly, into his Zen teachings. Where the five elements really come alive in modernity is either when you're desperately ill, or when you reach a certain level of awakening, that your scientific prejudices against religions begin to loosen and dissolve, and you begin opening your heart to ancient healing wisdom.

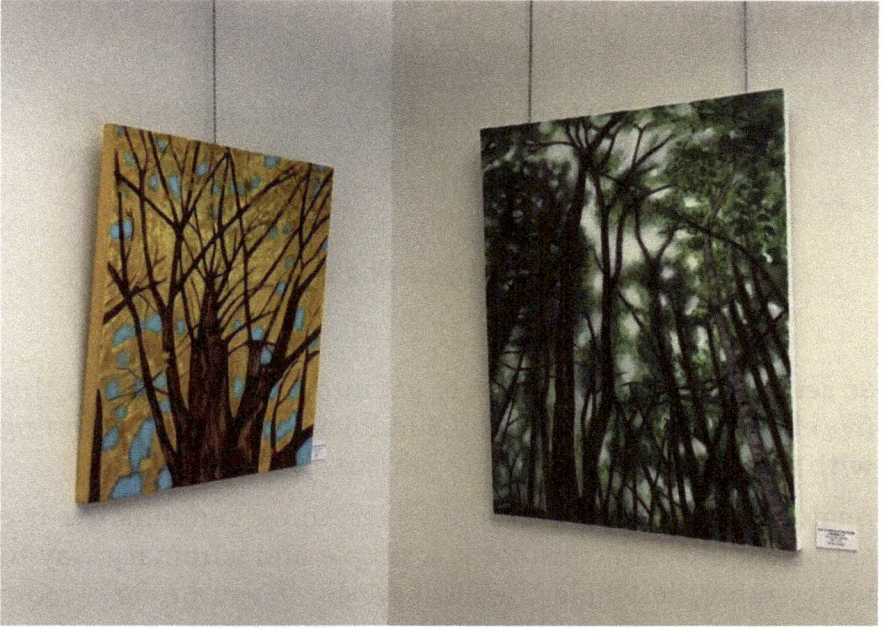

Janel's tree paintings on exhibit, Massachusetts Audubon Wildlife Sanctuary Exhibit, Belmont Massachusetts, 2016, Author photo

And that's enough for now.

Janel

There also a mantra for balancing the five elements internally, externally, and in your environment.

Five Elements Balancing Mantra

*Tibetan: Om Ah Hung, E Yam Kham Ram Lam, Shudde
Shudde, Ah Ah*

*English: space, wind, water, earth and fire, purify, purify,
body, speech, mind[40]*

So setting up further context to get into the five elements, this
five elements view is based on Buddhist cosmology, beginning
with the five elements of space, air, fire, water and earth.

Again, always keeping in mind everything contains the five
elements, one can consider it a simple and summary way to
understand the whole chemical world, if you prefer a more
scientific view. These elements we are made of come from
the universe, the dust of stars. All of life is interdependent,
nothing does not impact every form of life from the smallest
particles to the climate of our planet. All are impacted by
the delicate flow of changing seasons. This includes animals,
plants, humans, human systems. Nothing is separate from the
whole, and each of us is a complete mandala.

Sache

GOLDEN TURTLE / TORTOISE auspiciously positioned mountains or giant rock formations

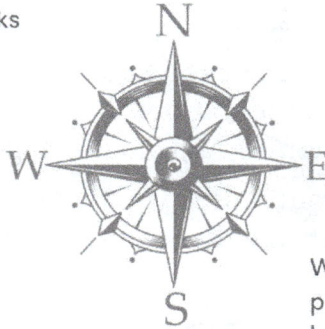

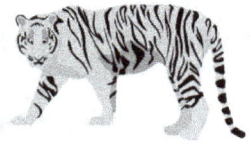

RED GARUDA / SPIRIT BIRD arrangement of trees, plants, or rocks

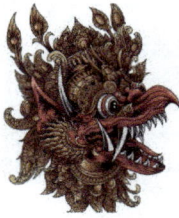

WHITE TIGER prosperity, vitality, happiness, and strength

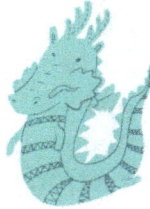

TURQUOISE DRAGON for positive energies of water

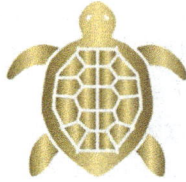

The way Sowa Rigpa is learned is quite fascinating. I'd like to share a synchronicity; as an artist, even since I was a child, I was always drawn to trees, and it was the thing that I depicted the most. I was always painting trees; I didn't understand why. So when I started studying Sowa Rigpa one of the first things they presented was how in Tibetan medicine people always learned, and studied, with all of the medical instructions mapped within drawings of trees. So part of studying remains drawing these tree maps of health, illness, and treatments. I was so surprised. I thought, oh, isn't that strange? As a child I didn't just think--I knew--I would be an artist and a doctor, and this fixation on trees, and then I discovered this synchronicity.

There are 99 trees of knowledge for studying Tibetan medicine and health. Trees show the different root tantras, they show different typologies, they show all different types of diseases. They show all different treatments. We were even instructed to draw our own trees, a method to study. Again there are 404 types of diseases. Because we're using a comprehensive, holistic view of health, we have a tree of diagnosis where one starts to work with observation, looking at the patient's tongue, and urine observation, also pulse reading is very important for questioning and diagnosing.

There's guidance around lifestyle, home and family care, and food is used as both medicine (and alternately, can also be poison).

There is also what in Tibetan is known as Sache, which is basically *Geomancy,* similar but not exactly like Chinese *Feng Shui.* The origins of this go back to pre Buddhist times in Tibet, the Bon traditions. Specific animals (white tiger, lion dog, dragon, Garuda) are major animals/mythical creatures associated with the basic directions.

Geomancy takes into consideration the many factors that determine the environmental balance of where one lives. For example, not to scare you all, but if your house has a front door facing north, with nothing blocking it if you have a neighbor blocking the north, this is a better situation, versus having vast space, open to terrain, considered inauspicious for geomancy.

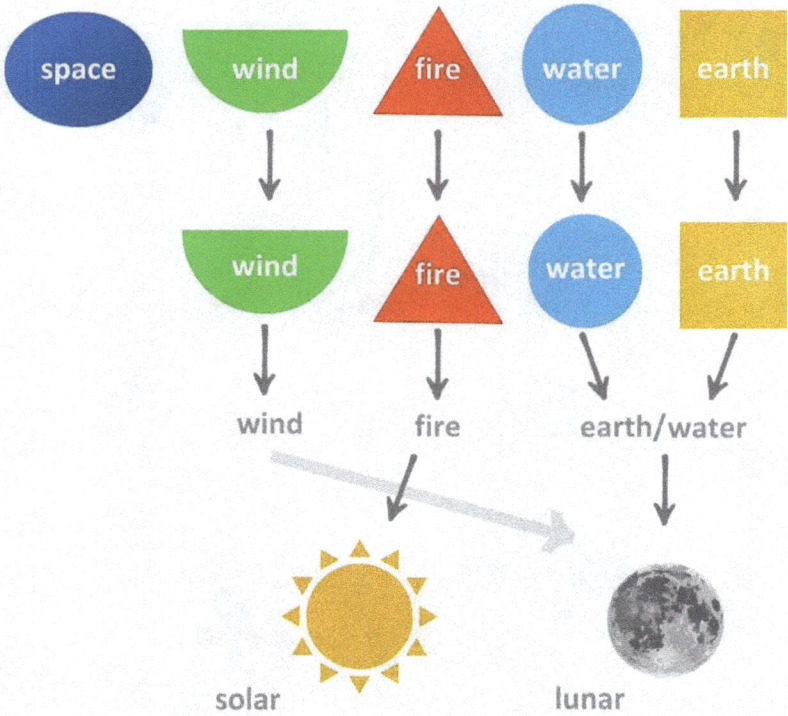

5 elements (jungwa) become 3 humors (nyepa) become two potencies

There are all these kinds of ways of working with one's environment, which are quite interesting, to work with the elements harmoniously, according to where you live. For example, it's very good to have some water element outside of your house as well as inside. In my room where I work, I have a little waterfall, which helps to support taking away disharmonious energies.

Sowa Rigpa also includes end of life care, spiritual healing, Tibetan yoga, which we'll start to talk about a little bit. I'll talk about provocations later, and meditation.

Getting back to the five elements, the way Sowa Rigpa typologies are explained is that we start with the five elements. Since everything is contained within space, the five become four on the right, and then they are further divided into solar potencies which are associated with the feminine, and lunar potencies which are associated

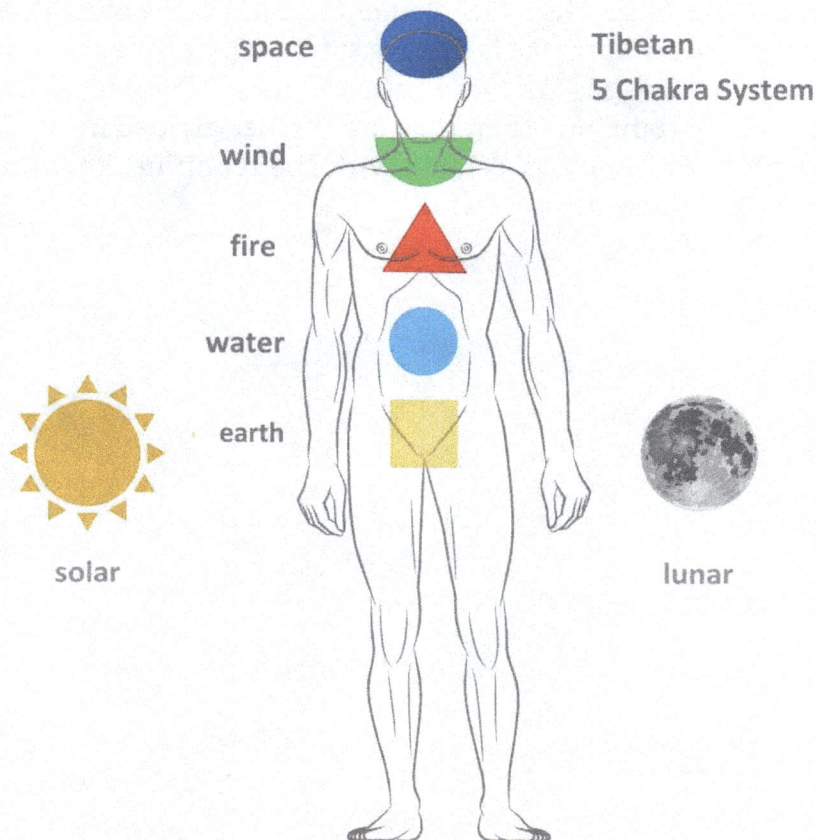

space

Tibetan
5 Chakra System

wind

fire

water

earth

solar

lunar

with the masculine. All of this translates into the Tibetan chakra system (five chakras) in the body, which is different from the Hindu system (seven).

So you may wonder in human conception, how these five elements become these three humors, called *nyepas,* which in Ayurveda are known as *doshas,*

First, people have an inherent typology that will dominate as their "natural" state, which is inherited from the parents, and whatever their typologies were (comparable to genetic inheritance from a scientific model). Most people's natural state is a combination of one or two typologies, less common are people with a combination of three.

There are different ways to determine typology, but what happens once you have determined what your natural typology is, we experience *life*. All different kinds of factors influence balance and imbalance within us, most powerfully, *the three mental poisons* (desire, anger, ignorance) which we will look at soon. Once we live and experience our lives, and let's say circumstances lead one to become out of balance with the elements, at a certain point, one will begin to manifest different symptoms. Some of the easiest ways to look at this is, let's say you're a dominant fire type. Fire is in its simplest definition, manifested as heat, and or inflammation. For example, in the summer, it's very easy to get too much *heat/fire in* your body, due to external conditions. Therefore, from the Sowa Rigpa elemental perspective, you would need to work with *cooling elements* (water can balance fire) which can come from different therapies or diet, herbs, lifestyle, Tibetan medicines, or you would do something to help you *purge* the fire (fire is the only element that one purges in excess).

There are many ways to treat imbalances within this framework, and if you are familiar with Chinese Classical Medicine, this approach is parallel in many ways. Getting back to the basic Tibetan typologies; water and earth are joined, to be called *bekken,* representing *phlegm. Tripa or treepa* is the name for the fire typology. Air or Wind, (which comprises a number of life force energies) connected to our nervous system and the physiology of movement in our body, is called *loong.* The winds arising, are connected to increasing conceptual, analyzing and discursive thought (to the extreme is overthinking, anxiety); the winds settled allow for non-conceptual awareness and experience of our natural state (Tibetan

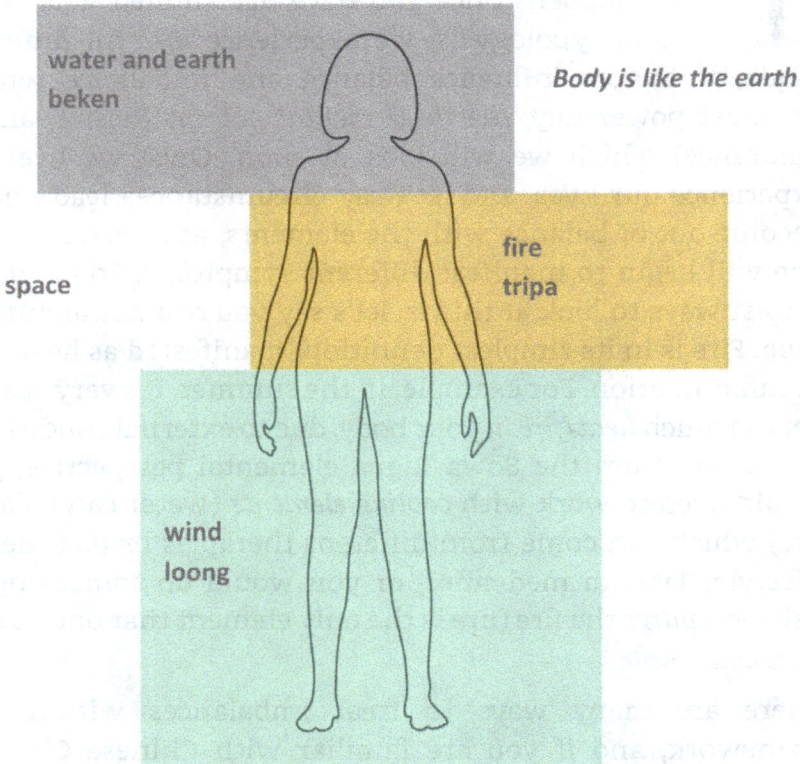

water and earth
beken

Body is like the earth

space

fire
tripa

wind
loong

rigpa.)[41][42] Space simply contains everything.

Taking all of this in, it is natural to wonder, how do we stay healthy? We maintain health by adapting our lives, according to our unique typology, to an appropriate life

style and diet, to start. This is very simply summarized, but is actually an extensive system that anyone can work with, to return to balance and harmony, within a holistic approach which considers the interdependencies of all of life, and is much more focused on the prevention of disease, versus an approach that works from attempting to cure or resolve acute symptoms, without much consideration of prevention.

I n Sowa Rigpa I find the study of Embryology particularly interesting. It is taught that certain factors are required for a successful conception and development of a fetus, becoming a baby, resulting in birth. If all of the factors (or criteria) are not present, then the fetus may not survive, or grow into a healthy child. What is required from this framework is first healthy sperm and egg, and this is where the typologies of the parents are passed down to the children. Next, is the entry of a unique consciousness, which includes *karma,* so that's karma from past life/lives. Past life does not necessarily mean human, it can be another life form. Also entering are the afflictive emotions, the three (or five poisons). Then, a proper combination of gathering together of the five elements with *subtle* consciousness, and *gross* sperm and egg. Sowa Rigpa teaches that the baby becomes aware of its consciousness around the 5th month of pregnancy and can then sense feelings with the mother.[43] This is all part of a framework cycle of reincarnation, where after physical death the consciousness exits the body later, and when a consciousness enters a body, it is said that the fetus can recall some awareness of past lives. We are microcosms of macrocosms, so it's just endless interconnection.

When you learn about these systems in detail, our body is similar to the Earth, in that different areas of our body are connected to these typologies, and then also parallel to stages of our lives. When we're children, up to the age of 16, our typology is more *earth and water;* during our adult life we are more *fire,* and then after the age of 70, we become more *windy.*

Paralleling the earth, in the upper levels, water and earth are surface elements of the earth, while the core of the planet is molten fire. Then in our lower body, the planet is spinning and floating in space, held in space through motion and gravity which is similar to the wind. What powers movement? The air/wind element helps us hold our hips and legs up in space.

So for the typologies if for example, you're dominant earth and water (*beken or phlegm*) it means you will tend to have these earth and water characteristics, for example, a solidness and heaviness. You can be slow to change. Earth/water type health problems tend to be slow to develop, slow to heal, and there's a theme of stubbornness. Earth and water are associated with *cold*, so just to give you a few examples, we can be the example. Doshin is a combination of earth, water and fire. I'm a combination of fire and air/wind. Wind/fire types are sharp, hot, active. Fire is associated with being smelly, so body excretions tend to smell more. For fire types anger[44] is the dominant emotion (poison), whereas earth and water, ignorance[45] is the dominant emotion (poison). Fire is associated with inflammation. So if you look at different kinds of headaches, an earth and water headache would be stubborn, heavy, slow to come on, maybe even a migraine. A fire headache is sharp, intense focused pain (tension headache for example), or one that comes on really fast in the heat. Wind pain moves all over your body, and can change quickly. Earth and water, the heaviness is associated with depression. Wind has the poison of desire,[46] and is associated with anxiety, so there are different behaviors too, for example wind people tend to be talkative, social, maybe nervous, frenetic. Fire types tend toward clear, sharp thinking, smart and analytical. Earth types are associated with being calm, steady, even dull and sluggish.

The Third Power Chakra, Solar Plexus

power, Sanskrit Manipura

eighteen months to 3 - 4 years, Integral Red

beginning of "me", first person perspective

- Location: Front of body solar plexus, back between L2 & L1
- Essential functions: Power, will, agency, language
- Meridians: Stomach-spleen, liver-gallbladder
- Areas of body: Mid back, the digestive system, diaphragm, lower chest cavity, stomach and spleen, liver and gallbladder
- Developmental stage: 18 months – 4 years**
- Development: We start to build a rational, intellectual-based understanding of our world, declaring I, me, mine

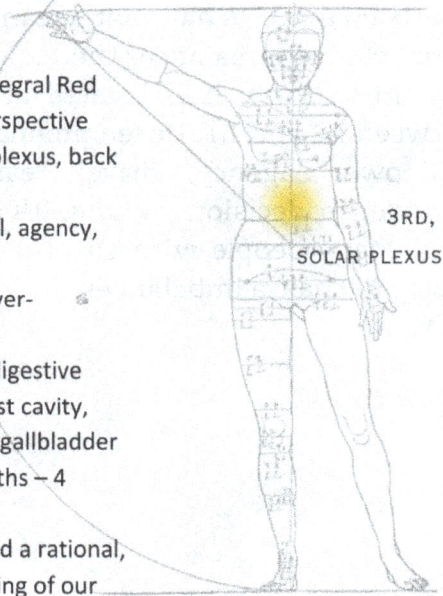

3RD,

SOLAR PLEXUS

ALBRECHT DURER

WOODCUT

C. 1528

third chakra themes

Language - Will Power – Drive – Reason – Motivation – Courage - Confidence – Decision Making – Agency

CHAKRA

SUPERIMPOSED

We have reached the third chakra, the power chakra. It's a big leap here developmentally. Doshin mentioned earlier, we go from Pre-pre, and pre-first person perspective, to first person perspective. This is where the child declares, " I, me, mine!" This is where the child generally starts using language. With language also comes the ability to remember more clearly, once we are able to speak.

This is roughly from 18 months to three to four years

Integral Red. It's really important and is building on what has happened with the first two chakras. The first two greatly influence how the third chakra development goes. Also the third chakra is also connected/paired, to the third eye chakra (sixth chakra). What that means is imbalances here, often connected to imbalances there.

Placement wise, it is located at the solar plexus, the back between L2 and L1. Developmental themes include language, willpower, agency, drive, reason, motivation, courage, confidence, decision making. It's quite related to the digestive area. Many people with chronic digestive problems seem to have 3rd chakra imbalances.

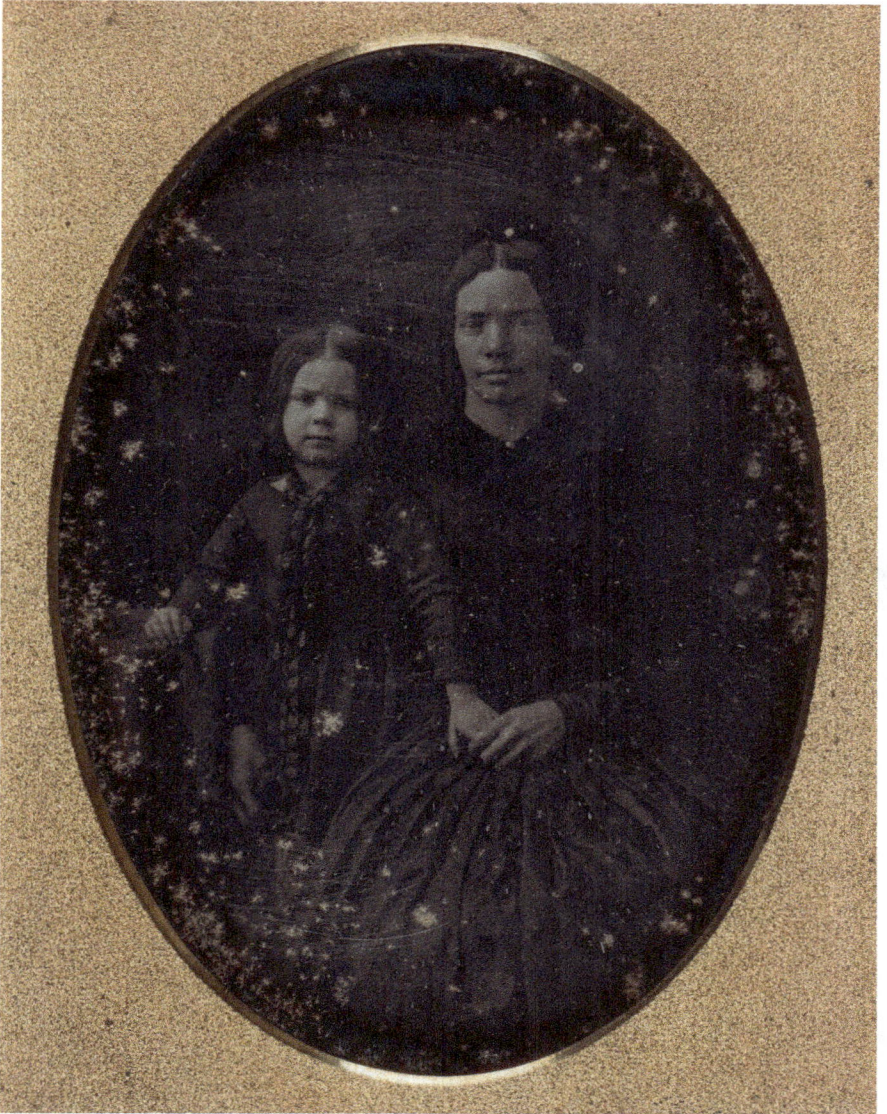

Daguerreotype. Fontayne & Porter. American, active 1848–1856. CC0 Public Domain Designation. The Art Institute of Chicago. Creative Commons Zero (CC0). Additional data about artworks in the collection is available using our public API.

This period is when we start to build a rational, intellectual based understanding of our world. I also tell people this is where we can develop, and you can choose different names for it, both an *inner critic* and an *inner advocate*. And when I mention this, this is something to keep an eye on, because if you keep in mind every time you hear these voices, to be healthy, there ought to be some indication of balance. There are a lot of people who seem to have inner critics on steroids, and have little to no inner advocate. (It can also be the opposite.)

An inner advocate is something that we may have to develop. Keeping this in mind, how we can bring this more into balance, is very useful for 3rd chakra work. (This also relates to negative/positive anima and animus, but that will be addressed in later courses.)

At this stage, what is healthy is the child wants to discover and develop their agency, themselves (with aware caretakers watching for actual threats and dangers as they explore). They explore this in their family and environment. A relatively healthy family is going to be aware of this happening in the child, and will adapt to support their growth (including encouragement AND setting necessarily limits). It can often be hard for busy parents, because children are so slow to do things, and I have people I work with who can clearly recall, telling their mother *"do it myself"*. It's very important for a mother to help support this, versus always taking over for the child, not giving them a chance to develop on their own. This is also so interesting how this varies culturally, whereas recent generations of parents in America are often criticized as being too protective of their children, I recall having lived in Japan seeing very young children given extremely sharp objects to learn to use, and how shocked I was watching this, but that by and large, the children learned quickly!

Very important to consider are the power dynamics within a family, which set a mold/patterning within us. When I'm exploring with people one-on-one, I ask them to really look and ask, what are the rules of power in your family? Not just your immediate family, but your extended family. So when you start to look back, generationally, there are important patterns that impact families and individuals. I hear stories of powerful grandmothers, matriarchs, just as there are patriarchs. The more you investigate, the more you may see patterns that go way back, leading to the present. Only when patterns become conscious, is there potential to interrupt what is unbalanced (creating harm for the individual and others), and take steps towards healing towards what is more balanced, and beneficial.

Starting to see all these power patterns (and of course all kinds of family and relational patterning) is really important because these patterns, you know, are established within. Also a lot of people lack awareness of the nuances of feminine power, so I often have to really guide them to look more closely at how women have been powerful in the past, and how women use their power now. Because it is often not the same kind of power that men use and have used. (It can take some real reflection). Just as well, all this is not just true for the power chakra, but for all of our development, so looking not only when there were and are conflicts between parents, but conflicts with other people. You may have lived in a different kind of household with more interaction and presence of aunts and uncles or cousins, for example. Conflicts in the family, in my observation, are internalized within us, becoming internal psychic wars. Specifically in terms of conflicts between parents, also conflicts *within* each parent themselves, also seem to manifest as conflicts within us. It also appears that this is first and generally, unconscious. Most people just carry on continuing these internal wars, expending and exhausting lots of energy in internal unconscious battles. I see parallels between what I'm describing here, and what Gregory Bateson[47] described as the *double-bind* that he theorized could contribute to schizophrenia, where paradoxical messages that he was focused on as mostly mothers to their sons, as an origin for a schizophrenic split. This is when the parent is communicating both directly and indirectly paradoxical, opposing messages to a child, (for example, a parent saying they love the child, contrasted by embodying somatic or visible emotional signs of disgust, hatred or rejection) that are impossible for the child to integrate psychologically, potentially leading the psyche eventually to schizophrenic split. It seems that while that is a relatively extreme example of what can happen, that most people experience minor versions of splits, in childhood, that leave residues of internal conflict, that likely are unconscious but experienced as anguish, tension, depression, anxiety, or other problems, including a general lack of peace and wholeness.[48]

So *really* seeing and examining what happened in your family is important. Can I identify the struggles, signs of the internal struggles of family members, my parents and others? Bringing this into consciousness, is a huge, first step. Another big step is, we could say this is going to a Zen view, where we accept that *things simply are as they are.* Acceptance, versus experiencing the conflict in resistance, in that strain, us fighting within, conflicts that we really just inherited from our families before us. Accepting all of this as parts of ourselves, because it has become part or parts of our habitual behavior, parts of our patterning. From then, we may work to decide that as I look at this now, from a more mature and wise perspective, and acknowledging that, *I see this isn't working for me.* I'm just carrying this conflict around, to no avail, unconsciously doing it, in it, repeating it, spinning like a gerbil in a wheel. What if instead, I try to develop myself, maybe get some help to grow and accept, or make some other choices? I could create new habits, new patterns.

Power Exercise 3

power exercise 3

Identify briefly

- what were the basic rules of power in family dynamics in my early childhood family life (18 mos - 3 years)
- unusual events or trauma in my life from 18 mos to 3 years) months

Answer scale 0-5, 0 least, 5 most

Presently in my life do I feel powerful?

Do I feel accomplishing?

Am I a healthy agent for myself?

Where do I feel powerless?

Can I set boundaries skillfully (not too little, not too much)?

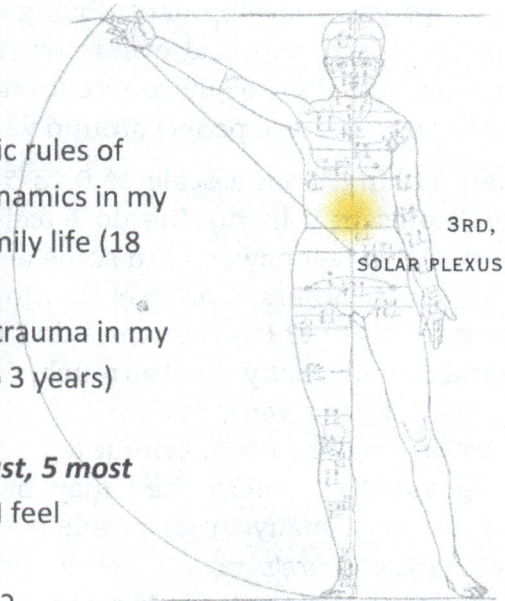

3RD,
SOLAR PLEXUS

ALBRECHT DURER
WOODCUT
C. 1528

CHAKRA
SUPERIMPOSED

Next is an exercise for everyone to do themselves. Again, we're just starting to explore this here. Look and try to describe the rules of power within the family dynamics of your early childhood, family life. You may not remember, however, assuming you knew your family, and if you can remember some things at all, and also assuming you have information about your family, you may be able to recognize certain patterns. All kinds of scenarios can dominate a family too, like addiction, anger, wealth, poverty, to name a few. If some situation was really preoccupying the family, (for example during war people could feel powerless against authority and be living under societal and political oppression), this could interrupt your development during this period as well, and this extends to unusual events or trauma in your life. Not just your life, it's the environment and culture and context of where you were and people around you.

Then looking from a scale of 0 to 5, *(zero the least, five the most)*, presently in my life do I feel powerful? Most people are going to feel powerful in some areas of their life, and not so much in others. Do I feel accomplished, am I a healthy agent for myself? In what areas do I feel powerless? Can I set boundaries skillfully (not too much, not too little)? Boundaries are such a buzzword, and so people often think, *oh, I need to set boundaries!* often only imagining their boundaries are being violated, where they may be the one overstepping, and, actually, many times people overdo boundaries. There's no nuance, there's no awareness of the impact on others. Boundary setting will likely be very influenced by the power dynamics that were modeled in your family (which were likely a variety of dynamics, even contradicting patterns). Being able to skilfully do this requires a lot of awareness of self and one's impact on others.

Doshin

Yes, that is something I'd like to say a few things about because it's been a major part of the shadow work I've been doing with people for years, particularly as this culture has shifted to more and more postmodern values and beliefs. Moral values that are focused on social justice and equality are not necessarily healthy. These values are coming in conflict with previous sets of moral values that are more traditional and modern. These conflicts are often described as culture wars. For example we find in this postmodern culture that it has become problematic to express any anger. So the children are taught from the earliest age not to have an outlet for any expressions of anger. Anger is first expressed by the child as the power chakra begins to come online in the red level of ego development. Expressing this anger is essential for the child to learn to set boundaries. If the child can't get angry, they can't learn to set healthy boundaries and won't mature into a healthy adult. Children must learn how to set boundaries. If their parents, caregivers and teachers teach them to suppress and repress their anger they never learn how to set healthy boundaries. Consequently, the child who can't express anger and can't set healthy boundaries, is continuously victimized and bullied by

power
solo or group exercise

- Identify briefly, internal patterns of power, overuse, dominance, manipulation, avoidance, passive aggressiveness

- Can I identify unhealthy patterns and interdynamics related to power I adapted from one or more parents and family, that I unconsciously took on, that I may revert to in situations where a healthy assertion of power or agency might be better?

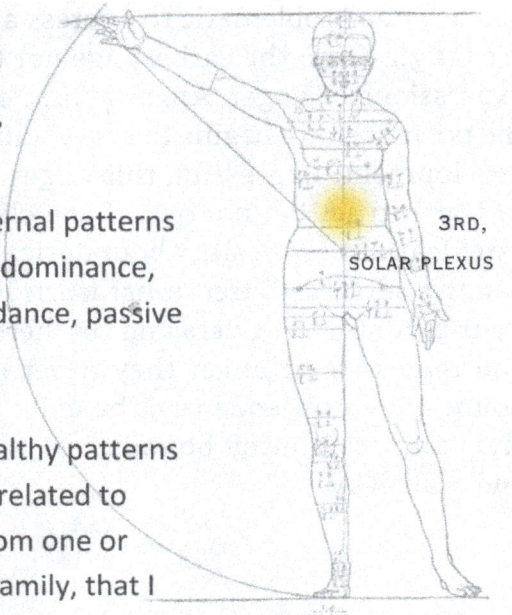

3RD,
SOLAR PLEXUS

ALBRECHT DURER
WOODCUT
C. 1528

CHAKRA
SUPERIMPOSED

other children. So a byproduct of our postmodern culture's antagonism toward anger, results in anemic boundary setting which is horribly unhealthy. Unfortunately this has grown to epidemic proportions in postmodern western cultures.

This inability to express healthy anger contributes to a condition of toxic shame, where the child feels something is hopelessly wrong with them. They develop feelings of helplessness because without anger, they have no power or no way of developing power. Children are much healthier if they are allowed to feel anger, and then taught how to manage it[49]. If a child is prohibited from feeling any anger they never learn to set boundaries or develop a sense of power to face life's difficulties. Working with those who have difficulties expressing anger, it is essential to help them understand that the anger that was suppressed at two or three years old, often comes out in a very immature way. As they are getting in touch with their suppressed resentment and feel their disowned anger in order to learn how to set boundaries, they need help. They often must start setting boundaries very carefully with someone giving them feedback as they learn. In our culture, in this postmodern culture, this inability to set boundaries and manage healthy anger is endemic.

Janel

Yes I forgot to mention passive aggressiveness, which is so common in postmodern culture. Again, whatever style of parent of power you may have experienced in your family, and people can actually have more than one pattern of using power that you just copied unconsciously (for example you might model behaviors from two different parents that come out in different situations), and you're not even aware of, as Doshin was talking about. We will be doing this much more in the next course.

I'd like to mention, when people start to experience the conditions for a pattern of *victim mentality* in the second chakra, this almost always creates an unhealthy relationship to power in the third chakra, and it can be very hard to get out of that if one remains in that mindset where there is always something or someone to blame. It can keep people terribly stuck and disempowered far beyond a time period where a victim works through to heal or come to terms with a situation to some degree, and then recovers to become a survivor. It's not impossible, but it can be very hard for an individual to even see that they're in this pattern. Again we will talk about this more later.

For the next exploration, identify briefly, internal patterns of power, such as over controlling, manipulation, avoidance of the use of power, passive aggressiveness. Can I see unhealthy patterns and interdynamics related to how I use power? Patterns I adapted from one or more parents, and family that I unconsciously took on? That I may *revert* to in situations where a healthy assertion of power agency might be more effective?

Another expression might be if you learned that you had to seek power using covert means. This may be unconscious. Remember if being direct wasn't allowed

power - on your own

- *identify someplace in your life where you feel powerless*
- *if you recognize you feel powerless, increase your power, try a new external or internal martial arts class*
- *mentor someone with something you are good at*
- *become more conscious of power dynamics by assisting refugees, volunteer for something that is really needed*
- *make a conscious effort to empower others*
- *identify where you were most courageous in your life*
- *Do something you've been procrastinating; see how you feel before and after*
- *look at the factor of interdependence in the challenging areas of your life, versus being the victim or blaming another, watch the roles you take on and reflect on this*
- *be aware for when YOU are manipulative versus direct with power, for example passive aggressiveness. As awareness increases, experiment with being more direct instead. (try requesting what you need and start with, "could I make a request?")*

in the family as a child, it may be very hard for you to be direct about what you need and what you want, and standing up for oneself. These can be signs of some imbalances. Or you could be the opposite, prematurely pouncing on others to protect your own power. There are many possibilities.

Next, this is your homework. This is "power on your own." Identify some place in your life where you recognize that you feel powerless. Then, do something to increase or develop your power. There are a variety of empowering options here. Try a new external or internal martial arts class; we're going to review some varieties of internal martial arts in the next few classes. Next, mentor someone for something you are good at. Let's also remember the higher, the evolution of power, is once healthily empowered, one empowers and mentors others, so this is a mature expression of this. This applies to all of the chakras, and this is very healing for oneself. Become more conscious of power dynamics by assisting refugees or volunteering for something that is really needed, which can be a real eye opener. Making a conscious effort to empower others. Identify where you have been most courageous in your life? This is one of the questions when I'm doing power with people. Really looking back, when was I courageous, or and then also, when did I fail to be courageous? Very important. Or where might I need to be courageous now?

Do something that you've been procrastinating. This is empowering! See and really look at how you feel before and after, really observe internally your body. I know if I think about something I need to do and I'm procrastinating, it just grips me physically with a kind of dread and aversion. Watch your whole body through this process. Look at the circumstances that brought you to this course, this moment in your life. The choices you made to end up here, and see the interdependence of all things. Be aware when you manipulate instead of being direct with power. For example, with passive aggressiveness, as your awareness increases, try requesting what you need instead, you can practice asking, could I make a request? That's an easy way to start being more direct.

I'd like to talk about some connection between areas of our body corresponding to development, and energetic channels. This is related to *TCM*, Traditional Chinese Medicine (differentiated from Classical Chinese Medicine, which I'll talk about later). This is also something for people to do on their own. Many people now, this is quite relevant for Westerners, can look at their early life and recognize that while they were *cared for* in a practical sense, but recognize an experience of some deficit in receiving expressions of love or being in what felt like environments lacking in warmth and affection, or play. Often there has been an absence of *play* in childhood, or atmosphere of supportive, loving energy.

Ancestry is connected to locations in the body in Eastern systems, and the interpretation of this varies (eg Daoist, Buddhist, etc..) The tendency–and this is not black and white–but what I see in working with people who grew up in Patriarchal cultures, is the right side of the body tends to be impacted by the male male ancestry, whereas the left side of your body tends to connect to the female ancestry. I want to say explicitly here, there are many ancient systems that map out the body differently–it is not one is right, the others are wrong, situation. One can employ different systems and work within those systems separately, but generally if you are studying or practicing something, I advise it's good to keep the number of systems you employ to a minimum, by choosing a system or systems that you respond well to, and stick to that. Again, it does not make other systems wrong! That is the fallacy of first tier Integral confusion. If you don't understand that, it's fine for now, in other words, be curious and keep an open mind. Different systems work better for different people. Different is not necessarily wrong.

Getting back to somatic blockages and ancestral connections, I recall recently doing a balancing self-care exercise, which focused on this lack of play and gentle loving support when young. I had been experiencing non-specific back pain for quite some time (several months) and I was not sure what the origin of it was. So as I was doing the exercise, all this pain just moved up from lower in my body to my mid back and released. I had no expectations of this.

It's very easy for me to recall many people in my family that were burdened by all kinds of life and karmic situations and were not able to experience a lot of play. Poverty, the

Depression, life as recent immigrants, war, and just fate/karma. Fateful situations where people are forced to grow up a lot earlier. Then you know their developmental level... (Janel starts to cry), sorry, this really breaks my heart open. Because even more for myself, my family, I just see that some of them did not have enough play in their life, so just giving this attention to one's body, and recalling the connection to ancestral energies and channels, brings it into consciousness. Whether we are aware of it or not, to some degree, these histories will be stored in your body. I will say more about this further on.

Part of healing is simply bringing our reflections and self and familial inquiries into consciousness and allowing ourselves to release what we may be holding onto by tension, bracing, obstructions, pain. From a Zen absolute view (the relative, and the absolute), one can also help heal those who are no longer physically on this earth, your family, or anyone. Prayers can reach them, prayers, practices and presence.

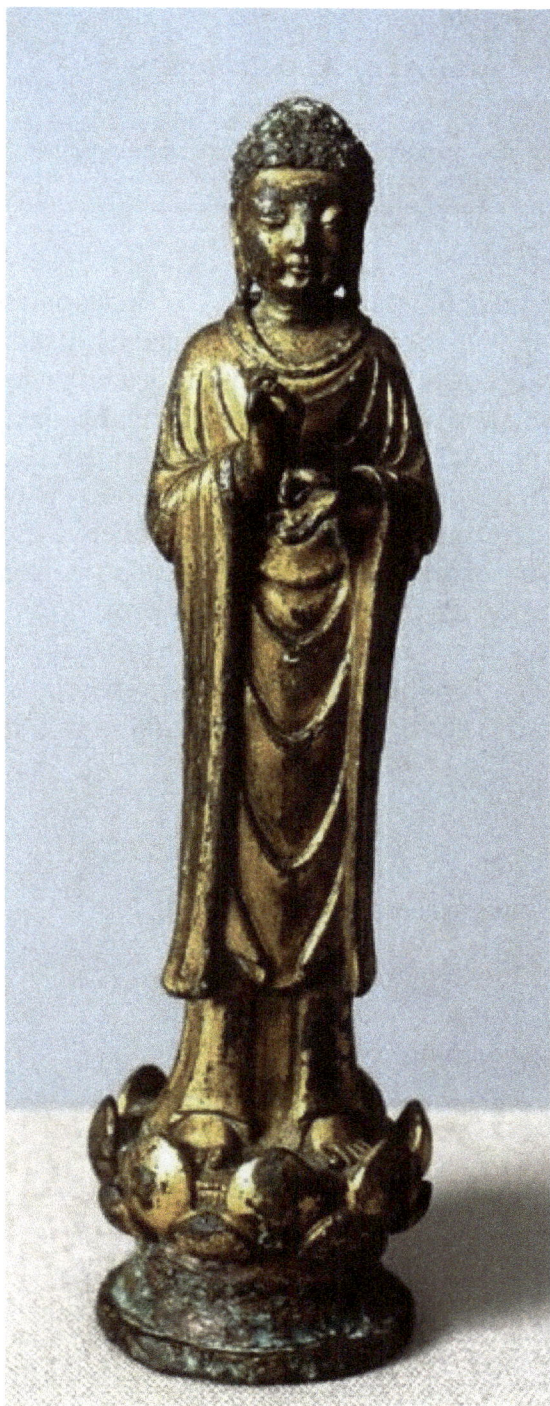

Mudra of Appeasement

Chinese Buddha, standing, in Vitarka Mudra, 7th Century, Gilt bronze. University of Michigan Museum of Art, Museum purchase for the James Marshall Plumer Memorial Collection, 1964/2.97

Next is the mudra of appeasement, An-i-in (Japanese), An-wei-yin (Chinese) and Vitarkamudra (Sanskrit), used in ritual, it appears throughout the world and history with variations. It's usually associated with some kind of incantation, some kind of speech as a ritual.[50] Generally it's done with the right hand, even though it's shown like this, generally the right hand is lifted, the thumb touching either inflected index, middle, or ring finger forming a circle, and it also generally is done with two hands. It's for consoling and protection of the body. What's interesting is because I'm super sensitive to the energy moving in my body and what I notice when I do this is that the circle brings the energy back within the body. Try it yourself and see.

Doshin

Great. Does anyone have any questions?

Janel

Or want to share insights?

Doshin

Anything that happened during the exercise that was noticeable, worth sharing or moved you in some way.

Questioner

Hi, Janel. I'm going back to the body types, the fire, the earth, water and air. Are there particular body types associated with each one?

Janel

Yes, very specific characteristics. When I work with people, this is part of the evaluation to determine what your natural typology is. But it's not always just body appearance for example. For example for fire, my appearance with red hair and reddish complexion is typical for fire types. Tall people are often earth and water. It's a bit like the Reichian[51] *Masochist* typology build, earth and water. Shorter people are connected to being a wind type. There's a bunch of different characteristics, I can give you more information later.

Question

Well, that's fine. Thank you.

Doshin

Anybody else have anything you'd like to ask or share about the power chakra, it is such a juicy chakra. These first three chakras are so foundational, in Jungian dream work, dreaming of houses, are symbolic of the individual psyche. The house is the part of the psyche that is above ground that you can invite people in, how you present yourself to people. The basements, the subterranean areas are the preconscious, pre-egoic structures that don't become conscious like the persona does. There are methods and ways of working the dysfunctions in the first and second chakras that are healing so they don't continue into the third chakra causing further dysfunctions there. Trauma work and insecure attachment work, are modern ways of working with these dysfunctions. If this is done in a modern therapeutic environment, where the therapist is trying to *repair* the "machine"- as if a patient is a machine that could be repaired it can be problematic. I don't know about you, but I am not a machine, I am a living, breathing human being who is complex and must heal, versus being "repaired." This modern metaphor is misleading from the start. Then there are the deeper Karmic levels of issues that are in the sub-basement in what is called the storehouse in Buddhism and the collective unconscious in Jung's Depth Psychology. There are no methods of treatment in Western psychology to deal with these. Religious practices are required in order to find and heal the karmic latencies and patterns. There's nothing in Western psychotherapy that will go deep enough to heal the karma.

Also I would be cautious. I didn't include Reichian character types in the sub-basement, but Reichian therapy is one way of dealing with a lot of these pre-egoic dysfunctions. Reichian therapy has developed some tools to identify and work with the early dysfunctions but they don't seem to have many tools to deal with shadows once the personality begins to become more complex. There are not any sophisticated shadow tools in Reichian therapy that I have found. When aspects of personality, the sub-personalities actually go underground and become unconscious, you need to have methods of working with human relationships that involve human beings interacting and projecting their shadows on each other. You might say that suppressed and disowned personalities have deeper roots, but they only become visible in relationships when they are projected onto someone else, and conflicts arise. I love what Byron Katie says, she says that we don't actually interact with each other, we don't talk to each other. What we do is we talk to each other's projections, but only 99% of the time. And that's often the case in my experience. You know, one projection arguing with another.

Developmentally, you have to have the capacity for a 2nd-person perspective for shadows to form. Second-person perspective starts at the heart chakra in the amber level of ego development around the age 5 or 6.

Before that, the child only has a first-person perspective. With a one-person perspective, there's no shadow. There may be a lot of dysfunctions in the first person perspective that develop into later shadows, but the shadow or sub-personality can't actually emerge and then be repressed until the 4th chakra.

When the second-person perspective emerges, it's a really important evolution. In my experience with Reichian therapy, it is really helpful at revealing some of the early dysfunctions, especially the ones that are connected to the body, connected to the root chakra and the sacral chakra. But the third-person perspective shows how those dysfunctions carry into the first-person of ego development. This type of therapy doesn't have tools when you start seeing how these early dysfunctions evolve into disowned sub-personalities or shadows that become suppressed and begin acting autonomously as if they have a mind of their own, coming into conflict with the other sub-personalities. And collective shadows have another level of complexity that little is known about and there are as yet no tools whatsoever that have been developed to deal with them.

Janel

I'd like to mention that it really does seem that if you're only addressing issues in the upper chakras, you're actually not going to get to the the drivers of those issues in the lower chakras, so it's like upper chakra problems are just going to keep cycling round and round endlessly. You have to return to the first three, don't you think Doshin? It seems like that.

Doshin

Absolutely, and you actually have to go deeper than that. You have to dig into the karma and that's where the work that you're doing Janel, is so powerful. You're asking questions that are extremely effective. You are not using the sledgehammer that I use. You're more gently asking very penetrating questions that make people curious and really look deeply. What was going on when you were born? What about your grandmother? Do you remember her? My God. What about your grandfather? And when people start exploring these areas, the insights start to flow, and the energy that is stuck in the body starts to tense up and once it tenses up, then you can learn to release it, but you have to find it first. You have to bring it into consciousness before you can release it. But once you start releasing it, then you have to become conscious of the suppressed dysfunctions that grow into disowned sub-personalities. These shadows and what underlies them have to be seen, brought into consciousness. Then they have to be healed before they can be integrated into the whole personality. This is a lot of work, but it's even more work if you don't do it.

How much do you need to suffer before you begin?

Question

You might have already been speaking to this. One of the thoughts I had was how some of these dysfunctions, such as my passive aggression, inability to set boundaries and those things... I guess it also occurs to me, can those also become superpowers that can be used for good? It's like some of the strategies are the signature of all these kinds of dysfunctions. I don't know if it even has to always be conscious. You could just think, oh, I'm really good at connecting and healing, but it comes from unhealed stuff there, so I'm curious. Any thoughts about that from either of you or how to work with that? I was also seeing it as I was getting overwhelmed, you know, with these questions. I thought, wait a minute, when you ask, where did you have to grow up early? I thought, wow, you know, I always think of myself as so, so regressed, and it's like, wait a minute, you know, maybe there was a part of me that was like being masterful, trying to dance around that family of mine, you know?

Doshin

You know, that's really an important question, and this is where it's really a delicate balance. Some people use the term *golden shadows*. I don't like to use that term, although I can see a perspective where there's some truth to it that is pointing to what you're asking. Not only do we have negative shadows, we also have undeveloped and positive aspects to ourselves that we haven't owned, claimed or developed. Very often, in ancient lineage traditions, there's an understanding that the more you awaken, the more you develop superpowers, *siddhi* powers, they call them. But if you're not awake enough, or not healed enough, then when you use those siddhi powers, these so-called magical powers, in ways that are not pure, they can be used in ways that are poisonous. If you use them selfishly, with greed, anger or ignorance, or for the wrong reason, they create great suffering, especially for you. Think of all the stories that have been told over the ages about white and black magic. So this is where it is a delicate balance. First, know if you are passive aggressive; then there is a hidden opportunity to cultivate a sensitivity to help people. Often this is caused by growing up with a dominant parent. In order to survive, you had to be secretly aggressive. You survived, but if you don't see and own your passive aggression fully, it's going to be a crippled, dysfunctional superpower. It's going to be a siddhi power that has control of you and you are going to in a sense, be a slave to it. If you haven't learned to fully face your passive aggression, it will create unnecessary harm and generate a false pride in something that isn't complete.

So if what you're saying is very true, it's important to become conscious of it. In my experience, it is far more useful to start with the negative shadows and then once I become conscious of them and their underlying dysfunctional foundations and integrate them, then the positive siddhi powers aren't usually a problem. But if an individual begins to awaken without becoming conscious of the shadows, now that is another matter entirely. As our personalities have become more and more complex this is more and more likely to be the case.

Questioner

Yes.

Doshin

It's the negative shadows that are a problem. Those are the ones we're projecting onto other people. If I look back at the teachers that I've been fortunate enough to have, who for God knows what reason, were willing to teach me, I could call that an example of golden shadows. There was a transference and countertransference. That could be viewed as my projection of superpowers onto them, or I could say siddhi powers. I was attracted to people who had the very qualities, the seeds of which I possessed, but they weren't fully developed enough in me. So I projected a "golden shadow," onto them. They projected their ideal of a good student onto me. Again, the golden shadows aren't the problem. The true gold is becoming conscious of the negative disowned qualities of the dark shadows I am projecting on others.

This is again where balance comes out and this is where from my perspective of seventy some years of life experience and wisdom, I see the critical need for both awakening and healing. We go to a Zen retreat or some kind of a retreat, and we wake up a little bit. Then from this higher vantage point, we look at ourselves and now can see more clearly how unhealthy we are. So then we focus our attention on healing, maybe we find a healer or a therapist and we focus on the healing. But then from a healthier perspective, we look at ourselves and now we can see how unawake we are and how shallow our insight is. So then we go to another Zen retreat and we start waking up a little more, and then we look back and say, Oh my God, I have to heal that! Where can I find another healer? So this is what is so important and even though from my perspective it feels like ratcheting up two things, healing and awakening. It is really a spiral, a vortex spiraling out.

It's important to include both positive and negative. But the positive aspects aren't usually a problem. Take you for example, your sensitivity makes you a wonderful healer. It's a siddhi power that you have. You can sense people's tension in their body. You are a magician. I've watched you work with me and others. Every time you worked on me, I walked out of your office an inch taller. My body just expanded! We laughed about it. But it was measurable and deeply experienced.

Now consider passive aggressiveness. It is the dark side of that sensitivity, and that's a shadow that you need to become conscious of, and heal the underlying dysfunction and integrate that disowned, unseen self into your personality, so that you're not poisoning people with hidden, poisonous aggression. You know what I mean? This is something we all have. We all can find times and circumstances where we are being a little passive aggressive, if they're not totally in shadow, or we are not totally ignorant of it, we all know exactly what I am pointing to. Anything else?

Question

My passive aggression will defeat your passive aggressive aggression. (laughter)

Doshin

No it won't, we will both cause suffering.

Question

Thank you.

Doshin

That's a little personal joke.

Question

Hi. So what you said you know about growing up, children growing up without opportunity to play, what is the function of, what are the effects of that? Are there markers of that? And as adults... what happens when they're adults?

Janel

Yes, one of the things I've seen in people is sometimes an internal saboteur will squash down any signs of play. When people are trying to focus on certain things, work, tasks, sometimes the part of them that wants to play will interrupt their work, and the person will feel compelled to do something silly, thus sabotaging the seriousness and focus with distractions. For example if you've got this inner dialogue, if you're always trying so hard, *I've got a schedule!* and *I'm going to study this, this, this and this, and then I have to go here and then I have to go here.* It might come out as compulsive distractions, an internal self-saboteur of the over serious, over taxed parts of you that are pushing too hard, or have too much agenda. Or it can show up as great stress, depression, anxiety, all kinds of mental poisons. Also sometimes you can see sub-personalities or archetypal drives forming a Peter Pan complex, which Marie Louise von Franz describes magnificently in her book, *The Problem of the Puer Aeternus*. Have you ever seen that? Yes.

Questioner

Of course yes.

Janel

I mean also avoiding responsibility, running away, drugs or whatever. Yes, each person will have their own version. Their own flavor of doing it. It can be a lifestyle. Avoiding commitment. Both women and men do it.

All of these things can just play out in all different ways. I would also say you can see a lot of sadness in people who weren't able to play enough as children.

I wanted to mention that our last Questioner has these healing abilities where he's very sensitive. There's lots of people who grow up in situations where they act or behave in certain ways out of a need to get attention, and they confuse that attention for love. Then they get in the habit of internally thinking *I have to behave in this way in order to be loved by people*, and that's not true.[52] You can exhaust yourself to death playing these roles, replicating the family dynamics they grew up in that were unhealthy. One first needs to see these family dynamics as an object (this is a big step). Once this happens in time there's a potential to learn to step out of old roles, to say no to harmful behavior, and recognize that just in one's own essence, each of us deserves love; being able to say to oneself, I am lovable. I don't have to do XY and Z, or behave in an unhealthy role, to be loved. It can be very hard to break these patterns. There is tremendous liberation in the process of seeing all of this and freeing yourself from it. First of all, is just seeing it, seeing what is, and then also realizing we can make different choices. We can live differently. We don't have to be a slave to all of this, unhealthy conditioning.

Question

I still have a problem understanding the meaning of the five elements. When we talk about these elements like Earth, is it in literal sense, or fundamental forces in the universe and these five are just the representations of those forces? How can I understand it better?

Janel

I would say it can be understood from the elemental gross to the subtle, to causal. It can be understood in all aspects, which I hardly said anything about. I know it must be confusing to some, I don't even know what you all think when I give this very brief presentation. You can learn much more about this in so many ways.

Doshin

Janel just barely scratched the surface of a teaching and an oral tradition, and then a written tradition that's been around for thousands of years. This is like trying to understand what I mean when I say meditative mind. There's no way I can intellectually define it in a way that would help you deeply understand it. If you want to understand it, then you really need to study with a teacher that already understands it. It is experiential learning versus intellectual theory. This is why at the beginning of this session, I emphasize that this is not like learning in a classroom. We're not going to present information that you write down and take notes, and then you spit it back to us on a test at the end of the course. This is a presentation that we are providing for you to experience. If you try too hard to understand it, you won't be able to receive it, to take it in experientially. So if you find the five elements confusing and nothing resonates with you, let it go. But if something does resonate, if it bothers you that you don't understand it, then there's a reason to really dig into it and find a teacher that can help you experience what the five elements are in a way that is useful to you. It is not about intellectually understanding the five elements, it is about experiencing something that will help you understand yourself and others. Once you experience them and then begin to understand them, you will have a *felt-sense* of what they are and how they can be used. Then you begin to understand a little more, and use them in your own healing or working with others. That's what's required here. So just receive it, and if it bothers you, or if it resonates deeply with you, then go further on your own or get help. Make it a project that you can explore more deeply.

It's like a koan. A Zen *koan* is an enigmatic question that the thinking mind can not answer. Most people immediately start thinking the minute I present the koan, which means that they're so busy thinking, they never actually hear the question. Then they're trying to answer a question they have never heard. So of course they fail. The thinking mind cannot answer a koan. Thinking-mind cannot experientially understand the five elements and how useful they are. The elements can be a tool that you use to deepen an experiential learning project. But it's not enough by itself. I hope that's helpful.

Questioner

Yes, definitely. I was trying to understand them intellectually.

Doshin

You must be a good student.

Questioner

Yes.

Doshin

You must get good grades.

Questioner

Yes.

Doshin

And you're probably very smart.

Questioner

Thank you.

Janel

Anybody else?

Questioner

Yes, if I may say something. When the question was asked about play and then Janel was responding, I felt that I probably could say something about play that could help everybody in the process of healing, because in my experience, playing is a medicine because it helps you not take things too seriously. I don't know in terms of the chakras because I don't know anything about chakras, but it seems that having a playful attitude towards life and towards your own healing is in itself something that could heal. The only problem it seems though is that in order for you to be playful, some people just don't seem to know how to be playful. In thinking, everything is taken too seriously. It seems that in order for you to be playful, a little play is required. One of the ways to heal that was mentioned, it said find the time to play or be playful.

Janel

Yes, it was dance and put on music, dance and look foolish. That was the assignment, and I heard from people, I heard from someone who said they did it, and it just felt so great. They loved it.

Questioner

So yes, I just wanted to say that keeping a good sense of

humour and a playful attitude could have, in itself, powerful healing properties.

Doshin

Absolutely. And thank you for adding that because you have learned how to play and you probably had to play a little too much to learn how to play just the right amount, didn't you?

Questioner

Exactly because then you get like too much.

Doshin

You get addicted to playing and it becomes poisonous. That is again where balance is really important.

Questioner

Yes, it's good that you brought this up because I asked this question to Janel the other day. When, when do we stop? Is there an end to this process? It seems to me that there is no end to this. You can always heal deeper and heal even deeper.

Doshin

When I disappear and my body returns to dust. Something continues, I don't know what it is, but I know that my body's gone and I suspect my ego is gone and most of my memories are gone. But I know that karma continues. The karma that I was born into, that I parachuted into, like a sandstorm that's been blowing for 5,000 years. That storm is inside another sandstorm that's been blowing for millions of years. Storms within storms. And when my body returns to dust, I'm sure the sandstorm will continue blowing. An enlightened being can become a karma eater. First I have to heal my own karma and then I can begin healing the karma of all beings; karma eater. For eternity it seems. But there's no time. That means there's no beginning and no end. Everything is now. Don't think about it, thinking will just twist your thinking into knots. Then the thinking stops and there is room for a sudden realization, a flash of insight into Buddha Nature.

Janel

A good level of confusion to leave everyone with.

Doshin

Stick with a sense of humor, as my Zen teacher JunPo used to say, one of his most useful teachings was: "When you've lost your sense of humor, you've lost the way." When you can't play and laugh when nothing is funny, you will know that you have become poisonous. That is when you will need medicine for that poison, and the medicine for the poison of no sense of humor, according to JunPo's teaching, is "sacred laughter." Ego inflation, ethnic inflation, religious inflation, nationalistic inflation, and individual and cultural pride are all poisons caused by taking ourselves too seriously. One of the medicines is laughter and another is fun. So go play and laugh. Not too much, just the right amount.

Janel

Not an agenda. Play cannot have an agenda. I think that's good for this week. Yes.

Doshin

Absolutely, okay love y'all. See you next week.

CHAPTER FOUR THE HEART CHAKRA

Doshin

Wonderful, here we go week four. How quickly time flies when we're having fun. So again, please remember this is an experiential course. Not a class. It is our intention to use the chakras within an Integral Framework, while at the same time presenting a broad overview of many healing lineage teachings that have been around for thousands of years, and include both healing and awakening. I haven't seen anything in Western medicine that takes into consideration the state of awakening. There are great things in Western medicine that are powerful healing technologies and methods, but from my perspective as an Integral Zen teacher, full awakening is impossible without healing. Complete healing is impossible without awakening. These two things are critical, and this is what's new about what is being presented here. What you won't find in modern medical views is the state vantage point of a Zen master, and what you won't find in the traditional lineage views is the Integral Framework. The importance of both healing and awakening can only be seen clearly from a particular Kosmic Address. Once we are able to see and realize how to use the Wilber Combs lattice, we recognize that there are two things going on simultaneously. There is an interrelationship between them, but they are different things. They're not the same thing. We have to parse them apart, seeing them as separate things, and then see exactly how they are interrelated. This is not something that everyone is able to do. It requires a certain level of structural ego development, and the attainment of a certain vantage point of state awakening. It requires a certain Kosmic Address. So, listen and trust that you'll take in what is helpful to you, and just let the rest go. There's nothing you need to argue with here. There's nothing you need to fight. Just let things be as they are. If it doesn't resonate with you, just let it go.

T his is the heart chakra. The root (again), involves grounding, rootedness, physical safety, security and protection. It involves survival and Mother Nature, the earth, connection to ancestors and Karma. There's a physical identity with the body. This is the infrared level of development in Integral Theory. Now the heart chakra is roughly equivalent to the amber level of development, as we're using it here. The heart chakra and the amber stage of ego development marks the emergence of the second-person perspective. All of a sudden, it's not just *me*, suddenly I can see *you* too, and suddenly, I have the mental capacity to be indoctrinated. *Me* has the capacity to be indoctrinated into a *we*, into an ethnic group. The indoctrination into the safety of the tribal ethnic rules and roles; this is where it happens. There's an identity with the collective values of what is right, and what is wrong, and this provides a critical sense of safety, belonging and protection to a developing child. They belong to the group, they're protected by the rules and the guardrails of the group. Remember that developmentally, we all need very clear rules, defined roles and guide rails at this age.

Now, interestingly enough, there's a deep interconnection between the root chakra and the heart chakra. If there is no safety, if I don't feel safe, then the heart cannot open. The heart stays closed, and the heart is the center of these 7 chakras. The heart is also connected to the 7th chakra. So if the heart, for whatever reason, cannot fully open, there is no liberation in the 7th chakra. So this is just something to keep in mind as we move forward. So it's not just the root chakra that's in intimate relationship

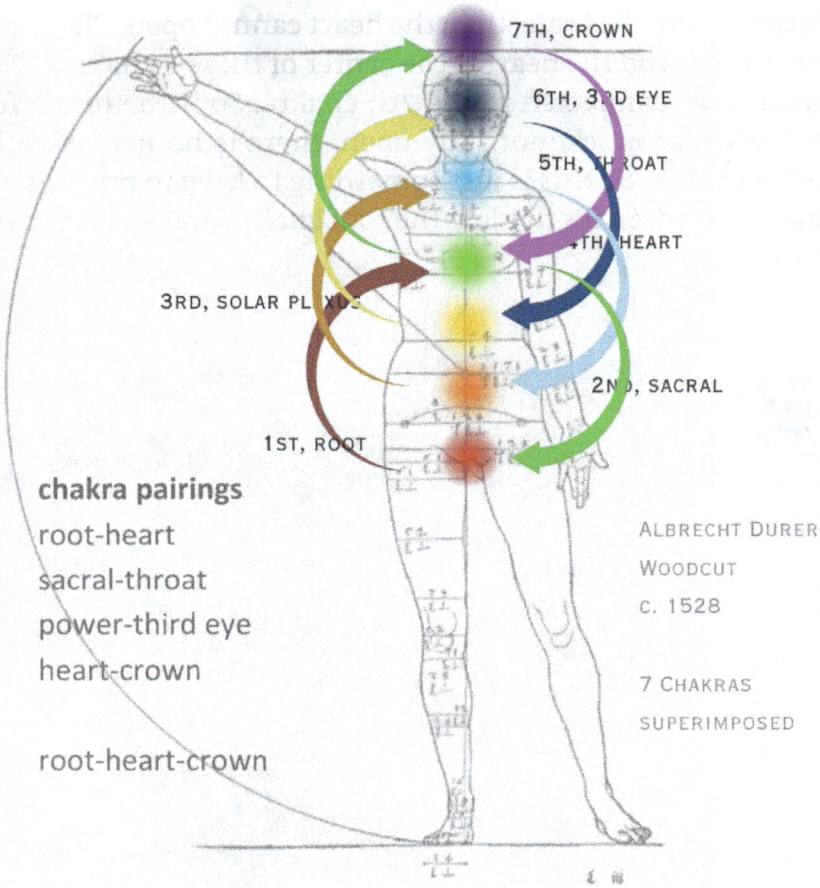

7TH, CROWN

6TH, 3RD EYE

5TH, THROAT

4TH, HEART

3RD, SOLAR PLEXUS

2ND, SACRAL

1ST, ROOT

chakra pairings

root-heart

sacral-throat

power-third eye

heart-crown

root-heart-crown

ALBRECHT DURER
WOODCUT
C. 1528

7 CHAKRAS
SUPERIMPOSED

with the heart chakra, the heart chakra is in relationship with the Crown chakra.

Another pairing is found with the sacral (second) chakra in relationship to the throat chakra (fifth). So these magical experiences that begin to emerge with the energizing of the second chakra will have a relationship to the ideology that we take on later when we start approaching puberty, when 3rd person perspective starts coming online and is available. The emotional and spiritual values that we develop when the

4th person perspective begins to emerge–that is only *if* the culture that you're born into and raised in supports it. Just as well, the 3rd chakra, the solar plexus, the power chakra has a connection to the third eye (sixth chakra). So if there's a dysfunction in your power chakra, if you have too much or too little power, that dysfunction carries over and it impacts this development of the siddhi powers and the opening of the third eye, which to me is the intuitive eye, the eye of direct knowing. Carl Jung defines intuition as "direct knowing."

Five Elements View
primary cause of disease, the three mental poisons

desire, greed
wind element
loong

Rooster

Snake

ignorance, confusion
earth and water elements
bekken
masculine lunar

anger, hatred
fire element
tripa
feminine, solar

Pig

Next, the three poisons (desire, anger, ignorance) are a fundamental teaching of Buddhism. The path of awakening begins with becoming aware of the poisons, the effects they cause, and then learning how to stop poisoning yourself and others. This also is fundamentally important for healing, which Janel will go into in a moment. Here is something that usually doesn't get noticed or mentioned. There are many descriptions and interpretations of the three poisons. They can loosely be arranged into three catagories, corresponding to the three turnings of the Buddhist Wheel. The first-turning of Buddhism, Hinayana,

Mahayana and Vajrayana. There is of course, much common ground, as well as some significant differences between these different Buddhist teachings, which have found their way to the West. Examples of the 1st turning teachings would be the Theravada schools. Mahayana schools would include Nichiren, Chan and Zen. Vajrayana schools would include the many schools of Tibetan Buddhism and Japanese Shingon. You really need to study them all, to get an overview and felt-sense of the three poisons, the negative emotions, the mental dysfunctions, and then there are so many different interpretations due to differences in language translations and structures of development. All this is beyond the scope of what we are doing here, which is just scratching the surface.

This picture is universal to all schools of Buddhism. This picture includes the rooster, which is equivalent to desire, greed and attachment; the snake, which is equivalent to aversion, anger and hatred; and the pig, which is equivalent to ignorance, confusion and delusion. Even at the very beginning of a human life before there is an ego, the capacity for pulling objects toward us, pushing them away and just outright ignorance is here for each of us. As a sense of self naturally develops, there's an increase in emotional intensity. As intensity increases, the attachment moves into liking. Now this self starts liking somethings disliking other things and to somethings it is just indifferent; completely indifferent, doesn't even register on the radar. So if we turn up the intensity of these three poisons a little more, then we have a sense of agency. This would be a first-person perspective. So now there's lusting after what we like, a loathing of things that we dislike, and a conscious or unconscious ignoring of other things we are indifferent to. Turn up the intensity a little bit more, and there's great intensity: you have loving, hating and deluding. Ignorance is said to be the most poisonous of all the three poisons, and in Buddhism is recognized as a basic ignorance of our own Buddha nature.

The Three Poisons &
Emotional Intensity

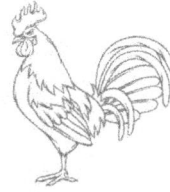

Animal Symbol	Small Intensity	More Intensity	Even More Intensity	Great Intensity
Rooster	Attachment	Liking	Lusting	Loving
Snake	Aversion	Disliking	Loathing	Hating
Pig	Ignorance	Indifferent	Ignoring	Deluding

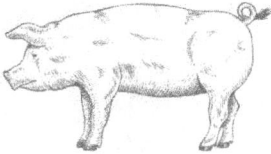

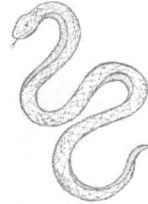

Poisons	Primordial Wisdoms
Pride	Wisdom of equanimity
Ignorance	Reality wisdom or state of phenomena wisdom
Attachment	Discriminating wisdom
Jealousy, envy	Wisdom that leads to achievement
Anger, disgust	Mirrorlike wisdom

This comes with just being human. Another form of ignorance would be confusion. When we start trying to think about things we haven't experienced or don't understand, we're just confused. Ignorance as delusion is when we start believing that our own delusions are the truth. In Buddhism, when we start thinking I am a separate self, then we start believing all the delusions that arise from this illusion that I'm here, and you are there. The more we delude ourselves and each other, the more complex the personality and all our relationships become. The more lies we tell ourselves, the more delusions we come to believe.

From an integral perspective, we can see that the greatest

intensity of the poison of attachment is an addiction to something. It becomes *something we can't live without.* The poison of aversion turns into an allergy against something. It becomes *something we can't live with,* something we would rather die to avoid or kill to prevent having to experience. The delusions are largely unconscious. When collectively shared, they take on a dark demonic quality. This is just an introduction to an Integral Zen view of the three poisons, and the way they polarize as they become more intense.

Janel

Thank you Doshin. So I'd like to present a traditional Tibetan Buddhist, Sowa Rigpa teaching of the poisons, the three mental poisons. From a health standpoint, we're going to go through a few exercises, and it should be said upfront, that the three mental poisons are considered the primary cause of imbalance in health. They're the first cause or origin of how our health becomes out of balance. Also if you add pride and envy, that makes 5 mental poisons, while these poisons don't directly cause disease, they do create the conditions for disease. They are called *long distance* or *indirect* causes. As Doshin pointed out, ignorance is considered the worst, and our *fundamental* poison, the ignorance of our Buddha nature. And so when we're born into a human body, this ignorance comes with it (until and only if we realize our Buddha nature). So it's considered the number one poison.

So what constitutes *indirect* causes of disease? For example, if we eat sweets, we desire to eat more and more, this will cause our weight to increase. This can then lead to diabetes or metabolic problems. Drinking too much alcohol and smoking can lead to health problems, and that can also lead to lifestyle imbalance problems. Too much desire, attachment, creates too much attachment and more, and more. The more you fulfill your desires, it's generally not that you are satiated, it's more that you fuel your desire to fulfill your desires until you

become a slave to your desires. Too much thinking creates
anxiety, and leads to wind/*loong* energy

Sowa Rigpa, three channels in the subtle body

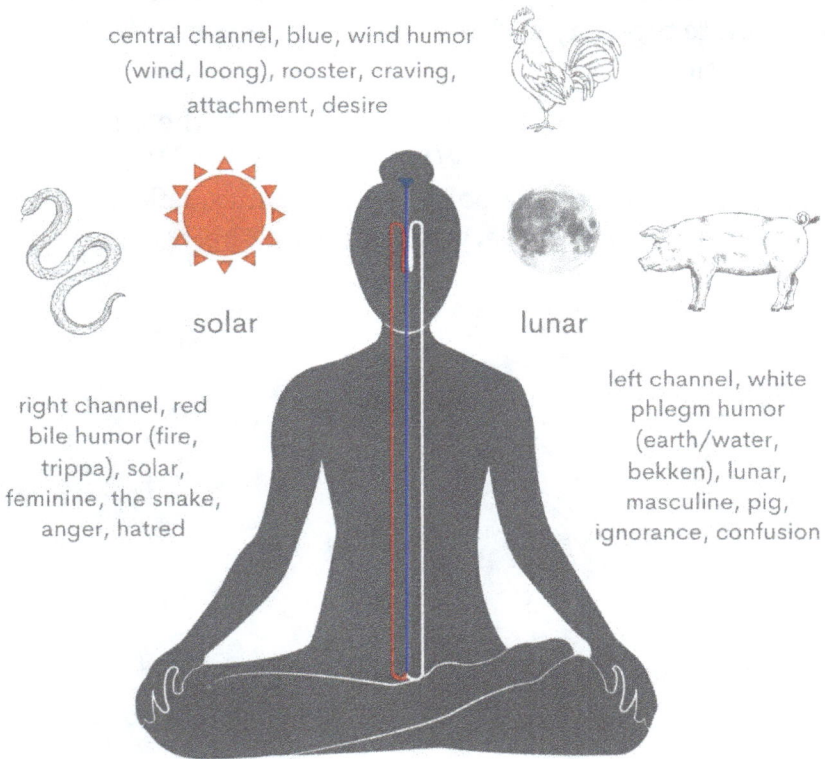

central channel, blue, wind humor
(wind, loong), rooster, craving,
attachment, desire

solar

lunar

right channel, red
bile humor (fire,
trippa), solar,
feminine, the snake,
anger, hatred

left channel, white
phlegm humor
(earth/water,
bekken), lunar,
masculine, pig,
ignorance, confusion

disorders. Overthinking, in this framework directly leads to, not just imbalance, but also cuts back your vital life force, related to the length of your life. Aversion or too much anger leads to bile, fire/*tripa* disorders. These directly correlate with physiological functioning. Laziness is a tendency when a person has too much earth and water/phlegm type, *bekken*, connected to ignorance, confusion, earth and water imbalance.

Sowa Rigpa starts by recognizing that human beings all experience these 3 poisons. Remember we talked about how at conception you inherit your parents typology. Each of their typologies are going to be either dominated by one of these, or a combination. Each person has a combination which creates their innate typology and as a result, tendencies, which begin at conception.

First we see ourselves as individuals, but then this is all of course interconnected. When humans lose the ability to control their own inner poisons, it becomes reflected in the outside world, which is very evident now. The

Five Elements View

self assessment for basic health

rate 1-10, 1 is low, 10 is high

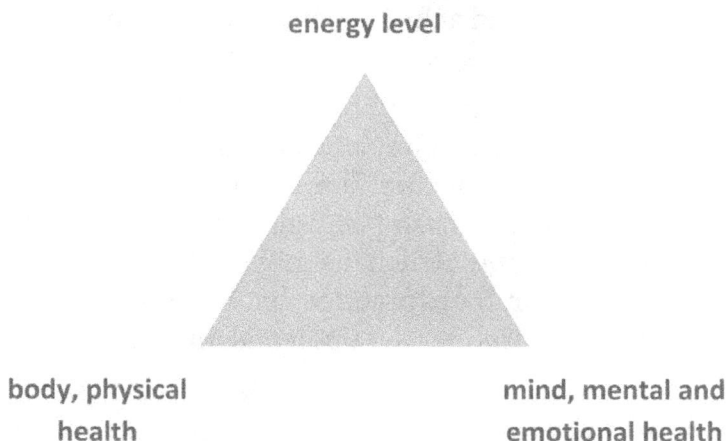

energy level

body, physical
health

mind, mental and
emotional health

more we disturb nature, the more we receive disturbance for ourselves too.[53] Our individual imbalances, lead to interconnected imbalances with others in relationship, lead to imbalance in our home, lead to imbalance in community, lead to imbalance in society, in culture, and we are now in, you know, exactly this kind of a global imbalances (this is especially evident in the environment.)

To bring us back, we have to deal with our inner individual poisons *first.*

"With wisdom, everything can become a medicine. With stupidity, everything can become a poison."

Dr. Nida.[54]

I n traditional medicine, hazardous substances can act as both poison or medicine. When used skillfully with mental poisons, emotions, the five poisons, can be mitigated by 5 primordial wisdoms, which express pure and positive aspects of mind, and serve as *antidotes* to the poisons. When we can learn and acknowledge that some of the poisons predominate within us, we can meditate on the connected primordial wisdom to mitigate effects.

This whole system in Vajrayana can be used in a secular way too. Represented by the five Dhyani Wisdom Buddhas, traditionally there are these five poisons, and then there are the *primordial wisdoms* which usually with the guidance of a teacher, and your own practice by meditation, there are ways to learn to *transmute* these poisons into these primordial wisdoms.

We have been introducing a number of different subtle energy systems. In Sowa Rigpa, when we view our body, our energy body is how we view it, with three energy channels. This is different from our gross body of form and matter–the energy body is not visible in conventional appearance, so when we practice and work with this, we visualize the body as non-material, the shape as crystal clear, and empty inside. If you can picture for yourself, how you experience your energy, your emotions, these are considered part of the subtle body.

So we visualize what is a central channel that is translucent and blue. Again our body is clear. There is a right channel that is red, (tripa) it is the solar channel, associated with bile fire, the snake, anger and hatred, and the feminine (some Tibetan systems have the red on the left). The left channel is the lunar channel white, associated with masculine, bekken, phlegm or earth and water, and the animal symbol is the pig. The central channel, which is blue, is the wind humor loong, representing desire or greed, attachment, symbolized by the rooster.

There's some of you who have practiced Tibetan Nejang yoga with me, which we do on retreat, with a breath purification method, called ninefold breathing. This is not only done in Sowa Rigpa, but by other Tibetan Buddhist lineages. Anyone can do this, it's a breathing practice that purifies the three poisons in our subtle body (which impacts the gross body as well). People do experience really beneficial mental, psychological, physical, and spiritual health benefits doing these practices.

Now we're going to assess ourselves. So I'd like you to consider these three poisons, and what you think may predominate for you? For each poison, confusion, desire, anger, rate yourself on a scale of one to ten; one is low, ten is high. Looking at your life, how much have you been ruled by desire? How much are you ruled by anger? How much by ignorance and confusion? So take a minute to reflect, and write down, for each of these. A number from one to ten.

This exercise, which comes from Sowa Rigpa, we evaluate in this way. First of all, each poison, if you rate below four, rates as relatively healthy. Anywhere above five is considered where you need to work on, and is likely to be your inherent weakness and typology.

Next we will self-assess basic overall health from a Sowa Rigpa perspective. First consider *energy*; do you have enough energy to do what you feel are the things you want to do, at this point in your life (reasonable expectation for age and life situation)? By now you should have some general sense of your potential range, we are estimating ourselves the same way on a scale of 1 to 10, 1 being I have almost no energy, to 10 being I am extremely energized and can do everything I want to do. Next is *body* in terms of physical health from 1 to 10. Then *mind* considering mental and emotional health in this respect. So I'd like you to all assess yourself, from one to 10.

One of the first things I want to say is that Dr. Nida emphasizes that for young people mental health is the number one priority, and impacts the other two aspects, energy and body, more significantly than when we are older. So when working with or considering younger people, we need to prioritize mental health.

Next is understanding that we are primarily impacted by the mental level, and secondary is physical. This is generally true for everyone. So let's look at how you rated yourselves. Any estimation above six is considered healthy. Less than five, this is where you need to focus. These estimates can be revisited, and kept as a diary, and can be quite useful to look at over time.

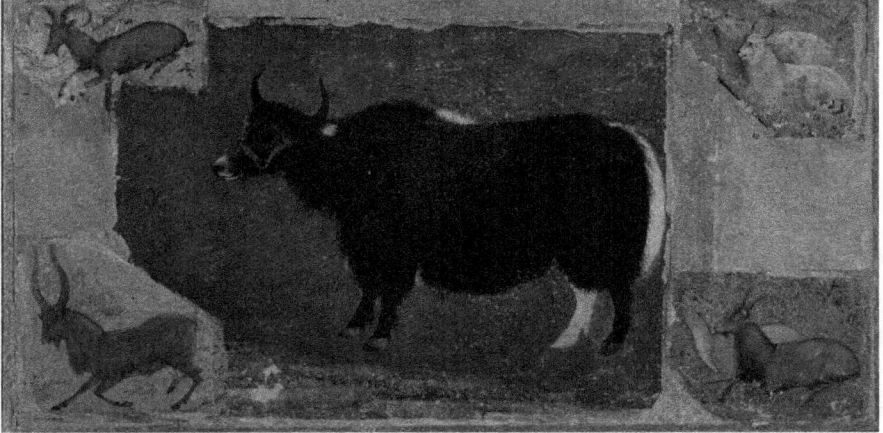

Attributed to Abu'l Hasan, Tibetan Yak with Vignettes of Animals, Harvard Art Museums / Arthur M. Sackler Museum, Gift of Stuart Cary Welch, Jr., Photo © President and Fellows of Harvard College, 1999.291

So just some more framework for the Sowa Rigpa system. What is considered balance in this system? The Tibetan word is *neluk*, which is our underlying unchanged natural state, which is one of health, so this refers to the typology that we were born with as the baseline, so to speak. If you were working with someone doing this practice, including me, we would work together to first determine what your natural state is, which provides us with the starting point. Let's say you were earth and water, phlegm, or *bekken*. That means you're always going to be more earth and water than the other two types (fire, and wind). Considering that as we age and live longer, the general tendency is that we become out of balance. In knowing your basic typology, you know you always have that as the reference point, that's where you're looking to bring yourself back to balance, a balance of body, energy and mind.

Imbalance is *nezhi*, our changed state of disease. What first may begin as being deficient or excess, can lead to disorder, and eventually disorder can lead to disease.

Secondary causes of disease

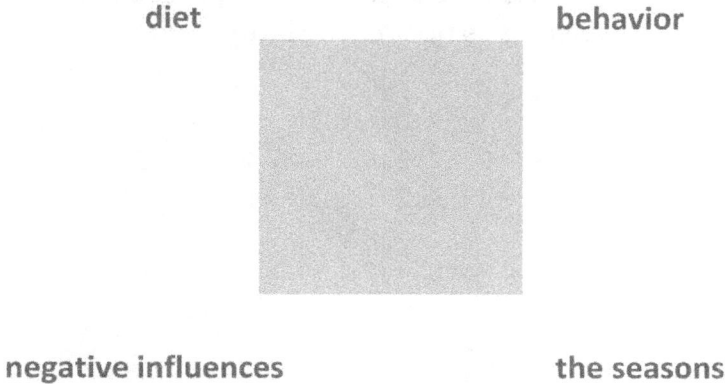

diet   behavior

negative influences   the seasons

Initially, the signs of imbalance are very subtle. In this tradition, and in medical systems that include working with subtle energies, imbalances can be sensed long before more gross symptoms start to manifest. Sowa Rigpa works in this way and is much more focused on preventative health. Indicators of imbalance come much much sooner and subtler and are more visible in these traditional approaches, than signs and symptoms that register as problematic in Western Bio-medicine.

Looking back at accounts of the Buddha's health later in his life, it was historically noted that he had a wind disorder, a loong imbalance/energy imbalance, and one of the treatments for this was the *three Peppers*: long pepper, dry pepper and Szechuan, these peppers are herbs that *kindle* the fire element. There's also an account of the Buddha commenting on an emaciated monk, and the Buddha saying that *the monk should eat some fat,* which would have referred to animal fat.[55] This is historically notable because a lot of people just assume all Buddhists are vegetarian, not knowing that the Sowa Rigpa system of diet generally is not vegetarian.

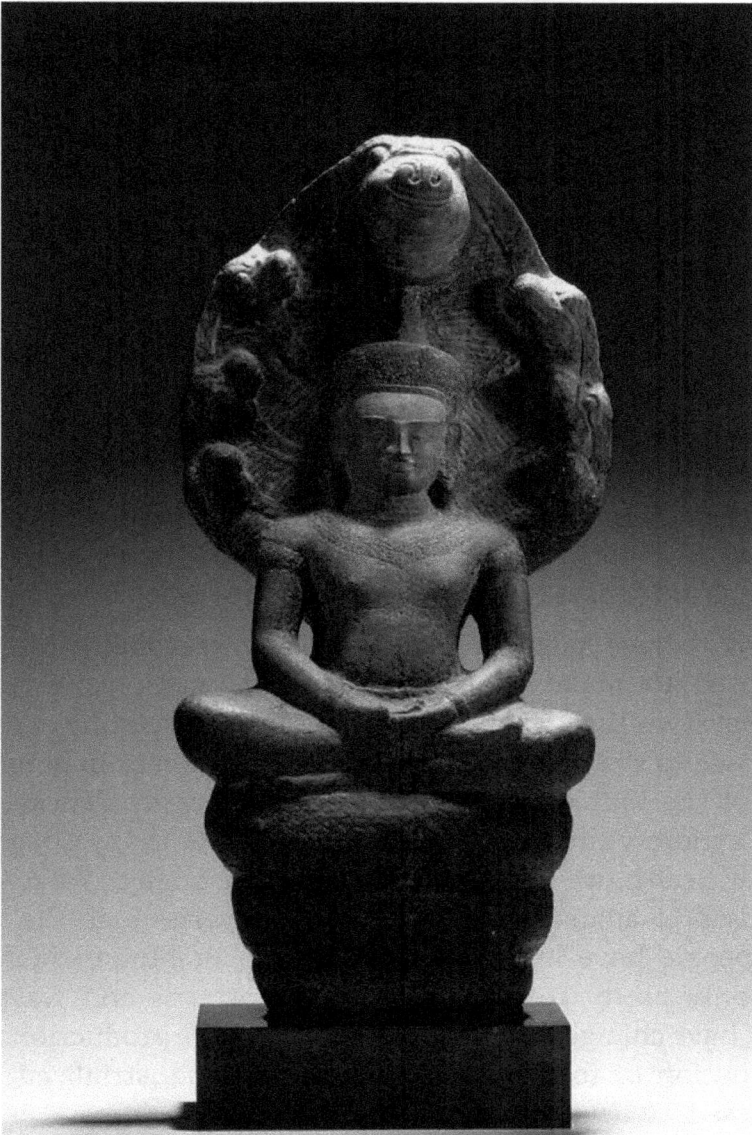

Crowned Naga-Protected Buddha, Cambodia, *ca. 1150-1190*, Stone (arkosic wacke), traces of lacquer and gilding, The Walters Art Museum, Baltimore

First of all, the region where the Dalai Lama comes from, the same region where Dr. Nida comes from Amdo province in

Tibet, very few vegetables grow because of the severe climate. Most people eat predominantly yak and yak products, yak butter and yak milk. Herbs as well are important in the Sowa Rigpa system. The overall view is very much that food is seen as medicine (and potentially, poison.)

Also worth mentioning, wind/energy/*loong* imbalances are common. This gets back to what was mentioned earlier when we talked about Zen disease, or meditator's disease. Once helpful dietary remedy for wind imbalance and wind types, is including more fats, in particular animal fat, and animal bone broth in the diet. These are considered very important for healing these imbalances.

The secondary cause of disease after the three poisons, is divided into four factors. Diet, behaviour, (that's lifestyle), negative influences (provocations) and the seasons.

I think I have talked here about how seasonally, we are supposed to make adjustments to the ways we eat and the ways we live. For example winter (Yin season), we are supposed to sleep more. There are also two weeks in between each of the four seasons, where health is really delicate, so there's more vulnerability to getting sick. Is it any surprise, for our health, we are supposed to eat seasonally? We're also supposed to adjust our lifestyle. This is very much the way that people have lived for the duration of human history. It is only pretty recently that these patterns and ways of living have changed so much, especially as the production and distribution of food became increasingly industrialized and processed.

Negative influences can be referred to as provocations[56] or *Dön* in Tibetan, which I mentioned before, but I didn't say much about. Part of the world is not just seeing beings visible to the eye, but realizing there are unseen beings. From the Sowa Rigpa and wider Tibetan Buddhist, and originally Tibetan Shamanic Bon traditional view, there are all kinds of beings. There are naga water spirits living below the earth, spirits in the clouds; earth spirits are very much affected by environmental imbalance, so if we consider this from a scientific framework, this can be "seen" as climate disturbance. Another example are global pandemics.

There's a whole framework and system for viewing these factors, which integrates all beings' interconnectedness. Stepping back, this is a framework of health through balance. The aim is to balance the three humors; wind (loong), fire (tripa) and earth and water (bekken), and in working with the five elements, we can develop individualized treatment, starting from each individual's unique constitutions and personal imbalances. It is a holistic approach that recognizes that body and mind are not two. Dietary recommendations are a big component of this, and the importance of supporting digestive health, again this is considered an essential aspect of healing. There are herbal supports for generating digestive heat (some of these are very common kitchen herbs). Our metabolic heat is connected with the fire element. I know digestive problems are very common with people I work with, so if this is something that you struggle with, there are easy over the counter herbs and herbal supplements that are worth trying, which don't have the side effects and problems of Western pharmaceutical drugs.

There is also lifestyle modification. I mentioned before the 8-8-8 pattern, sleeping 8 hours, working 8 hours, then another 8 hours that you decide how you use; even pausing to review how we use our time, is an important reminder that *ultimately we are in control of those 24 hours*, so, to remember that, and adjust accordingly.

Exercise for body and mind: each of the typologies are better supported and suited by different types of exercise intensity. There are energetic balancing methods which we will talk about more next week. Respecting the sense organs is also emphasized; I've talked about this a few times, which means taking care, control and responsibility over how you treat your sense organs, for example what you look at, what you listen to. What you do with your orifices, a *conscious* relationship with all of your sense organs.

Other health supports in Sowa Rigpa, include what are called *external* therapies, Moxibustion (a heat therapy) can be very helpful, cupping, massage, herbal compresses, herbal baths. Hot Springs are known to be extremely healing, also baths with Epsom salts. Preventive measures, building healthy habits, mindfulness, and rituals all contribute to prevention and treatment.

This also gets into the realms of deities, demons and unseen beings (Dön). People feeling they may be under the influence of curses. Sowa Ripga has a framework that includes all of this area. At the same time it's possible to work with people in a secular way, a scientific way, but sometimes there are karmic patterns and problems that people face where conventional approaches don't help, so one may need to be creative and explore other possibilities. Ritual healers are common in Buddhism in general, they are generally people trained and have developed siddhi powers to support others with unusual problems that normal health support can't resolve.

Vajra Breathing

You may recall that "mantra" translates to *mind protection*. The mantra "Om ah hung" is considered the mantra of all mantras, for body, speech, and mind purification. The seed syllable "OM" includes all mantras itself, encompassing everything, all sounds of the universe.

I'm going to introduce this breathing exercise. So the OM

is in this tradition and in many others. OM is associated locationally with your head, so that's your third eye and your head (Dr. Nida calls it the head chakra), and it's connected to white light, which we visualize emanating from our head. "AH" is connected to the throat, and a brilliant red light. "HUNG" is connected to the heart, with brilliant blue light.

This version of the mantra and breathing, is called a simplified Vajra chanting and breathing practice, taught in Sowa Rigpa. It can really settle the nervous system, and it's simple to do. We can even do it simply by visualizing the lights.

Start by sitting with a straight spine, relaxed, with normal curvature. We're going to imagine as we are breathing in, visualize, a brilliant bright white light entering into our head, into our body, through the nostrils, and we're going to imagine the sound- you don't have to say it, although you can, just imagine the sound of "OM" and white light, and if you want, and it's easier, just a white light is enough. Once we breathe in, we breathe in through our nostrils deeply, and expand our belly as we imagine the light going all the way down to where the energy channels meet about four finger widths below the belly button, and four finger widths in towards the spine. Once we've breathed in we can pause as long as is right for us, and imagine the light changes from white to red (you can imagine the origin of the red coming

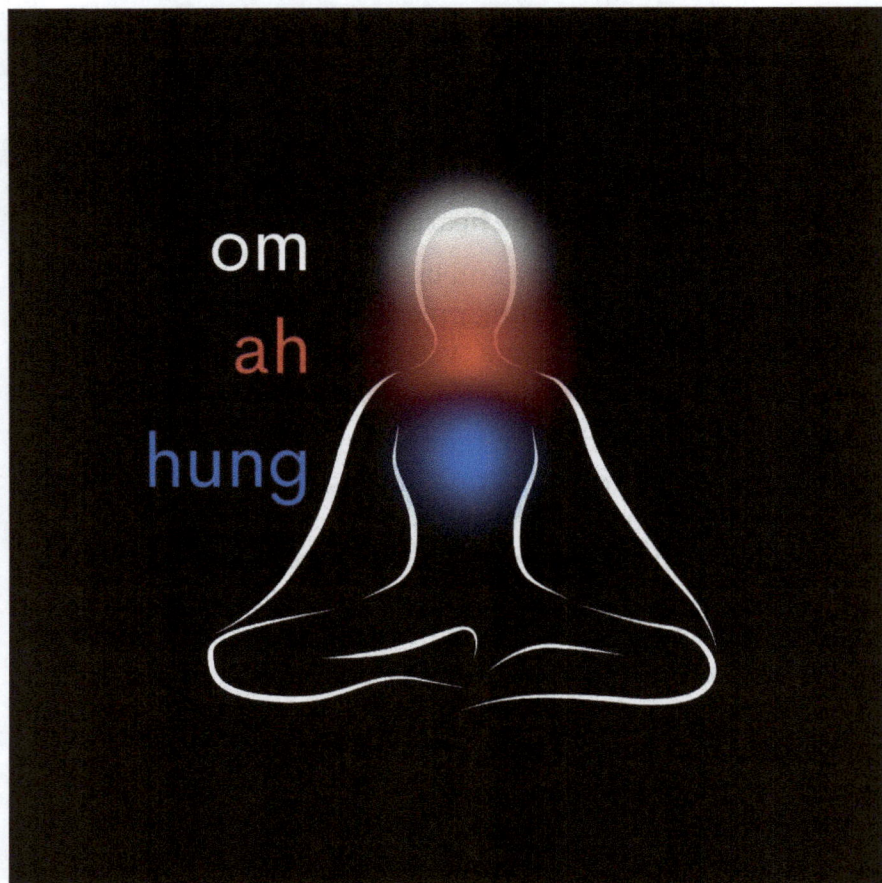

from your throat), expanding through to fill the body.

We retain the breath according to our capacity and ability, maybe just pause, and after expanding the light to fill our whole body with brilliant red light (with the sound AH). Then we can breathe out through our nostrils, visualizing this red light turning into blue (you can picture the origin of blue at your heart if you wish) and we exhale and both breath, and light leaves our body.

These three locations, white OM at the head, red AH at the throat, blue HUNG at the heart, are the last locations from the view of this framework, from where our consciousness remains in our body, after gross physical death, until the subtle consciousness leaves (usually said to be 3-4 days after clinical death.) So initially the energetic areas that remain are at the head, the throat and the heart, even after you are declared clinically dead, these energies are still here, until the consciousness leaves, out of one of several possible locations.[57] So this type of breathing, which is a purification practice, is used in bardo related practice, to help people to prepare for death. I've been taught, and tell people that it's an excellent way to actually prepare for the end of life, to simply visualize a white light, breathing in a white light, then turning to red, and then exhaling blue. You don't have to think about the seed syllables.

So breathe through your nose in brilliant white light, at your head, moving the light and breath down to your throat. Brilliant red filling your body, even going beyond, and then you can exhale out, blue light, HUNG. Let's just take a few minutes and do this, you can shut your eyes if you want. If any of you have actually studied any of the bardo practices, as we are getting ready for the possibility of going into the bardos, if you recall, that original *red essence* from our mother, and the *lunar essence* of the father, that came together at conception, then separated, well then they come back together at death. Part of this awareness as part of dying, if one has generated enough practice to be aware throughout the death process, is experiencing this *Clear Light* experience, experiencing brilliant red and white lights. This is something we teach about in our course on the process of death, from traditional Buddhist teachings.

We've hardly mentioned anything yet but here are some traditional healing methods, not just in Sowa Rigpa. There are other traditions that can support not just your life, but actually, your preparation for the end of your life, which is an important part of coming into wholeness and balance.

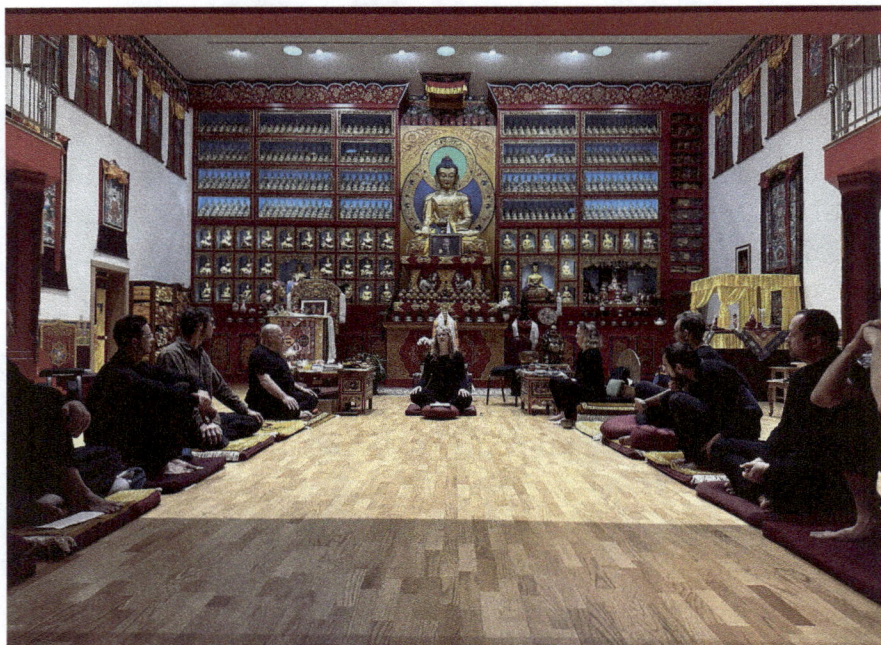

Janel preparing to practice Nejang Yoga on retreat in Crestone, Colorado

Now *Nejang* Tibetan yoga, which I introduced before, is a way that Tibetan doctors have worked with patients for centuries. Anyone can do this practice, religious or secular. It has similarities with advanced Tibetan Buddhist tantric and yogic practices including Tsa-lung, Trul khor, and Tummo, coming from the *Six Yogas of Naropa*.[58] These originated from the Indian Mahasiddhas Tilopa and Naropa around 1100 CE, although some of them precede this time.

I personally do Tibetan Buddhist practices (so reading prayers, practice ritual, recite mantras and meditate) under the guidance and instructions of lineage teachers and teachings, and what this means is that teachers were taught and approved by their teachers to teach certain things to people who are within the lineage, and then certain things if you are not in the lineage, cannot be taught to those uninitiated. From my experience when working with teachers who are presently engaged within a lineage, even if their teacher has died, if they still maintain connection to the lineage, there are rules (even if unspoken) of what is generally okay to share with initiates, versus non-initiates. Some traditional teachers open instruction to those who receive *empowerments* (where you attend a teacher's initial ritual and practice instructions in order to read, study or practice a formal practice), but may also offer teachings open to anyone. Some teachers may study with traditional teachers formally but then may teach people who have not made any formal commitment to a lineage. For example Integral Zen is a branch that came from the Rinzai Zen lineage, originally from Japan. Doshin Roshi teaches both to initiates (those who take Jukai) and non-initiates. Likewise I am an ordained Minister in Integral Zen, but I also received training as a Sowa Rigpa Counselor, approved to teach and do some ritual practices from Sowa Rigpa with permission and instruction from Dr. Nida, and I am empowered within a number of Tibetan Buddhist Lineages to practice, but I teach mostly non-initiates, in addition to those who have taken Jukai in Integral Zen. That said, there are practices I have learned that are fine for me to practice, but not appropriate for me to teach. I thought it would be helpful to explain this, because I think it can be quite confusing for people.

Having said this, until one is *approved* by lineage teachers to teach certain things, it is my understanding and belief that you do not teach these things. Why I am talking about this is, there are a lot of people and teachers and teachings where people are taking material that was not meant to be shared, and sharing it, without approval from their teachers. I know I keep repeating this, but for your own well being, be aware of who you're studying with, to have a sense whether or not they've gotten an "okay" to teach. It isn't necessarily that these people have bad intentions, it's just that teachers generally wait until their students are ready, to encourage them, and request them to teach; not before. One needs to wait, because teachers who have higher state vantage points, are going to see things most people can't. Doshin often jokes something to the effect that you don't want to go to someone for brain surgery, who just decided they are a brain surgeon based on a weekend workshop at a hotel, but who is obviously not a brain surgeon.

Since we're on this subject already, it is also worth mentioning with the seemingly endless online teachings available now, caution is warranted to be aware and concerned regarding where, from whom and what teachings one is participating and more often *consuming* these days. With increasingly sophisticated AI tools many people with a lack of ability to see karma, have jumped into the production of YouTube videos, blogs, and endless social media content, where they basically can take other primary content and manipulate it to produce something that may appear to be something, it is not. It's important to consider what the kosmic address may be of whomever (if in fact, human and not machine!) is making any content or presentations? Because that's part of what carries through of what is created, the kosmic address. Also, remember this--if you listen to dharma from a teacher, you will get a very different transmission than from a layperson teaching. The exact same thing applies, so again, I listen to more recordings from *primary* sources versus *secondary* sources. There is a BIG difference. Like listening to a book *about* Jung versus listening to an old interview *with* Jung. Like listening to Krishnamurti himself versus something *about* Krishnamurti. Listening from a Rinpoche versus a scholarly or secular accounts *about* Buddhism. Very different teachings and transmissions.

Next we're going to introduce some Chinese practices. Before that I do want to mention Hatha Yoga. The definition of "hatha" is yoga in which physical methods predominate. The Sanskrit word हठ haṭha literally means "force", alluding to a system of physical techniques.

Hatha yoga is very useful for healing, working with the chakras, for physical practice, and preserving and channeling vital force life energies. It traces back at least to the first century in the Hindu sutras, and it's also mentioned in Buddhism's Pali canon. The oldest text I have read about is an 11th CE century text from Tantric Buddhism. As a system it is designed to purify, balance, strengthen and transform the body. Again, I always encourage people to study with teachers who have trained within a lineage, if this is an option. I had one yoga teacher with a deep spiritual practice who really helped me on a path to deeper transformation and healing, and I still practice some hatha yoga today.

I'd like to mention the book *Mind of Clear Light* by the Dalai Lama as a good introduction to death awareness and preparation from a Tibetan Buddhist perspective. Also the book *Sacred Passage* is by a woman who worked in hospice who studied Tibetan Buddhism and adapted some of the traditional Tibetan Buddhist approaches to death for a more secular audience.

The Fourth, Heart Chakra

heart, Sanskrit Anahata

5-7 years, Integral Amber, second person perspective

- Location: Front sternum, to the right of the heart, back between the shoulder blades
- Essential functions: Moral indoctrination, rules, group relationships, love – the center of balance, the point of integration of of lower chakras 1 – 3 and higher chakras 5 – 7
- Meridians: Lung / large intestine, pericardium / triple heater, heart / small intestine
- Areas of body: The skin, heart, lungs, upper chest, arms (outer upper arm, elbow joint, forearm, wrists, hands), between shoulder blades, shoulders, lymphatic, fascial, nervous system can be connected to subtle heart practices
- Developmental stage: 5-7 years**
- Development: Our understanding of love, our initial indoctrination to morality and groups, initial experience of us and them, discriminating dualistic mind emerges (70% of the world is in an Amber perspective)

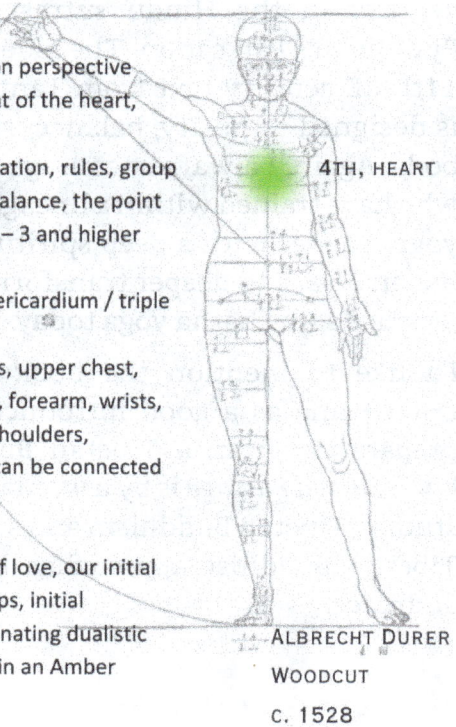

Heart Themes

Love – Family – Groups – Rules – Compassion – Devotion – Community – Forgiveness – Grief – Moral Indoctrination

4TH, HEART

ALBRECHT DURER
WOODCUT
C. 1528

CHAKRAS
SUPERIMPOSED

As we start the Heart, Doshin provided us with an intriguing introduction. It's really important, to keep in mind that the heart is the center, the *unifier* between the lower and upper chakras and in Tibetan Buddhism, where it is taught that everything that's important about your life experience is stored in your heart, which includes ancestral content (the *kunzhi*)[59]. Again, this is one of the last places where our consciousness remains before it leaves our body. The heart is critical to everything in your being.

The corresponding developmental stage is roughly five to seven years (this can vary person to person). It is Integral Amber, entering second person perspective. I will say more about that in a little bit. As far as the body, it's not just the area of your heart in terms of energetic location, it includes your arms and your hands. So if you have physical issues with your arms and hands, this can relate to heart channels. We've talked about how in the Sowa Rigpa view you have 72,000 channels; you also have powerful channels that run up both arms related to higher powers, going from the center of the palms, to the heart.

This developmental period is where the child experiences moral indoctrination, where we learn the relative rules of our family, community, culture, which we are ready for at this time. This means we're *not ready earlier.* It also means that we actually need this amber framework as part of healthy development.

Amber also relates to group relationships, love, which is a complex area, relative, and unconditional love. The heart is the center of balance. It's connected to the small intestine in Tibetan medicine, also the tongue. It also can be considered as connected to the skin, and fascia. The fascia is a whole other complicated area, I would say is yet to be well understood in the West. The development or understanding of love, and our initial indoctrination to morality in groups, and the initial experience of *us and them,* the emergence of discriminating dualistic mind. Presently, I believe you said 70% of the world is at an amber perspective, Doshin?

Doshin

Ken Wilber says that, and I think that's very important to keep in mind. I personally think it's higher, because in today's world at the amber stage of individual development, children are indoctrinated into amber, orange or green collective values and beliefs. They are still amber even though their values and beliefs might appear to be orange or green.

Janel

Interesting. Heart themes relate to love, family groups, rules, compassion. Devotion is hugely important in Vajrayana and Tibetan Buddhism. Devotion is something that's often forgotten or left out in what I would say is a green biased, postmodern interpretation and adaptation in contemporary Buddhism.

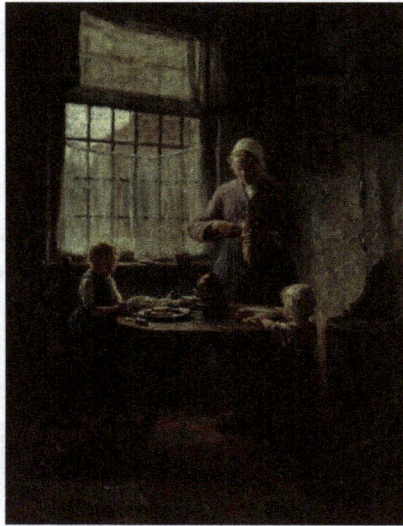

Evert Pieters, A Family Meal, 1890-1899. The Art Institute of Chicago. This information, which is available on the object page for each work, is also made available under Creative Commons Zero (CC0). Additional data about artworks in the collection is available using our public API

Now, consider community, forgiveness and grief. For your heart to open, to heal, you really need to forgive everyone and everything that needs to be forgiven, including yourself. You need to grieve everything that needs to be grieved. That's not just death, that can be grieving outgrown situations, relationships, or our youth. Everything that needs to be grieved.

Also, the chakras become more complex as they go up. Remember, they're working with the other chakras too, it's all dynamic. I am quite sensitive energetically, and I can experience a somatic, visceral experience if something triggers me in the heart. If I'm in a group being triggered, I can feel my heart shift suddenly. The walls come down metaphorically and energetically, so palpably, with a strong sense of separation from others. Whereas when my heart opens, there is wide open compassion, and the experience of this is when I see or even think of other people, I see them in the most compassionate light. When you are grounded and balanced you are available for the heart to open to others. It is clear in working with people when they have *root* issues, they often have *heart* issues, when you are aware of the signs, it's pretty easy to see the connection.

When I work with people one-on-one and I've worked with many of you here, when we get to the heart, I try to help people extract and define what their individual moral indoctrination was. We look at what you actually learned at this age, what were the *rules* (spoken and unspoken?) Where did you go to school? Do you remember your first teachers? Did you go to a church or synagogue, or mosque, or temple? Did you have a relationship with God? It's fascinating to hear how some people can remember as children, clearly having an active relationship with God. That they spoke to God, they prayed or they questioned God.

One thing I started to notice as I worked with people is if you grew up with more than one parent, that it's rare that both parents are equally aligned completely in their belief systems and backgrounds. Therefore if your parents had two quite different views, the child also learns and internalizes this, which can lead to internal strife and confusion.

Then there are the collectives (integral speak, holons). There is a cultural environment, ethnic, culture, time and place, so the child is learning all of this as well. If you're growing up in a kind of complicated scenario, this too can create a confusing amber stage of development.

So what does this actually mean as we grow up? If we're confused in this period about belief systems, and what is *right*, what is *wrong*? In looking at individuals I would say, the confusion generally continues. I also notice that for a lot of people, unless someone can point to it clearly (as an object), they won't see it themselves, or they may see what happened, but can't see the impact on them in the past and present. (Doshin says *we can't see the waters we're swimming in*). The Amber period also relates to rules in general, and I suspect organizational capacity is connected to this too. What I've observed is that if a child is in the amber stage exposed to paradoxical, conflicting scenarios and models, they can struggle with these themes, and creating their own organizational models for their life. Also, finding their way through moral challenges. Even simply the direction of their life, management of their life, intimate relationships.

This is where identifying your own early moral indoctrination is important. For example, if you lived in post-war Germany, since I work with a number of people like this. Following the war as children some people were exposed to some traditional, still conservative teachers, older teachers on the one hand who still adhered to past rigid moral and political models (and indoctrination) on the one hand, and then people may have also had younger teachers who were trying to just abandon all the history that had happened (WW2, and at that time there wasn't much discussion of the prior history to children, but it was in the collective air, no question). Meanwhile, whether people are talking about the bogeyman in the room or not, children absorb all of this atmospherically (the collective unconscious), and so there's so many varieties of ways this can play out.

I work with people whose parents lived through war situations or had to emigrate. There is all the baggage that comes with that, the psychological trauma, a statistically notable increased vulnerability to mental illness, financial difficulties, loss of cultural identity, loss of social status, the karma and impact of which, is passed down. It's not just your grandparents' situation, it's been *passed down to you*. The more we explore this, the more we find it's quite complicated. By laying out what happened, you can start to look at it, which we'll do more in the next class and book. Looking at your indoctrination and then, next is (as we move into the throat) how much of this do I still believe, or have my beliefs changed? Until you do this kind of work, a lot of this may be unconscious for you. So Doshin you may want to say some things about this.

Doshin

I do want to say some things about this. This is an area where things appear to be much more complicated, and the more complications increase, the more developed people get, or think they get, then the more developed they think they are, the more they come to believe and feel they are better, more advanced than others. Of course there is some truth to that and some unhealthy ego inflation as well. It's an area that can deeply benefit from an *Integral Framework*. We each can become more conscious in the context of an Integral Framework, and then we can develop the capacity to use it, *this can be earned with training, feedback and practice*. It can't just be learned, it has to be earned. It takes approximately four years, according to the majority of the experts in the field of development theory, to move from one level of development to another, and that is under optimal conditions. Remember, individuals *can't skip steps,* you can't jump over a step. You can try, but it doesn't work. It leaves a developmental hole that becomes dysfunctional, unbalanced and unhealthy. So this is an area where an Integral Framework changes everything. It makes so many things understandable that weren't understandable before. This is a process of both healing and awakening. Leave either one out and it can't happen.

When we get into the fifth chakra, the throat chakra, we start learning an ideology that's connected to the second chakra, the sacral chakra, where the individual's emotions, sexuality, magic and feeling of sacredness first emerge. In the Integral Framework, this is both the orange and green level of development. It's not just the moral values which emerged in the amber stage with fundamentalist, black and white rules and roles. As the fifth chakra begins to be energized, we develop a belief system that extends beyond our moral value system. In Integral Zen, we call this new combined system of moral values and ideological beliefs *"moral dogma."* At a second tier level of cognitive development, the capacity emerges to see our *"moral dogma"* as an object that can be observed. The practice of objectively observing and subjectively feeling it both at the same makes a huge difference. Liberation from the prison of our own *moral dogma* now becomes possible.

Once we begin to become conscious of that, we can start becoming conscious of what our *moral dogma* is currently, or was in the past. What the *moral dogma* is that we are indoctrinating our children into. This is a profound insight, and so many aspects of our problematic relationships with our children suddenly become clear and can be understood when examined in an Integral Framework. Healing now becomes a possibility and the heart breaks open. Keep in mind, too, that when we teach our children our beliefs and values we're providing the guard rails of what they should and should not do, what is right and what is wrong. We're indoctrinating them into a structure of development with our fundamental values and our beliefs, our *moral dogma*. It is at the amber stage of development, as the heart chakra becomes active that this can happen. Here, they have a second-person perspective. They will not yet have the third-person perspective of rational thought to understand all this. They will not understand the scientific method at five, six, or seven years old. That capacity doesn't show up until puberty, and *only if* the conditions exist in the culture. Only in an orange cultural environment, will the third-person perspective with a particular Western form of rational thinking develop. As individual human beings, we move from an amber heart chakra perspective to a throat chakra perspective with an orange and a green *moral dogma* (at least in the West). So that's why I say that worldwide most of the people are at an amber level of development. Ken says it's somewhere around 70%, I think it's even higher. Because so many of the people that appear to be modern are just parroting modern ideologies without really having the capacity to understand science or practice the scientific method. It's the same with post modernity, they're really stuck at an amber level of development, and have adopted green moral values and beliefs in an amber black and white, fundamentalist way. They are stuck in amber guide rails, shoulds and shouldn'ts, with green values and beliefs that they don't really understand, just mimicking them and parroting them back. So, if we take this into consideration, the true number of people that are at the amber level of development could be much higher, and they appear to be modern, postmodern, or even integral, but they're not. So that is a lot to digest. If you find it confusing or too much, just let it go, and if it resonates and is helpful, take it in.

Next, the AQAL framework can really help us make more sense out of things that we can't make sense of without it. Let's take the individual interior space where this young child is confused about what should I do? They've been indoctrinated into a nexus of collective moral values, "you shouldn't do this and you should do that" and this is what Freud called the internal structure of the *superego*. The voice in the head of the individual parroting back the *shoulds and shouldn'ts* of the parents and the grandparents and the teachers and religious authorities. So that is the little blue Angel and red devil that have been whispering in your ear. Does anybody have one of those?

The child is really looking for guidance: as to *what I should and shouldn't do?* Not giving young children adequate guidance and guard rails that are simple and black and white, does them a huge disservice. It creates great confusion and instability in their lives, in their relationships, especially their relationships with their parents, other siblings and their schoolmates. Each child needs to be given some simple fundamental rules to follow, some guide rails to stay within. If they receive different rules from the school, from the church, from the parents, and from their peers, then they are confused, disturbed and they are not able to develop in a healthy way. They don't know which set of rules to follow, which set of rules is the right one.

Heart Chakra in Four Quadrants

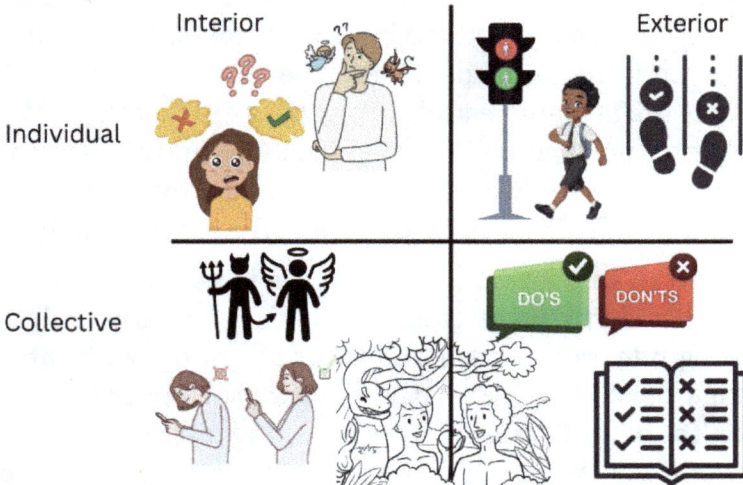

Then in the lower left quadrant, that is where the phenomena of the nexuses of the collective voices of different groups exist. In Integral terms, we speak of these groups as "social holons". These collective cultural voices are speaking to the individual saying: *these are the things you should do, these are the things you should not do.* If there are different groups with different rules and voices, it creates the perfect conditions for moral dilemmas, great confusion and suffering.

T hen there are the stories that historically teach collective moral values and beliefs, like the story of Adam and Eve. In the story of Adam and Eve, we find powerful symbols like: the tree of life, the snake, the apple and the knowledge of good and evil. These symbolic stories are part of the indoctrination process. These stories formalize and implant the rules, the dos and don'ts, the things that *are acceptable* and things that *aren't acceptable,* as well as the values and beliefs. Eventually in addition to these implicit rules, we end up with a more formal explicit written guidebook, which emerges in the lower right social quadrant.

Indoctrination into these rules with their guide rails is very important. Imagine what would happen if a young child has no inner guide rails and wanders into traffic without the knowledge of stop lights or the capacity or training to pay attention to them. That's what we're asking our children to do, if at an early age, we don't teach them in a way that they can understand, that *you have to stay between the lines.* This type of training provides a foundation that enables them to begin to learn how to make moral decisions.

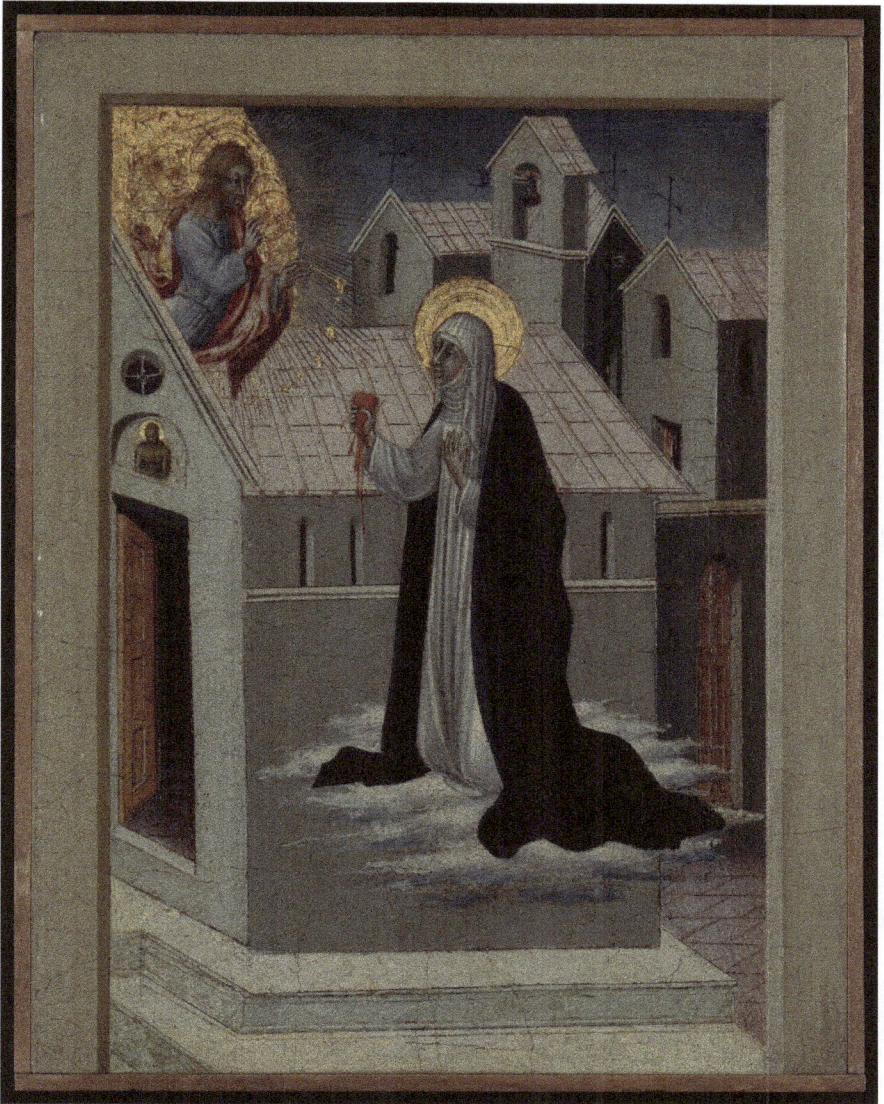

Saint Catherine of Siena Exchanging Her Heart with Christ, Giovanni di Paolo, Italian, Siena 1398–1482 Siena, Bequest of Lore Heinemann, in memory of her husband, Dr. Rudolf J. Heinemann, 1996, Metropolitan Museum of Art, New York, Public Domain

There's a saying in Buddhism that is very helpful. *The heart knows the way when the foot feels the ground,* so it's not enough to teach children what the rules are. You have to teach them to make moral decisions, healthy moral decisions, not just take twisted and poisonous egocentric positions. This is all part of the heart chakra coming online. It becomes so much clearer when you learn to examine the heart chakra in the Integral Framework in all four quadrants; they're all interconnected. Everything we experience is tetra-arising, in all four quadrants simultaneously, whether we are aware of it or not, and it all has an impact.

In every school of Buddhism, there are six *sense consciousnesses*. In my view, which is biased (I'm a Mahayana Buddhist) the Mahayana and the Vajrayana have not just six consciousnesses, they have eight, but I'm not going to go into that now. We're just going to deal with the sixth sense consciousnesses that are common to all schools of Buddhism. The six senses are broken down into three different categories. There are the sense objects, the sense gateways - the sense organs, and the sense consciousnesses. This is really important. To put it very succinctly, if a taste comes in through the gateway of the tongue, it's not the tongue that recognizes the taste, it is the sense consciousness.

It's the tasting consciousness that makes sense out of the taste and differentiates the sour taste from the sweet taste, the salty taste from the sour taste. The sour taste of a lemon would be the sense object. The sense organ of the tongue is the sense gateway. The tasting consciousness is the sense consciousness that processes the taste and makes sense out of it.

Six Sense Consciousnesses

sense objects	sense gateways (organs)	sense consciousnesses
tastes		tasting consciousness
smells		smelling consciousness
images		seeing consciousness
sounds		listening consciousness
touches		touching consciousness
feelings & thoughts		feeling & thinking consciousness

manovijnana -- discriminating heart/mind consciousness -- Jung's feeling and thinking cognitive functions -- like a "little black box" that processes all the information coming in through the six sense gateways

It's the same in all of the five of the physical senses. Take for example the sense of smell, the sense objects are the odors that come in through the sense gateway, the organ of the nose, and then all this is interpreted by the smelling consciousness. It's the smelling consciousness which learns from experience, and starts discriminating the many smells and making sense out of them. The images come in through the eyes and the visual consciousness makes sense of them. It's not the eyes that make sense out of anything, they are just the gateway, it's the visual consciousness which makes sense out of images, colors and shapes. It's not the ears that hear or the skin that touches. They are just the sense organs.

In all Schools of Buddhism, there are six senses. When it comes to the sixth sense, the sense objects are feelings, beginning with pre-verbal grasping and pushing away, and post-verbal conceptual thoughts. The sixth sense organ is the gateway of the heart-mind, and the sixth sense consciousness makes sense of the feelings and thoughts that come into the sixth sense organ of the mind. The sixth sense consciousness is difficult for modern westerners to grasp in the way it is understood in Buddhism. In Eastern Buddhism it's not the heart-mind that feels and thinks the feelings and thoughts. The feelings and thoughts are sense objects that are arising in the sixth sense organ of the heart-mind. This information- the feelings and thoughts, are the sense objects coming in through the sense gateway of the mind and are interpreted by the sixth sense consciousness.

I am using *"interpreted"* here in a loose sense, because in a traditional Buddhist culture, the sense consciousness just senses and perceives "what is," it doesn't really interpret anything. It is very useful in a modern or postmodern western culture to think of the sixth sense consciousness as the processing, interpreting, discriminating mind. In traditional Buddhist teachings that are pre-modern and pre-science, this is not quite accurate. For the modern and postmodern stage of ego-development it is more accurate. There is some interpretation going on in the mind. In a flash of insight, Choan, one of the teachers in Integral Zen, labeled it as, *"the little black box"* that is capable of interpreting and processing all six sense objects, this is *Manovijnana* in Sanskrit, the sixth sense consciousness, the discriminating heart-mind consciousness. This sixth consciousness has evolved in the west as the ego has further developed. Today in the West, it's more equivalent to a combination of Jung's cognitive functions of feeling and thinking combined in a package of what we might call "the ego's self-processing." This little black box that processes all the information coming in through all six of the sixth sense gateways. First you know the sense object exists, information comes in through the sense gateway, and then there's a sense of self that receives it, and there's a relationship between the subject and the object. This relationship involves emotional reactivity. It is a primary *Oh, I like that, soft and warm. Oh, I don't like that, it's bitter. Oh, this tastes terrible.*

This relationship between the subject and the object is what creates the poisons, and the poisons become more poisonous as the emotional intensity is increased. Just like we showed in the three poisons: desire/greed, anger/hatred, ignorance/ delusion. The fourth of the five poisons is pride and the fifth of the five poisons is envy/jealousy. All five are poisonous. In traditional Buddhist teachings they are the five *kleshas*, also known as the five *negative emotions*, or more precisely I would say, the five *poisonous emotional reactivities*. It becomes so simple when it's placed in a living, realized, Integral Zen framework at a certain Kosmic Address.

Heart Exercise 4

heart exercise 4

Identify briefly

- can I zen out what my initial indoctrination was at the age of 5 or 6, who was my "us", what were the "rules", can I see the "them" that was created opposing my "us"?
- unusual events or "developmental trauma" in my life from 4-6

Answer scale 0-5, 0 least, 5 most

Presently in my life do I generally feel comfortable in groups?

Who is my tribe?

When am I most open hearted?

When am I most closed hearted?

How tolerant am I of people very different from me, especially those whose ideas I find unacceptable or triggering?

Where and of what, am I most critical?

Do I have any regular ritual or heart opening practices?

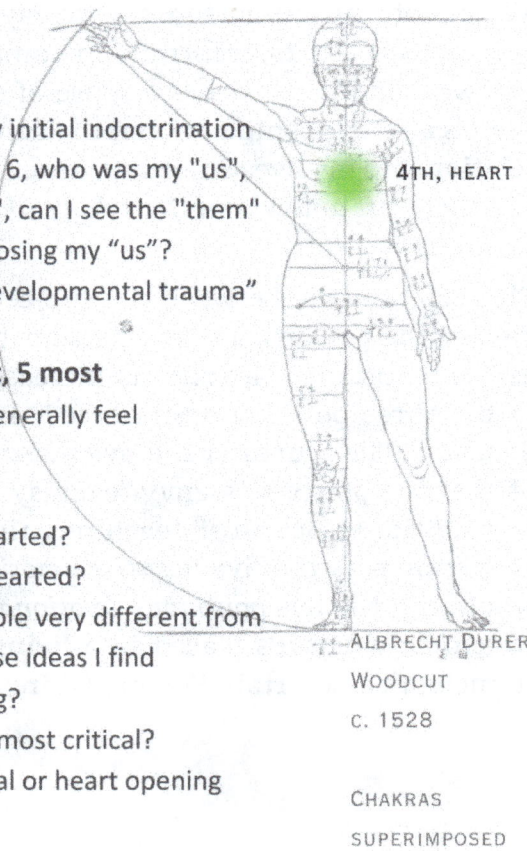

4TH, HEART

ALBRECHT DÜRER
WOODCUT
C. 1528

CHAKRAS
SUPERIMPOSED

Janel

Okay thank you so much for that Doshin. Next is a reflective exercise. So can you *Zen out*, (make it concise and simple) what your initial indoctrination was, at the age of five or six? Part of this is identifying who was in my "us" group (versus them).

What were the rules (*spoken and unspoken?*) Can I see the "them" group that was created opposing my "us" group, which might take a bit of reflection. Also consider unusual events or developmental trauma in your life from the ages of around four to six.

Then some questions for self reflection on a scale of 0 to 5. (*Zero is the lowest, five the highest*). Presently in my life do I feel comfortable in groups?

More questions for reflection: Who is my tribe? When am I most open hearted? When am I most closed hearted? How tolerant am I of people very different from me, especially those whose ideas I find unacceptable or triggering? Where and of what am I most critical? Do I have any regular ritual or heart opening practices?

heart

solo or group exercise

- *can you identify someone in your childhood or life who deeply touched you and helped you open your heart?*

- *have you done this for someone else?*

- *what stands out to you now about this?*

4TH, HEART

ALBRECHT DÜRER
WOODCUT
C. 1528

CHAKRAS
SUPERIMPOSED

We'll take a few minutes so people can take notes.

Next questions for group work, can you identify someone in your childhood or life who and this can be now, who deeply touched you and helped you open your heart? Or alternately, have you done this for someone else? What stands out to you now about this?

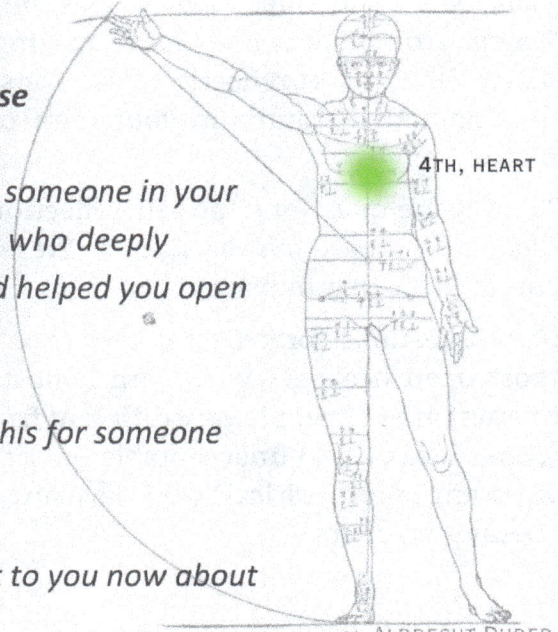

Now for the heart work on your own. We didn't talk that much about love yet. Part of opening your heart, really opening your heart, it seems to me, that this is actually a practice to really open your heart. You may need to do some heart muscle training, for generating selfless compassion.

Part of the practice for people to do at home and it does seem to me that if you don't exercise the muscle in this way, it actually may not develop much. Gratitude practice, which we talked about before, where you take time every day to take stock and appreciation for what you are grateful for. I think both in the morning and at night this is really beneficial.

We're going to review the four immeasurables. Then I'll talk about the sympathetic joy of practicing going out into the world and pausing to observe others and share, enjoying and appreciating others, with no expectation but to go within and practice genuine unreasonable joy, or rejoicing, in and for others. This is a very good practice to just go and do, you're not saying anything to anyone, but you are doing this internal practice simply appreciating and sharing in other people's happiness.

A Heart Opening Practice

The Four Immeasurables by Doshin Roshi

May all beings intend to attain liberation from the reactivity of self and abide in true equanimity and noble wisdom

May all beings heal and escape from the prison of their addictions to happiness

May all beings heal and escape from the prison of their allergies to suffering

May all beings awaken boundless joy that lies beyond all unconscious addictions and allergies

---

Another traditional practice is Tonglen, a practice of taking and giving, a meditation technique which people can research if they need instruction. Traditionally Doshin has updated an Integral Zen version of the four immeasurables. This is a quite fundamental practice for opening your heart, and his version, *May all beings intend to attain liberation from the reactivity of self and abide in true equanimity and noble wisdom.* The way you can do this practice is to

heart - on your own

- *gratitude practice - taking time every day to take stock and appreciation for what you are grateful for now*
- *4 immeasurables. Start with those you love, work towards specific others (one prayer for each) gradually work towards those you have difficult relationships or feelings for*
- *sympathetic joy - practicing going out into the world, and pausing to observe others and share internally in joy and appreciation, with no expectation but to go within and to practice genuine unreasonable joy in and for others*
- *tonglen practice - taking and giving meditation technique*

start to sincerely generate this heart wish for all beings, for all beings to be liberated, and to abide in true equanimity. First we start with *all beings*. Then, really feel it, wish it, put your heart into it. *May all beings heal and escape from the prison of their addictions to happiness. May all beings heal and escape from the prison of their allergies to suffering. May all beings awaken boundless joy that lies beyond all unconscious addictions and allergies.* So in doing this practice, after starting with *all beings*, then you can wish this for yourself, (may I..) and then, the advanced practice, is to start to work on genuinely wishing this for people that you may have problems with, or maybe are resentful towards, or have wronged. Then for the *really* advanced practice, would be for the people that you may even despise. If you keep doing this really from your heart, this is a genuinely heart opening practice. You can also use a traditional four immeasurables as well.

Doshin

The *Brahmavihara*, that's the first turning version of the four immeasurables. This advanced practice is not with your friends and even your enemies, it's with your family that is often the most difficult.

Heart Chakra Self-Care Practice #1

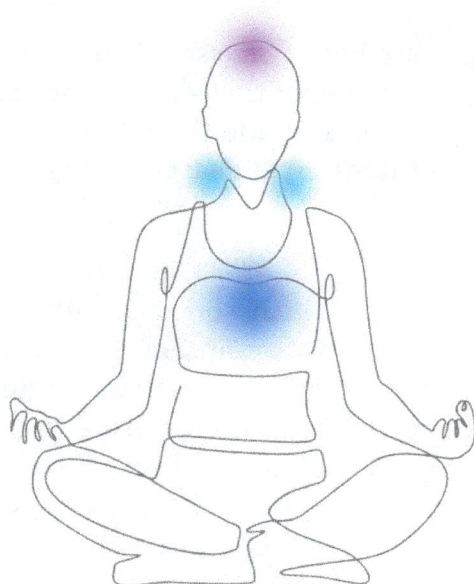

heart chakra self-care practice

- negative speech or hearing lies, can cause tightness and hardness in the ears, headaches and neck tension

- the heart protects itself as the energy tries to come downward - which leads to pain above

- release tension in neck by squeezing the sides, using one hand in the back of the neck

- fully massage ears, all parts, using opposite hands, simultaneously or one at a time

- massage crown rapidly using center of palm

Okay last for today, is self-care you can do on your own. As a reminder, in terms of looking at our sense consciousness, sense gates, senses, this is addressing the fact that when we hear negative speech or lies, this can create tension in our body. From our ears, our body doesn't want it to receive this down into the heart, so in protecting the heart, the body can experience tension and pain. There are ways to simply make the intention to release tension in your neck. First use one hand at the back of your neck, and consciously release tension. You can then massage your ears the way we do in Nejang Yoga, either you can do it cross-armed (opposite hands massage opposite ears) for balancing, but if that's too hard, you do the ears one at a time, and remember your ear, your whole ear, can be massaged with some strength, you don't have to be super delicate. The ear is a microcosm of all of the body, so this is very stress relieving.

For your body, your mind, your brain, massage the crown rapidly back and forth, using the center of the palm flat, so this is also a technique in Nejang. Doing this, and then doing your neck, and then just having this intention of heart opening.

Questioner

I was going to say it really hit me, with so many cultures crashing together like in the United States and globally, that when you're five or seven years old, it'd be very hard to figure out what group you're actually with. Then we have green and it's like it's rootless, and lacking a code to live by. Right? Like within your own families, ethnic groups that have come together and everything; very contradictory messaging to young people.

Doshin

The young people are growing up in culture wars and they are being indoctrinated into some system of values and beliefs. I hear some people say "I'm not religious" and I say, "my that is a very strange religion, an anti-religious religion, isn't it?" Then I hear other people tell me that they're spiritual but not religious, and I say, "my that is a strange religion." Isn't that interesting? Is it even possible to be Spiritual, without Religious devotion? We have just expanded the category of "religious dogma" to include: religion, anti-religion and spiritual but not religious. So, look closely at the religious dogma the children are being indoctrinated into. Is it the religious dogma of scientific materialism, scientism, or postmodern egalitarian pluralism? Is that what the children are being fed? What are the rules, the "shoulds" and "should nots" that the children are being taught at the amber structure of development? So, the children's amber values and beliefs are often either orange or green, and these are taking root in their hearts in an amber way. Or worse yet are they being taught that there are no rules, they are entitled to do whatever they want. This is moral anarchy and it is creating incredible confusion and giving rise to naive delusions and great suffering. It is also contributing to the increasing polarization and intensity of our current culture wars. It's very sad. It's tragic, actually. It's not likely to turn out well.

Question

Yes, I just want to say, I found it hard to find anybody in my childhood that opened my heart. Then someone in our group pointed out wisely, what about a dog, and I went boom, got me. There's something about a relationship with an animal. For you Janel, it was a bird. That this vulnerable being is dependent upon you, that is just rooted in your heart. It's just worth mentioning how we relate to animals as being our heart. Much like children, but I never had any children. Yes, that's fine.

Janel

Thank you, absolutely. These days, increasing numbers of people's closest relationship is with a pet. Naturally it can be devastating when we lose that pet, especially if we're not in close relationships with other people.

Question

Yes I'm just gonna sit with this connection between the root and the heart, and I really see how my lack of safety is keeping me from fully opening my heart in many situations in my life, and especially in my closest relationship, and so really doing whatever work I can with the root, will bolster the heart. Also you know it will bolster the 2nd and the 3rd chakras as well. I'm just really seeing that more clearly and I think I notice it in the heart, then I look back and I say oh, but it affects my ability to stand up for myself, to nurture, and you know, to be nurtured. Even those things. So that's what I have, thank you. Appreciate this so much.

Janel

Thank you. It's a good reminder this is again where the second chakra magic comes in, as well as at Amber at the heart. Religious and devotional practice is very important for healing the heart.

Doshin

It's foundational for the heart. We are religious, we have been for about 100,000 years. That brings up what Wilber calls the level line fallacy, which I'll save for another time. Anybody else?

Janel

Well, thank you all for hanging in there and we'll be back next week with the throat, which is really interesting. Thank you so much.

CHAPTER FIVE, THE THROAT CHAKRA

Doshin

Janel sent me a wonderful quote from one of our favorite Zen masters,

Dogen: He who can keep sane while the world is insane, is the Zen master.

So here's a troubling Koan for you; the world seems quite insane. Are you sane or have you joined the world's insanity? That can be a very disturbing question. Have fun with it. Well, let's jump right in, shall we?

So we are at Session five. So again, let me say it again in a slightly different way, Please remember. This is an experiential course. It is not an intellectual class, it's not food for your intellect. We're using the chakras in an Integral Framework, while also presenting a broad overview of healing lineage teachings that have been around for thousands of years and

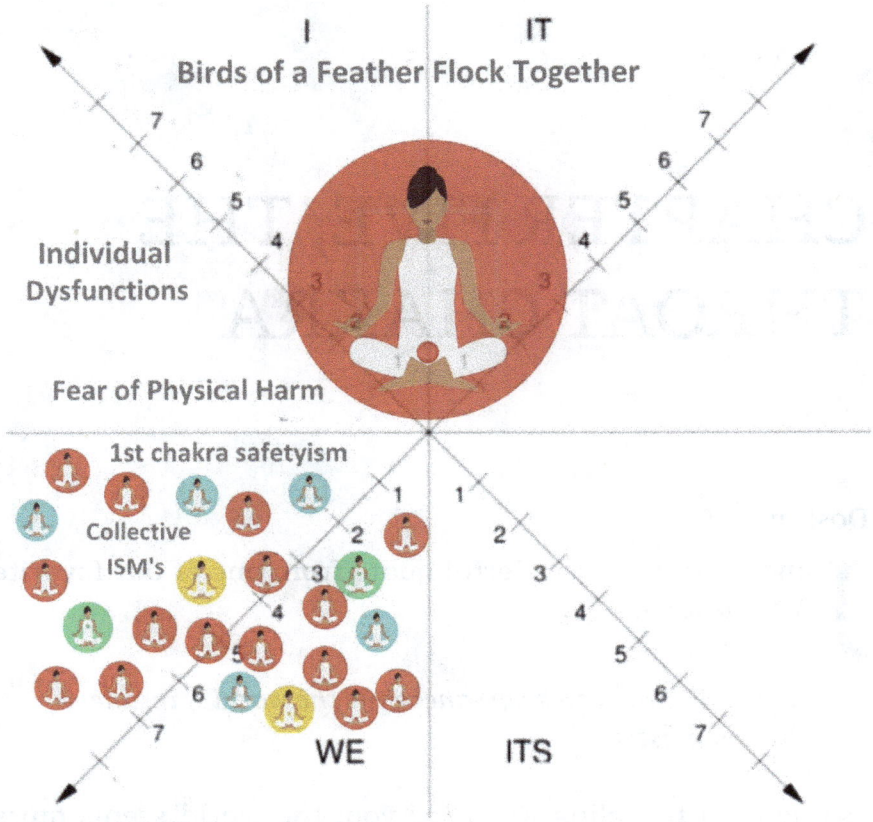

I   IT

Birds of a Feather Flock Together

Individual
Dysfunctions

Fear of Physical Harm

1st chakra safetyism

Collective
ISM's

WE   ITS

include both healing and awakening. Trust; just trust that you will take in what you're ready to receive. Stop trying to understand everything. Just receive what you can. When nothing can be lost, there is room to actually *receive*. Just empty your cup so we can pour you some tea.

The fifth chakra, the throat chakra is the voiced belief system. In Integral colors, the stages of ego development, it is both orange and green structural stages. Here, an integral understanding of *holons* is most helpful, perhaps even essential. Nothing else will substitute for this. Here's a brief presentation of an integral understanding of holons. Individual holons have a *dominant monad*. This is what we commonly call the ego. Don't get fooled by Whitehead's big phrase *dominant monad;* it's just a more technical term, describing what we commonly call the ego. The illusion of a permanent self. If there is no permanent self, then the ego is actually a perceptual illusion. There is something that relentlessly tries to process all the information it receives. Something that interprets all the information and fits it into a personal and collective view, a cosmology of what it believes to be real and important. It relentlessly attempts to control everything. It is what seems to make all the decisions in the territory of *me.*

Social holons, on the other hand, don't have a dominant monad, an ego or CEO of the corporation of me. Instead, they have a common *nexus*, a nexus of resonance. This holonic resonance often has an emotional charge and moral quality. It is the glue that bonds all the individual holons together into a social holon. It is the resonance of a shared collective "moral dogma" composed of emotional biases, moral values and beliefs that resonate with each other. This collective resonance can be positive or negative and lies at the heart of all culture wars and what I am calling *interholonic interdynamics.* Each social holon has this type of common resonance, but what it doesn't have is a heart, a body, a mind, a soul, a spirit, and most importantly, it doesn't have *a conscience.* The *we,* the miracle some call *we,* is a resonance of beliefs and delusions that *cannot directly evolve, heal or awaken.* This view of holons is a radical idea, a brand new way of looking at the world that begins to emerge with an Integral Framework. This is indeed, something to sit with.

For example, let's take the old saying, *"Birds of a feather flock together."* If we have an individual holon that has a dysfunction, say what we are calling a first chakra dysfunction, such as a pervasive unbearable fear that *I'm not safe.* Such a feeling can be an immobilizing, almost paranoid fear of being physically harmed. This is one of the first chakra dysfunctions. It lies in the same territory as the first milestone of attachment theory–Safety. Do you feel safe or do you not feel safe? If you never feel safe, then your heart is closed, unable to open. If many individual holons who share the same primal fear gather together, then this becomes a common nexus that connects them all together into a social holon. In a human social holon or "flock" the "feathers" are the emotional feelings, moral values and political ideas, the "feathers" of a group of birds that flock together.

When many people, many *individual holons* that have this first chakra dysfunction of "I'm not safe," then they gather together, *flock together like birds of a feather.* The common nexus is the emotional state and the emotional reactivity, the fear of not being safe, and a social holon of safetyism forms around this common nexus. Jonathan Haidt's descriptions of *Safetyism,* are excellent descriptions of this even though he doesn't seem to have the advantage of an Integral Framework, and isn't using Integral Language. This adds such incredible value and enhances our ability to see, understand and predict the insane interactions of individual and social holons in what we call *culture wars.* Remember that all this is tetra-arising in all four quadrants, and this is where we'll stop today. In the following more advanced courses, we'll go a bit further and really dig into this radically important material.

Janel

Yes thank you Doshin, one of the things in the next class we'll explore much more in depth with the chakras, in looking at individual and collective perspectives. Doshin is really excited about the collective. You know, safety so greatly impacts both individuals and their relationship with collectives for all further development. Safety actually is a critical requirement for not just the first chakra, but for children in order for them to develop healthily. They need to feel safe enough so that they can explore and make mistakes, fail and be creative. When there isn't a threshold of safety, it will impact all of their development through the chakras. A kind of stunting, or imbalance, developmental delay, will play out differently for each individual.

Doshin

I'd like to point again to the connection between the first chakra and the fourth chakra. If the individual never repairs or heals the first chakra disturbances, if they never feel safe, the heart remains closed, it cannot open and blossom, and further, healthy development in the other chakras is impeded, stunted and can become quite dysfunctional. This deeply impacts the ego's continuing development into more complex subpersonalities, which cannot happen in a healthy way. This is where we start lying to others in the orange stage and to ourselves in the green stage. This is also where problematic shadows or subpersonalities are split off and seem to develop a life of their own. Once the individual holon (person) feels safe, then the heart can begin to open. And if the heart opens completely, as open as the empty sky, then liberation becomes possible. The whole channel must be clear for the Crown Chakra to open.

Janel

It's also worth saying, however, if you did not have healthy circumstances as a child, you can still experience secure attachment at any time in life from any individual. So it's not if you don't get it in the early development it's game over, not like that. We'll talk about that more next week.

I'm going to shift direction and talk a little bit about the origins of not just Zen and Chan traditions of healing, but we're going to go back and just talk a little bit about China and then Zen Master Hakuin Eikaku, the figure considered responsible for revitalizing Rinzai Zen in eighteenth century Japan.

Hakuin is a really important figure for obviously Rinzai Zen and also for healing, which I talked about a little bit in one of the prior Sunday Dharma talks which you can go back and listen to on our website, and I think in the future at some point we will explore more. However in order to look at this in general, first we need to go back to China and Chinese healing.

Chinese Healing

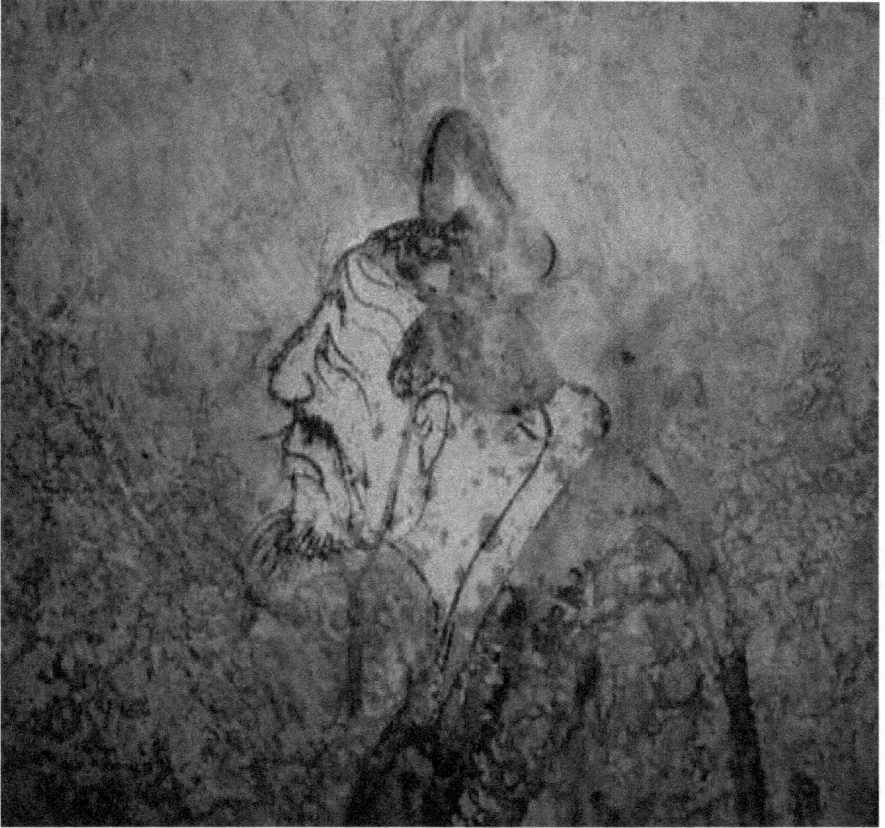

Photo of a fresco depicting ancient Chinese philosopher and educator Confucius (551 B.C.- 479 B.C.), found in a tomb in an old residential yard in Dongping County, east China's Shandong Province. Public domain US

Chinese healing originates during the prehistory of northern China. Generally if you know anything about Chinese healing, the history goes back to a text called the *Neijing*, the *Huangdi Neijing*, literally the *Inner Canon of the Yellow Emperor* or *Esoteric Scripture of the Yellow Emperor.* Like the name indicates, this was established at the time of the Yellow Emperor, C

2697-2596 BC, with the earliest written record from around 200 BC. The oldest copy of the complete work comes from the Tang dynasty, allegedly compiled by Wang Ping in 762 AD. Most Far Eastern modalities for healing originate from the *Neijing*. To start looking at China we would be remiss not to mention the early figures of whom established the roots of Chinese heritage and philosophy.

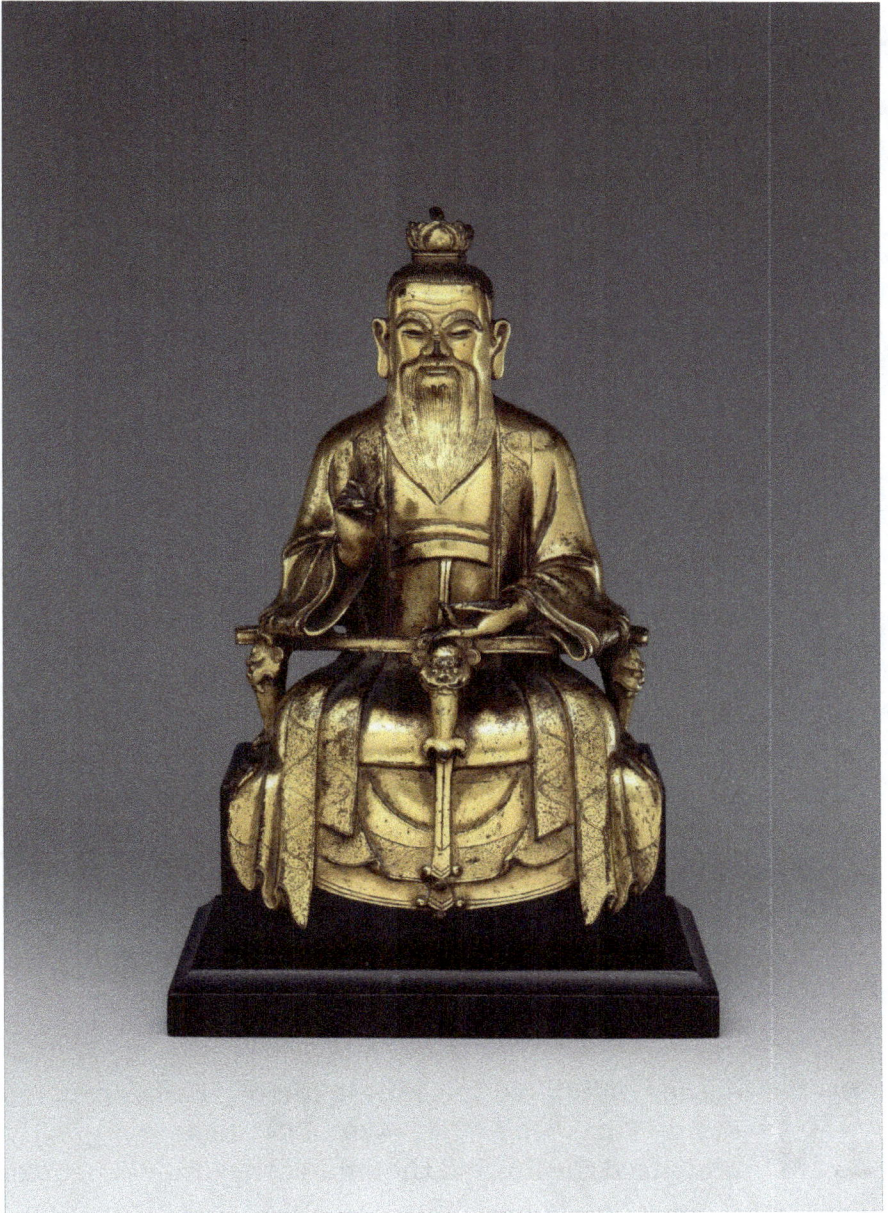

Daoist immortal Laozi, Chen Yanqing (active 15th century), 1438, Purchase, Friends of Asian Art Gifts, 1997, Metropolitan Museum of Art, New York, Public Domain Open Access

The first figure is Confucius, and there are a series of texts generally considered the pre-Confucian classics,[60] the most important body of literature traditionally accepted by Chinese as forming this basis of heritage from ancient times. These books are generally not believed to have been written by Confucius himself; like the Bible, scholars surmise that while Confucius might have worked on some of this, most of it likely predates him, and the *I Ching*.

Divination practice is mentioned in records from thousands of years back, archaeological evidence and descriptions give us a picture of what was used and practiced.Looking back at these books, forms a picture of what ancient Chinese culture was like, for one thing there was a lot of ritual, especially described in *The Book of Rites*.

Looking at the basic early beliefs of Chinese people, to summarize a few, was a belief in a supreme deity or moral force which ruled the world, which took a strong interest in humankind. There was belief in the existence and power of numerous nature spirits and ancestral spirits, who needed to be served and placated by sacrifices; belief in divine sanction of the political order and the heavy responsibility of rulers to fulfill moral duties to heaven and its subjects. These early beliefs are still very powerfully active today.[61]

No other individual in Chinese history like Confucius (Kong Fuzi, 孔子 551-479 BC) has so greatly influenced the life and thought of the Chinese people. It's interesting, when you go back and study this history, you can read in texts, the calls for a *return* to virtue of the past. It's kind of amusing to see how far human civilization has *not* changed in this expression. Looking at the *Analects*, or sayings of Confucius,

"There were four things that Confucius was determined to eradicate: a biased mind, arbitrary judgements, obstinacy, and egoism." (IX:4)

Sound familiar? Has much changed?

After Confucianism, Taoism (Lao Tzu/Laozi) 老子/Tao-te-ching 6-5c BC, is the most important, influential native philosophy of China. While Confucianism emphasizes a *grave solemnity* of social responsibility, Taoism is more unconventional, with a vision of transcendental worlds of the spirit, mysticism and poetry. The Daoist school, often referred to as *The teachings of the Yellow Emperor* or Lao Tzu, and Chuang Tzu. Taoism and Confucianism, even though they could be at odds with each other, did integrate, along with Chinese Buddhism, forming an early base that influenced, and continues to influence, so much of life throughout Asia, and now throughout the world.

Tao Te Ching:

"You look at it, but it is not to be seen;

Its name is Formless

You listen to it, but it is not to be heard;

It's name is Soundless.

You grasp it, but it is not to be held;

Its name is Bodiless

These three elude all scrutiny,

And hence they blend and become one."[62]

Yin And Yang

Yin and Yang are fundamental to Chinese philosophy and medicine

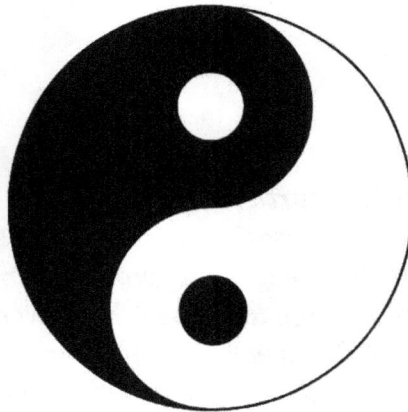

Yin	Yang
night	day
dark	light
cold	warm
negative	positive
passive	active
female	male
solid	hollow
liver	gallbladder
heart	small
spleen	intestine
lungs	stomach
kidney	large
	intestine
	urinary
	bladder

Good health can result from a balance of Yin (negative, dark, and feminine) and Yang (positive, bright, and masculine)

Taoism includes working with the balance of Yin and Yang. These are fundamental ideas, concepts, ways of being, for Chinese philosophy and medicine. Throughout time the characteristics of Yin and Yang have not changed. While gender perspectives have shifted through time due to cultural, political and relative historical change, the basic characteristics of Yin and Yang remain entirely relevant for every individual's health, which when combined reflect a balance of the whole. I do say in working with people, the legacy within one's family relationships, with masculine and feminine ancestry, relative histories appear to significantly impact people's health in their body, heart and mind. We will explore this more in further seminars.

Continuing to look at the context of China, it is widely believed that Buddhism arrived in China during the Han period (206 BC-220 AD). As time passed, the early healing arts and other arts became integrated with traditional Taoist cosmology.

Qi 氣

> "Before heaven and earth had taken form all was vague and amorphous. Therefore it was called the Great Beginning. The Great Beginning produced emptiness and emptiness produced the universe. The universe produced material-force (Qi) which had limits. That which was clear and light drifted up to become heaven, while that which was heavy and turbid solidified to become earth … .When heaven and earth were joined in emptiness and all was unwrought simplicity, then without having been created, things came into being. This was called the Great Oneness (Tao)…he who can return to that from which he was born and become as though formless is called a "true man." The true man is he who has never become separated from the Great Oneness."[63]

Huai Nan Zi (c. 122BC)

T he body traditionally in China is both part of and considered a replica of the Dao, which is the base of all creation, *the essential productive power of all the universe* causing everything to come into being; nothing is actually *separate* from the Dao. *Qi* is the human's vitally individual yet cosmically connected energy. *Daoyin* are healing movement sequences documented in Chinese antiquity that have come down through the ages as various techniques, as the origin of and closely related to, contemporary *Qigong*.

Some of the different modalities derived from the Neijing, include Tui Na, acupuncture, Gua Sha, Tai Chi, herbal medicine, acupressure, acupuncture, and moxibustion among others. Cupping is a modality also used in Tibetan medicine.

One of the things that I think becomes increasingly important for health as we age are embodiment practices which return our energies into balance; these are done in *internal* (eastern) martial arts. In contrast to what are known as the *external* martial arts, for many as we are aging physically it is a natural shift, to go from the external to the internal. So these practices offer a focus on spiritual, mental or Qi related aspects versus an external approach focused on physiological aspects. *Nei jing* is developed by using *nei gong* or "internal changes", contrasted with *wài gōng* 外功 or "external exercises." *Wu Dang Guan* reflects a specific grouping of internal martial arts associated with the Taoist monasteries of the Wu Tang Mountains, connected to *Hubei* and Chinese popular legend.

Naturally there are many different traditions and schools. Criteria characterizing the internal martial arts as we know them today, developed in the 20th century, after Mao Zedong stripped what is now called *Classical Chinese Medicine* and other traditions to create a *martial* themed system congruent with Communism, generally referred to as *TCM, Traditional Chinese Medicine*, removing the sacred and spiritual. Especially since the late 19th century in China (but true throughout history), so many profound Chinese teachings went underground because they threatened political power. Therefore, getting information has been, and remains relatively difficult, and just not that accessible. This is connected to the need for systems of *secret teachings*, where a student/disciple has to demonstrate long-term commitment, loyalty, and fealty to a teacher, lineage and tradition, in order to even be considered to receive higher, protected teachings, which one is *never* simply entitled to.

Internal practices versus the external, martial, generally have an emphasis on training the mind to coordinate and use the support of the relaxed and energetic body, versus coming from exclusively physical strength. Generally speaking the aim of practice focuses on the internal development, and circulation of Qi, the vital energy.

Doshin

My experience as a humble student of Tai Chi, is observing the master's confidence, humility and extreme skill all at the same time. The same energy to heal can be used to destroy an opponent. I have heard it said that in America yoga is too yin, and that external martial arts are too yang. A Tai Chi Master models a living balance of yin and yang that is dynamic and adapts immediately in the moment to changing conditions. I can testify to many of the health benefits I am experiencing, and I am amazed by the whole experience.

Janel

Yes, so as we get older, I mean just for self-care these practices become more important. Doing healing and energy work with people, I know that understanding internally what is happening can be difficult to determine at times, since people can many factors that impact energy balance. Part of coming back into balance which we can do for ourselves–which is very important, that fact that we can do it ourselves–are practices like this. For your own self-healing, having a reliable regular practice is incredibly beneficial. It can bring one back into balance quite quickly, and actually there are a lot of relatively younger people that are training now with more lineage traditions, as the world is more interconnected, and there's actually more potential in recent years to be able to study with lineage teachers. It had been much harder in the past to have such opportunities.

Doshin just mentioned Tui na. It's not only massage, but it's focused on energy and health balance using different techniques from Chinese classical medicine origins. It was first mentioned in the Nei Ching, but archaeological evidence dates it back to about 2700 BC. I have a body worker who many years ago just ran into a Chinese master in Tui na who he studied with, that had just come from China, and in the past they called them *bone setters*, since they could just set a bone relatively painlessly. I believe you need to study under a master for at least seven years to do this.

Tai Chi Ch'uan includes the interplay of yin and yang, it is an internal martial art for health balance and self-defense, where awareness is a practice through movement versus stillness. *Qi gong* as it is known contemporarily (again the categorization is modern) was derived from Daoyin practices going far back in history. There are variations to help regulate body, breath and heart, mind. As Doshin was mentioning about his teacher who could use the energy to harm, there's different ways of working with the Qi. For longevity you can learn ways to circulate it through the body. And for medical approaches people do this specifically for healing. As a practitioner, you actually learn to store up Qi, and then you use it to work with patients, which I'm doing some kind of equivalent, although the lineage I'm connected with is a Tibetan lineage, so my daily practice is doing practices that help so that when I work with people I have the energy to work with them.

Hakuin and Japanese Healing

Getting back to Hakuin. Those of you who know me may know I lived in Japan for ten years, so I know a lot more about Japan than other East Asian countries, even though now I'm teaching mostly about Tibetan health methods. In Japan, the connection between the Nei Jing derived arts with Zen healing is generally described as dating relatively late, and whenever I see this, I always think no, that's not right. This seems to me something one sees a lot which is a gulf between popular knowledge and practitioners. I actually know that for a lot of the teachings in Zen in Zen healing, the transmission has been primarily passed down orally in Japan, my sense is written sources may have had less exposure outside of Japan.[64] I also suspect from people I've talked to, some of the things I've read that much has never been translated from Japanese to English, in terms of documented, solid connections.

You know, they say in the time of Hakuin, but if you live in Japan, the 17th century is actually considered not far from contemporary culture. I worked for ten years as an antique dealer in Japan, so I would always talk about antiques, I would be buying and selling with Japanese dealers, and if you talk to a Japanese antique dealer, they would preface about objects, *oh, that's not old.* (Unless they thought you knew nothing, in which case people would try to con you, something that happened less frequently but did certainly happen, and say *oh yes this is old!*) The Japanese antique dealers start considering things of value, authentic, *old,* from the 15th century and before. So old and new are relative within the culture.

So back to Hakuin, he was called Chuko no So (father of restoration) of the Rinzai Shu sect, and he's credited with revitalizing Rinzai Zen in 1710. He learned a healing method from a hermit, a Taoist sage called *Hakuyu,*[65] in north Kyoto. Hakuin had been suffering from Zen disease, called *Zenbyo (byo* means illness) attributed as a result of too much asceticism and too many koans.

So in the Chinese view Zen disease, or meditation sickness, can develop for different reasons, often called *Qi stagnation* or *deviation*. This is again why the way you meditate is so important and having a straight spine (not overly straight but with natural curves) because over time, as you practice, if you progress in a positive way, your Qi moves more upward. If you are sitting and your spine is crooked, it can lead to all kinds of dysfunction and health problems. So Hakuin's teachings of what was called the Naikan-ho method is presented in the account *Yassenkana* which you can read translated into English (There are a few translations).

The Japanese approach using these ancient methods, and specifically acupuncture, was based on a master interpretation of Chinese Han dynasty texts. So if you really know Asia at all, you know there were millenia of trade, contact and wars between different countries. Naturally over time, each country would assimilate what was introduced from other countries, in their own style (ironically what is now referred to as *appropriation,* but if you study history you know cultures have an endless history of doing this). For example, Japanese often took ideas, objects, food (*tempura* was adapted from the food of Portuguese missionaries), from China and Korea especially, and then made their own versions. So one way that Chinese methods changed, is that traditional Chinese medicine relies more on indirect diagnostic methods than the Japanese traditional approach.

Some of the ancient point methods that derive way back from the *Neijing,* using acupoints and acupressure, variations of these methods were used in Zen temples around the world for the monks' own self-care and healing. Japanese tend to use *shiatsu* and the simple method of holding of points, and I use a method like this that has been powerful in working with people, in addition to several Buddhist healing methods I use, mostly from the Sowa Rigpa Medicine Buddha tradition.

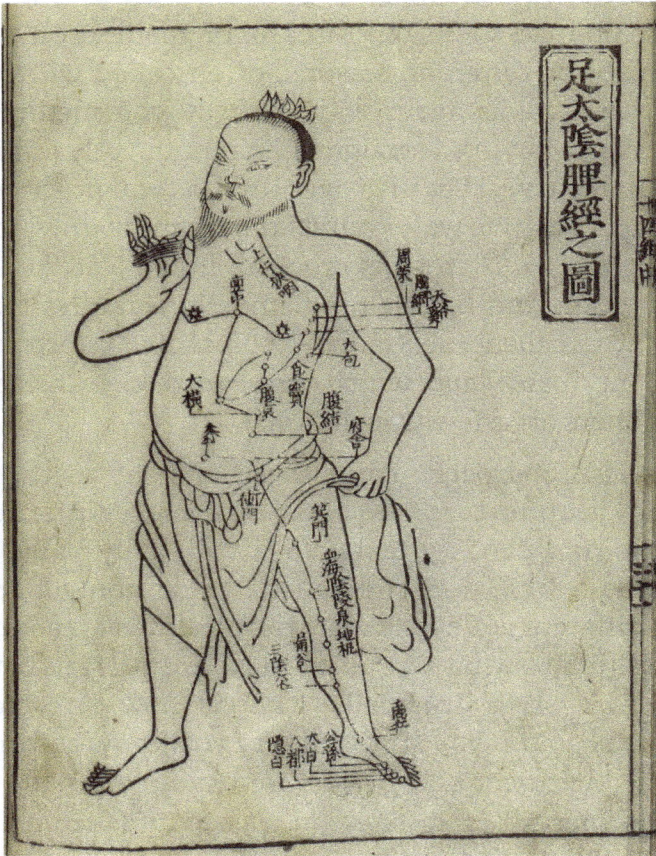

Hua, Shou, active 1360-1370, Jūshikei hakki, Expression of the fourteen meridians, Inoue Shoten Bunkyō-ku, Tokyo, Japan, Isseidō, Suharaya Heisuke kankō, Kyōhō gan, 1716, Public Domain

As I have said, in Japan, the methods were and still are passed down orally. Japan has a rich history of samurai arts, and in Japan they use the word *Ki* instead of *Qi*, so there's *Ki* focused internal and external martial arts, which we may explore more later. Old handbooks for practitioners illustrate acupuncture points and channels.

Also *Anma* 按摩 is a Japanese therapeutic massage treatment that still exists today.

Visually impaired people were the ones who often did these massage techniques in Japan (I believe this was true in Korea too) until other educational options became available. Before this, the profession was limited to those with visual impairment.

The Fifth, Throat Chakra

throat, Sanskrit Visuddha

early adolescence early adulthood, Integral Orange-Green

third and fourth person perspective

- Location: Front, center front of throat, back, center back of neck
- Essential Functions: Truth, clear and truthful communication, the ability to communicate personal truth and true beliefs, emotions, feelings and needs through use of speech, writing or artistic creativity. Ideology and affiliations with us and them groups.
- Meridians: No meridians associated with fifth chakra
- Areas of body: Throat, mandible and jaw muscles
- Development: The problem of what is "truth". Experiential versus conceptual truth. Needing to grow beyond our family and community's ideological indoctrination

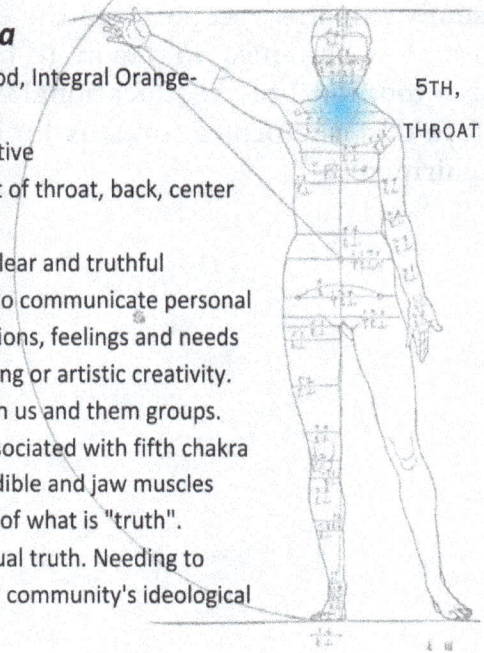

5TH, THROAT

Throat themes

Voice – Differentiating Relative and Absolute Truth – Creativity – Communication – Ideology – Speaking with Integrity and Authenticity – Listening – Self Expression – Silence

ALBRECHT DURER
WOODCUT
C. 1528

CHAKRAS
SUPERIMPOSED

Let's return to the throat chakra. This may not make much sense to you, but the throat represents the end of the first-tier of three developmental tiers of the Integral Framework. The age range for this can range from late childhood, adolescence and early adulthood.

Doshin

It of course varies greatly in different systems, but I place it at the beginning of puberty. In our modern/postmodern culture, this is where the third person perspective starts showing up and we start beginning to differentiate our own beliefs from the beliefs we were indoctrinated into, which is a long process.

Janel

In terms of location in the body, this includes the throat area and can include the jaw. Incidentally I want to remind people the way we are presenting this again; we are presenting a similar framework to what Ken Wilber presented in *The Religion of Tomorrow,* but there are differences, and we are expanding in some areas he doesn't cover.

I also want to say that different energetic systems can work independently, and *that doesn't make other systems wrong.* This is very much critical to the Integral Second Tier view, where there is a capacity to hold multiple perspectives, and to find there is usually always some truth in different perspectives. A characteristic of the structures of the first tier is "I'm right and you're wrong", and an inability to see this. I see teachers sometimes, for example I heard a teacher recently (Western) coming from a Chinese tradition saying things like "there are no such thing as chakras!"...which one might argue reflects the traditional presentation in a relatively rigid ancient framework, where the Chinese systems doesn't account for chakras (but there is still is an energetic system). A reminder, when we get into esoteric teachings, subtle and causal realms, archetypal forces, these do not follow the rules of gross, form and matter appearance. So maybe this is more a word to teachers, we can know what we know, but we cannot know all that is unknown. Humans, limited by life span and relative time, also have a limit to how many topics they can study in depth. I encourage humility, and flags go up for me when I don't hear a teacher acknowledge that they don't know everything. Red flag!!

I just wanted to remind people of this. Another thing, so the chakras, the developmental structures, as they're going up from the bottom, are becoming more complicated. The second chakra is connected to the throat, and we're going to talk more about that. It seems that for example if in the gross physical area of the throat, one might experience all kinds of physical throat problems, and a vulnerability or proclivity to sickness, injury, in that area will often have connections and origins with something going wrong developmentally or something not being given enough space developmentally in your history. This can show up as gross problems here.

The throat is obviously connected to the voice. The ultimate, higher expression is silence. The throat is connected to truth, to clear and truthful communication, and an individual's ability to communicate personal truth. Also in differentiating relative and absolute truth. The ability to communicate emotions, feelings and needs for the use of speech, writing, creative expression. Like with the second chakra, creativity is a big theme in the throat. But then, really, so is ideology and affiliations with *us and them* groups. So at the heart, you have your first, initial indoctrination. The age of five and six. From there, you start (generally) becoming more exposed to the outside world, developing as a child. Then, as an adolescent, you start exploring different groups, different identities. It is a normal natural stage of life where you're exploring different ideas and learning about the world.

A big question for me when I'm working with people in the throat is I ask them what kind of teenager they were, because it's normal for kids to start to individuate from their family of origin at this age, it's part of healthy development. Were you really obedient and just trying to be a great student, and perhaps, didn't challenge your parents, or any type of authority like at school, just accepting everything? Were you a little rascally, testing the waters and experimenting? Or extremely rebellious? Were you experimenting with drugs, were you getting arrested, running away from home? This is important information and what is actually healthy, some version or expression of finding your own way reflects healthy development at the throat. If it isn't done in the appropriate developmental period of your life, it is likely to have some consequences for you as an adult. For an individual to develop, they will need to go through that development at some point, if not at that time, or parts of them can remain immature, stuck, delayed.

Back to the throat themes. The question of *what is truth: experiential versus conceptual truth.* Needing to grow beyond our family and community's ideological indoctrination (remember, much of the world never moves beyond amber, so not everyone evolves here). Differentiating between relative and absolute truth, creativity, communication, ideology, speaking with integrity and authenticity is a huge theme for people, so your early environment at home is really significant to this. Listening, your ability to listen; self-expression. Again I'm going to say if there's some disruptive thing that happens during this developmental period for you, which could be anything, this is likely to impact your development in this period. That's the first thing to keep in mind. Second is the communication style in your family. How did your family communicate? How did they allow you to be, as a teenager? Could you challenge them? Was there open communication at home or, or not at all? Then you go out in school and here in late adolescence, many begin to move from orange to green, if you went on to further higher education. Then as an adult, you start connecting with other groups, then your relationship to groups evolves and changes. Sometimes we have to leave groups, sometimes groups regress. There's so many themes going on here, relationships with systems, the ability to see systems, so I'll stop. Doshin you can jump in for now.

Doshin

This is what makes this so complicated. As the *Weirdest people in the world*[66] began to emerge in the scientific age, the traditional religions are rejected as irrational. Then more recently, a new secular anti-religious form of spirituality emerged. The one that is now "spiritual," but still "not religious," in the form of postmodern egalitarian pluralism. In order to make sense of these new complexities, an Integral Framework is extremely helpful, even perhaps essential. If we look at the chakras and individual ego development after the emergence of the modern social holons of rationalism, industrialism, and scientism, we can divide these new meta-social holons into traditional religious, modern scientific, and postmodern egalitarian categories of distinct social holons each with its own moral dogma. This more advanced and complete Integral Framework, begins to enable us to see the specific changes and differences in these complex systems of collective values and beliefs. Each individual is indoctrinated into one of these meta-social holons with its differing world view and different moral values and ideological beliefs. We remain part of the culture we are indoctrinated into until we outgrow and transcend it. That's all I want to say now. Just pointing to the powerful tools that an Integral Framework can bring is a beginning, which will help make all of this more understandable and accessible. But this is only true if you've attained a certain Kosmic Address. Exploring this would require much more than a course in itself. So I think that's where I'll stop. With this framework, it is confusing at first, and then becomes exponentially more understandable and useful once you are able to place all this complexity into a simple Integral Framework. With that, we move on.

Janel

Okay getting back to the second chakra relationship with the throat. So in observing people, unmet needs of the second chakra developmental period, can greatly impact the fifth chakra and manifest as unhealthy, imbalanced drives, addictions, allergies, in structures and states from gross to subtle. So in your second chakra, where we first needed to be nurtured and our emotions and senses come alive, if we did not get our needs met to a certain degree, the effects will vary. If we're not conscious of this in the lower second chakra, we might for example, develop a *hungry ghost,* where we're seeking out gross desires of the senses. That might manifest into insatiable seeking and desire. You know, it could be sensuality, sexuality, it could be addictions to drugs or alcohol. But then just note, so that's an example of a relatively lower level sense drive. It can also go instead of the gross, towards subtle seeking. Then we might have a hunger for meaning (up in the throat). What type of meaning? Well, it's going to be different for different people. If the person has an integral orange center of gravity, they might be obsessed with status or status objects (on their "altar", as a replacement of god). If someone's center of gravity is green, one could be addicted to seeking different kinds of meaning. There are other versions as well. This can play out with all different kinds of ideologies in the throat chakra, not just green, it could be someone fixated on a conservative ideology. It could be any kind of extreme view, a fixation where the need to really communicate, as the expression says, you know, results in one *shoving* one's ideology down people's throats. (This can be amber orange, which is common, the mythology of the individualist, libertarian ideology, for example). These unhealthy drives for each individual will play out differently, *unless it becomes conscious,* and we are able to slowly change. Unless you see the origin of this, developmental disruptions, unmet needs, neglect, unhealthy attachment, etc, unless you have a way to deal with it, a way to work on healing or just getting help, these drives and energetic patterns cycle and spiral and it's not just these two, the energies disrupt all the chakras, and all of your energies will be out of balance. We're not trying to pathologize this, but it's more just describing what is. Karma, cause and effect. I want to emphasize, if you don't see this, don't have the perspective at the least, then really the way we can describe it is: *one is driven, one is not the driver; one is driven.*

It is useful therefore to know and inquire, as to what one might be driven by? Wounds, dysfunctions, confusion, greed, desire, etc... When ruled by these drives - there is also an increased vulnerability of the potential for *archetypal possession* in the upper chakras, which one becomes more vulnerable to. This will be explained more in further courses.

Throat Exercise 5

throat exercise 5

Identify briefly

- from late childhood into adolescence, was I supported in finding my own way to express myself, and communicate, or was the home environment not supportive?
- unusual events or trauma in my life late childhood to adolecense

Answer scale 0-5, 0 least, 5 most

- In my life have I explored and questioned my beliefs?
- Where and how do I lie to myself?
- Are there issues I feel very passionate and driven about? Have I explored the opposite view?
- Which groups (us-es) do I belong to? Which thems are opposing them, can I see them?

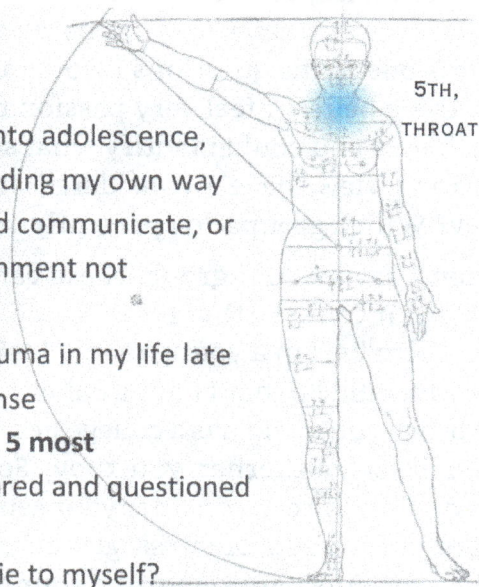

5TH, THROAT

ALBRECHT DURER

WOODCUT

C. 1528

CHAKRAS

SUPERIMPOSED

We're going to do our first exercise. Take several minutes and look, identify briefly. From late childhood into adolescence, was I supported in finding my own way to express myself and communicate, or was the home environment not supportive to this? Were there any significant, unusual events or trauma in my life or in my family environment, late childhood to adolescence. And then from a scale of 0 to 5. In my life have I explored and questioned my beliefs? Now a lot of us think we may, but when we start going through these exercises, one can be surprised how much of it is just unconscious (meaning just beliefs of the groups you were indoctrinated in and affiliated with, versus beliefs you have wrestled with through experience and reflection). Where and how do I lie to myself? This is one of the questions I work on one-on-one with people. Are there beliefs I feel very passionate and driven about? And you know, you could identify what some of those are. If I have a strong view, have I considered and explored the opposite view? Which groups do I presently belong to? Us versus them.

When I say an "us" group, these can be, well, they're kind of endless. It could be that I feel I'm affiliated with Integral Zen. It could also be, I'm a young man, I feel an affiliation with young men. It could be that I have a college degree, I feel an affiliation with everyone who has a college degree. I grew up in the South, I feel like a Southerner, you know. So many different ways you can do this. We can consider your sense of identity. I'm a parent of young children, or I'm single or I'm divorced, so many. Then, which "thems" are opposing your "us" groups? Can I see? I realize you can't do this in a short time.

So did anything come up with this, anything you want to talk about, you observed? We're asking if you've ever examined your belief system. Just looking back at your time during this developmental period, did this bring anything into awareness such as no, my parents did not encourage my communication. Or did someone come from a family where it was really supported, exploring and finding your own way?

Questioner

OK, I can say something. In my generation, when I was young, there was no talking in the family. Of course, practical things were shared, but only practical things, so I never talked about myself. I had two older brothers, but they left home when I was two and four years old, so I was only with my father and mother. They were rather old, I think, I thought. And well, I never thought about myself. Never shared something. Only the practical. Or maybe say, okay I did this in school, this exam or something? But other things, what was happening in myself I never shared. So it was not very supportive of my communication.

Janel

So when do you feel like you started to learn? Or it started to feel you were in an environment where you could develop that and share.

Questioner

When I started my studies, so from 17 on, but most when I got closer to 22, 23.

Janel

Yes, I know in many places there's such a high respect for the instructors that the students not speaking is encouraged. What was the culture like? Did it vary from instructor to instructor?

Questioner

It was 1986, so the authoritarian system was cracking so we could say a lot, but OK, but then, it was not about my inner self. We talked in class and we talked about the subjects and issues, and so on, that was okay. We tried to influence the whole university system, these kinds of things. That was the time for student protests so a lot was happening, but it was not about my inner life, you know.

Janel

So I'm curious, with your own children. Were you aware of their self-expression? What was that like?

Questioner

I tried, but I think I was not too good at this. I have good contact with my youngest daughter, so I could have talked with her more also about what she experienced, but I think I was not so good for my eldest daughter. I think I was still struggling a lot with myself.

Janel

I understand. Thank you.

Questioner

Yes. The question about when you start examining your beliefs or something, yes, I remember that much later in life, I became conscious that I never had a proper thought about anything, that everything was just beliefs from others. That I learned when suddenly during a quarrel with my husband, I heard my mother speaking, rather than me. And I said, wait a minute. From then on, it started developing. At the age of 6, I was walking by a quarrel between my mother and father, I couldn't make a sound, I felt very guilty. I decided, I remember that very clearly, that I can never ask for help, or never tell them anything. So from the age of 6, I never told them anything but, surprisingly, I'm still alive.

Janel

How did you survive?

Questioner

I survived, yes. Yes, it's a big subject and it's very helpful to go and dig in. I was very surprised because we had this exercise to do at home and so I did it today, and you discover many things that, I think when you are not looking at, there was someplace where you lied to yourself. If you're unconscious, you lie all the time. Nothing real, does one ever say to anybody. Universal truth. That's all.

Janel

Thank you, wonderful.

Questioner

I was going to say. I came of age in the early mid 70s and there was so much rebellion of the younger generation against the older one with the Vietnam War in the United States and the race riots, all that. And so I think as a generation we were maybe a lot more rebellious against everything, religion, all of that. I remember confronting my parents quite a bit when I was coming of age, and it was maybe in fashion at that point to be questioning belief systems. But I think that has dried up, or it seems to me it feels like it has, but I did get support for trying to find my own way, and challenging, and my parents actually provoked us at times to be that way. And now I'm in with a bunch of heretics, so I don't know what to say.

Janel

Thank you. Sorry.

Doshin

So I want to share a perspective for you to consider. And this is how states of consciousness come into the picture. If our vantage point is looking out from a gross view, we are stuck *in the prison of me*. Everything that I'm presented with, I make a decision and it sounds something like this. "Oh, I agree with that." And that really means that I include it in my belief system. "Oh, I don't agree with that." And that means that I exclude it from my belief system, because it is antagonistic to my personal or collective beliefs. And "oh, I like these things." So they become a part of my personal belief system, and "oh, I don't like those things." So this is the way that we make decisions *in the prison of me*. And if we haven't become conscious of the prison we're living in, then we're stuck in it and we can't see beyond it, which is the case for all of us for a significant period of our lives. Some never escape this prison. I would say most never escape this prison, but let's say we move to a higher level, a higher state of consciousness, a higher vantage point, where suddenly we become more worldly, and this kind of happens automatically at the green level of development. Structurally at green, we move from a state vantage point of gross to a state vantage point of subtle. This happens naturally as the individual holon (person) enters the green, postmodern stage of development. As we join a social holon (a group), with a green nexus of emotional, moral and ideological resonance, then we begin to experience what feels like and is sometimes called the miracle of "*we*." Here, when we are presented with some information, it becomes more like this: "Oh, we agree with that." "Oh, they don't agree with us" and the social holons start to polarize into an "*us*" *against a* "*them*." Alliances can form with many different "us" groups, aligned against many different "them" groups. The significant thing to form an alliance is the common

throat

solo or group exercise

- *Look at your "me"*

- *What moral values (shoulds and should nots) were you indoctrinated into at 5 or 6?*

- *What ideological beliefs (think this way and don't think that way) were you indoctrinated into next?*

- *Which moral values and ideological beliefs stayed the same and which ones are different?*

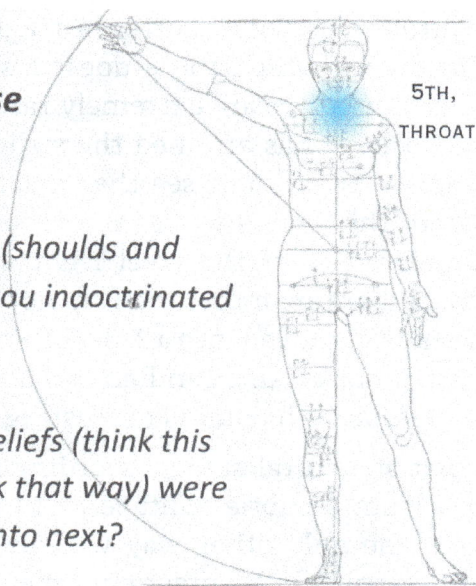

5TH, THROAT

ALBRECHT DURER
WOODCUT
c. 1528

CHAKRAS
SUPERIMPOSED

nexus of similar moral values and ideological beliefs. We're not limited, as Janel was saying, to just one us group.We each can belong to many different groups, each one a different world, a different social holon, each one with similar but slightly differing moods, values and beliefs. Each with their own belief system, their own moral dogma, their own combination of emotionally charged moral values and ideological beliefs. I have noticed countless members of the Integral social holon become true believers that they have attained the higher developmental structures of indigo and above which they have read about in *The Religion of Tomorrow,* or the integral yoga of Aurobindo. This is often a tragic case of delusional ego inflation for which there doesn't seem to be a cure. Those higher structures are extremely rare. I only know one person that I believe has attained the structure of ego development of indigo. We cannot see the structures of ego development beyond the one we are at. At best we might see some characteristics of the level right above where we are at. I suspect there are more, and I am not able to see them, because I have not yet moved into a 3rd-Tier structure. The only one that I believe has attained indigo ego development is Ken Wilber. He says that he has, and I'm trusting his judgement.

At that structural stage, according to Ken, we automatically move from a subtle vantage point to a causal state vantage point. The only other way we can move into a causal state vantage point is by practicing meditation for years, at least 20 years. First practicing preliminary types of meditation Shamanta, Vipassana and then more advanced methods like Shikantaza or Dzogchen. From the causal state vantage point, we begin to separate ourselves from the perceptual illusion of me and the perpetual delusions of we, we begin to step back and move into the higher balcony of witnessing mind.

So as you're thinking about the throat chakra consider also your state vantage point. Are you looking out from a *prison of me or a prison of we*? Individually liking and disliking, agreeing and disagreeing with everything you're experiencing? Are you identified with a group that is collectively liking and disliking everything that "we" see, and then collectively agreeing and disagreeing with everything that arises in "our" common experience. Or have you gone beyond the gross vantage point beyond beyond the subtle vantage point? Have you gone "beyond" the gross, "beyond beyond" into the subtle, or have you gone "beyond beyond beyond" into the vast empty void, where the causal vantage opens the way to crossing the great water to the mysterious other shore of Zen. Where you're free from attachment, prejudice and any bias for and against anything. This is the world that the Zen poem, *Faith in Mind* alludes to. So this is just something to consider as you're trying to answer all these questions. These are deep probing questions. And in future courses, we will be really looking in more detail at the early chakra development, where we really begin to explore the roots of me. All the way back into the karma. We will be looking from an Integral Framework. At the very root of being.

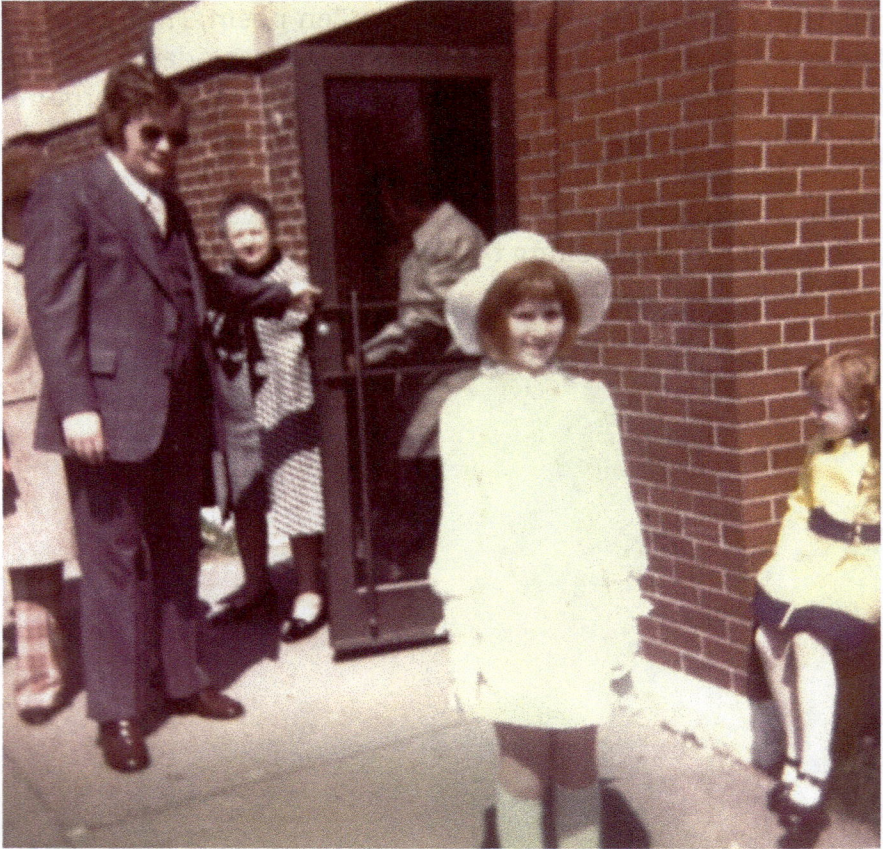

Janel, First Communion

Janel

For the next exercise, last week we talked about the moral values, the should and shouldn'ts that you were indoctrinated into at age 5 or 6. Try to summarize these. What ideological beliefs, think this way and don't think that way, were you indoctrinated into next? Which moral values and ideological beliefs stayed the same, which are different? Now this can take a lot of exploration, and you may belong to lots of different groups, but you may be able to identify some things that you really stepped away from, or held onto from that first initial indoctrination. Pick something simple from these options that you can work on.

So that you can just see a little bit how this can work. I'll talk about myself a little, so at the age of 5 or 6. My parents were taking me to a Catholic Church so we went to church, and then I had my first communion. At the same time, my father had been quite impacted by his Catholic indoctrination, probably more by the Catholic nuns in the education system (and yet I know he had positive experiences as well, with a high level of Jesuit education from Boston College High School, and then a short time at the Franciscan College St. Bonaventure but had to drop out I believe due to the cost) and was very angry, rebellious, and quite political. So while my parents were on the one hand bringing me to do these things, on the other hand, I was being indoctrinated unconsciously into all of his experience, which was the anger and resentment at the Catholic Church, but more broadly I would say against *untrustworthy authority*. Of course, I didn't see this at the time, but so my amber I would say was a little confused. It was saying, you know, behave this way. Definitely the environment was, I would say amber, coming into orange. So I have great respect for elders, for family, but then also there was mistrust of moral and civic authority, rebellion, and my personal family and individual trauma. So this led to a struggle, internal fighting or splitting in me. So as an adult, I can have both traditional views, but then I am also rebellious, challenging established norms. I can have a lot of mistrust of authority, but also respect for tradition. This is just one small aspect of how this can play out.

Also we're not just looking at the surface, the surface rules, or literal instructions you were taught (but if you remember them that's good too). So like I said, you know, I was brought to church. But yet, what else was I learning? Unconsciously, what was going on in your family, their ideological battles, were you living in a certain political environment that was for example, terrible, and your family was struggling? It's not just the explicit instruction, it's the implicit and often unconscious aspects.

Janel

Yes, go ahead please.

Questioner

Yes similarly, I had a dichotomy with my father as well, and just my whole family system. Where on one hand, the girls were raised to be like the poem, you know, sugar and spice and everything nice. And we were the ones in charge of always doing the dishes, taking care of the kids. The guys never had to do these things. So there was a strong message of traditional female roles on the one hand, and on the other hand we were always told that we were going to be strong and we were going to be successful. Also that we had to really pursue these achievement orientations and that if we weren't that, we wouldn't be good enough. Without both, we wouldn't be good enough, just being traditional, like my mother's role. But as life ended up, we wouldn't be able to really attain that level of masculine achievement orientation that we were raised with. At the sacrifice of being a good wife, good mother. It was really like we couldn't win. We couldn't be successful completely at one or the other, because there was always some polarity there.

Doshin

So, you actually were indoctrinated into amber values, good old fashioned family values that are quite traditional, and orange values that were success oriented, you know and the gift of that conflict. That's a culture war that you were indoctrinated into, that you took inside yourself, and this war continued within you, I suspect. You know, it's a wonder you came out as good as you did to describe it like you did.

Questioner

Yes, Sir.

Doshin

Blood, sweat and tears. Congratulations. I'm kind of curious, you survived. Do you know how you survived? How have you come to peace with this? How has this worked through your life over time? When did you develop this perspective that you're sharing now?

Questioner

It's been layers, you know, I think that it didn't really hit home until after I became a single mother. And the impossibility was just so stark. Like I really can't be the perfect mother who's doing all of what my mom did and also take care of us both completely on my own with my own money, because I had no support from the dad. So this was when I started to be like, wait a second. Something's not right here, it isn't all on me. But I do think it's been a work in progress and one big helpful component has been actually looking at it from a macro perspective of all the ways that we are raised to believe that anything masculine is better than feminine. I don't know, this could be perceived in different ways. Yang. But like doing and achieving is better than just being, who says? So just kind of looking at it from a broader perspective and getting a lot of good input from others has helped.

Janel

Thank you very much for sharing. Would you like to go?

Questioner

Okay so it's really blurred and I've got a lot of work to do to try and get some clarity, but just what comes up after just a few minutes of thinking, looking at these questions is like this huge elephant in the room, which is sex. I'm not sure if it was at 5 or 6 or or as a teenager, if we're looking more like the teenager and the ideology. There are all levels, but then when I was becoming a teenager, there was something. Even though I saw all my peers, particularly boys, showing and emerging and exploring and sharing sexuality. I had really internalised this, internalised it all, as if it was dirty and wrong. So actually, once a boy brought in a book in my class on Kama Sutra, one with photos on every page, and everyone in the class was fascinated by it and going to have a look in it and passing it around and talking about it and stuff. And I was of course interested and curious but I steadfastly refused to go and take a look. Then talking about culture war stuff really interferes in the sense of I had no way, no distinction between what's OK and entering, as it were, the sexual market. I have no internal distinction of what is okay, and what's predatory? And I internalized that anything I do, any advance I make is on girls and women is liable to be deemed predatory so, stay the **** out. I was terrified. Yeah, that's all.

Doshin

So do you see how this is a conflict between the traditional moral values that you were indoctrinated into at a very young age, hitting head on with a different reality that is presented to you in a non-traditional way at school. And, one of the things that's really involved here is peer pressure. Suddenly you're thrust out of that traditional value system into a social holon that doesn't share those traditional values. There's a conflict that emerges that you're not equipped to deal with because you haven't been properly prepared. This is a traumatic situation and it can be quite overwhelming to the point where you just can't deal with it. You're overwhelmed by it. So you shut down and you shut down that whole aspect of your life for a period of time. Until suddenly things happen that enable you to make your way through that conflict. Does that make sense?

Questioner

Oh, absolutely.

Doshin

So again, this is an area where you might ask yourself where do you go for help when you're overwhelmed like this? You know you can't go backward into the traditional. I mean, you could, but that would mean you'd have to suppress all these things that are arising in you as a teen. Suppress, repress and deny them, which is not really a good option, is it?

Questioner

No.

Doshin

Those hidden shadows and sub personalities are coming into the light. That's what is happening.

Questioner

Yes, yes. All true, And then it came out, and when I acted out and then I acted.

Doshin

Yes.

Questioner

Then it came out. They leaked out.

Doshin

Yeah, support is nowhere to be found, I suspect under those conditions.

Questioner

It felt like that.

Doshin

Yes my heart goes out to you. How many young people are in a similar position with nowhere to turn? It just breaks my heart to look at that.

Questioner

Yeah, it's very confusing, these times in the Western world, I would say. And we're still not over. We're still not, I think, like culturally we've got all this sex positivity and stuff, but we're still not over being stigmatized. Looking at what's what's right, what's wrong? What's OK? What's not?

Janel

Yes, you know, I'm obviously much older than you, but it's interesting because I came of age when the women's movement, women were really trying to support women's reproductive rights and when I was a teenager, I was given this book by my cousin, that became really political in the US, called *Our Bodies, Ourselves*. Since my family didn't talk about any of this, this was extremely, I would say it was pretty radical and it presented sexuality to women as if there was not much consequence. Which now I can say at my age, can do a tremendous disservice to people. The fact is, you know there are consequences when you become sexually involved with someone, even if it's, you know, very brief. There are emotional and physical consequences. The world we're in now in America is so different from actually the time when I was a teenager. Now these culture wars have gotten much more extreme. I have a teenage daughter, and depending on what state you live in, women are being put in jail for having a miscarriage. So now you know the idea of being somewhat free as a teenager looks crazy, some of the anti-abortion states are going after women or health care providers who support them, and some are attempting to prevent birth control altogether. So as a teenager, I was presented with a presentation that downplayed the consequences of free sexuality. Then now to add to all of the culture wars we also have these incredible identity politics going on. It is so, so confusing and so when I hear that children are having less sexual activity, you know, teenagers, it's totally understandable to me because I mean, my god, what could happen as the result of unintended pregnancy? My heart goes out to all the young people.

Questioner

Thanks. What came up for me was that when I was very young, I grew up very close to my mother and we are talking about 2 1/2 years old, and at that time she had cancer. That time, she knew that she was going to die because that was in the end of the 60s and they didn't have any treatments at that time. And I found from diaries and photo albums that there was a very strong close connection between us, she was a classical pianist and we played piano and sang. She taught me how to read and write before I was three years old. And she really taught me how to use my voice both in singing and also to speak up for myself in a healthy way. And she died when I was four, and I was growing up with my father, who had this sort of ptsd from the Second World War and he was not supportive. He had a very strange way of communicating, and his expectations of me were that I should be silent, perfect, whatever. And my voice totally disappeared, so much so, when

I was eight years old and I didn't tell anyone because there was no point to tell anyone because no one would help me. So I was screaming for my mother and they took me to the hospital and found I had, yeah, that I was quite close to death, the Doctor said. And then what was with my father? It was so difficult for me to raise my voice, but I had something really growing inside. When I was 11 I became a footballer and I saw again and those boys became my voice. I have to say that even if it is an environment it was very healing for me to be in a group and express rage and use my voice in that way. But after a couple of years I felt that that was not the right environment for me. So I stopped with that and tried to find better ways to express myself. So yeah, that's my story.

Janel

Thank you, this is really touching and it's also very interesting and I think one can see parallels for a lot of younger people that they are in that kind of connection with an environment where they are able to let out so much expression and emotion and and actually it does somewhat end up being a kind of healthy expression. It sounds like it was healthy for you at that time. It was a way for you to channel those energies. Doshin, would you like to say something?

Doshin

Yes I would. I'm just deeply touched, not only by the way you survived, and thatwas part of your survival, but I was deeply touched by the transcendental seeds that were planted. In your young heart-mind at such a young age, by someone who deeply loved you and how that love and the trusting the depth of that love has led you on a spiritual path.

throat chakra - on your own

- *sing with vitality, alone or with others, even if out of tune, join a singing group*
- *mantra practice (get a mala, 108 mantras to a mala)*
- *try a creative activity with a therapeutic intention of simply enjoying the activity and seeing what happens*
- *connect with a community out of your comfort zone with people who have quite different beliefs from you, with the intention of pure listening and practicing being present*
- *identify groups that you have left behind in the past, look closely why and see your growth*
- *volunteer in a situation where your role is to purely listen*
- *reflect in your life, is there something unsaid, that needs to be said, skillfully?*

Questioner

Yes I really think she planted a seed because she was, she really talked to me so often that she would always be my only guardian Angel, and always be there even after her death. And that's something I cannot say that I have felt, but I just, I know it. I think that it has a lot to do with pushing me on the spiritual path, at a young age.

Doshin

And that is such a gift you were given. In comparing that

with the stories that the younger people are telling us where they have nothing that they can trust. No seeds of trust were planted at that tender young age. When the ego began to emerge and before in the 1st and 2nd chakras that's such a difference and there's such a deep longing for something to trust that you were given. And the youth today don't seem to be getting that, that really breaks my heart open. And, I hope you can really hold up the gift you were given and be grateful for it, and make use of it to benefit all beings, especially yourself. Thank you for sharing that touching story.

With this, yes there's such a difference that I find in dealing with people that are a couple generations into what we are calling the *weirdest people in the world*. You know, when I deal with North Americans and Northern Europeans that have been indoctrinated into the modern social holon, the orange, and the postmodern social holon, the green, there's such a difference dealing with those people than dealing with people that still have a sense of spirituality that hasn't been negated and crushed. People from Mexico, South America, Eastern Europe, the Middle East, Asia and Africa. There's something still alive there, something that can be trusted that's greater than the "me," and greater than "we." It's some mystical force. Some magical force that emerges in the second chakra and continues on in the ego development. It is something that has been sterilized out of us in Western Europe and North America. It is a flame that has gone out and needs to be reignited. I trust that something is going to happen that will reignite it somewhere along the way. That gives me not hope, but solace that some mystery is almost ready to unfold. That the "readiness of time," is almost ready. Some slight spark of light in this great darkness that seems so insane, when I look out into the world.

Janel

Thank you. All right, so a few suggestions for *throat on your own.* Singing is very therapeutic for the throat chakra, alone or with others. If you want to be ambitious, you can join a singing group. Doing mantra, using a mala, if you don't know what a mala is, it's a number of prayer beads, typically it is 108 beads, you go through a whole strand. If you need a mantra, I have ones to suggest depending on what you need or practice. I can give you one specific for you. Doing creative activities with a therapeutic intention of simply enjoying the activity and seeing what happens; just trying something new and creative that maybe you've been curious about. You know, not with an agenda to be excellent, to just enjoy trying to do something fun and new. Connecting with a community out of your comfort zone with people who have quite different beliefs from you with the intention of pure listening and practicing being present. So if you do want to really transcend this throat chakra, then put yourself around people who you aren't ever around, maybe a very different culture.

This is a great practice to experiment with. Identify groups that you have left behind in the past. Look and inquire, why did you leave them? See your growth. We all have groups that we spend some time with and then maybe decide we've outgrown, or it's going in a different direction; really look closely. One of the ways you can do that is look at what the shoulds and shouldnt's were for the group. What were you okay with and what was actually a problem, or how did you change? Volunteer in a situation where your role is to purely listen. This is excellent practice. Reflect on your life, is there something unsaid that needs to be said skillfully?

Heart Self-Care Practice #2

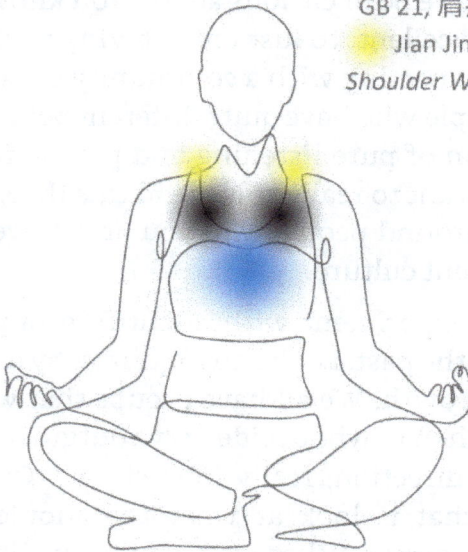

heart self-care practice #2

GB 21, 肩井,
Jian Jing,
Shoulder Well

- TCM gallbladder point GB21 and meridian related to frustration, anger, resentment and rigidity, bottled-up feelings

- gentle massage treatment of the trapezius supported with additional heart chakra focus

- warm the areas, offer yourself self-assurance, compassion

- loosen energies of loneliness, grief, sadness and despair, stored in gray areas of upper chest and between the clavicle

Here is another self-care practice. This is focused on the gallbladder points GB21. They are the yellow circles in the image, but we're also looking at these areas that go across the chest where a lot of loneliness, sadness and despair can be stored.

So in a patriarchal culture, most people feel the right side is associated with masculine energies, so your father and father's ancestry. The left side is connected to the feminine and the mother's side. My father died about a year and a half ago and it's so I've noticed much more pain on the right side for me now. My right side is what bothers me and this isn't a surprise. So all of these areas. Just again speaking to the body, acknowledging, making conscious loneliness, grief, sadness that may be stored still in these places?

Do we have any questions? Anything, is someone dying to free their throat chakra? So next session is our last one and we'll do it a little differently because we're going to do the third eye in the crown together. So this marks the end of Integral first tier, at the throat. Most people don't get beyond the gross third eye and gross crown. We'll do some more overall review exercises together and see what we're walking away with.

Doshin

No, I think that's sufficient for today. I don't know whether we put them to sleep or woke them up. I suspect mileage will vary among individuals. I trust that you took in what you were ready and needed to receive. And everything is perfect as it is. Deepest gratitude.

CHAPTER 6, THE THIRD EYE AND CROWN CHAKRAS

Doshin

Time sure has flown by quickly, hasn't it? Let's just jump in, are we ready?

Janel

Ready.

Doshin

Final week of the introduction. Again, I'm going to remind everybody please remember: this is best experienced and not intellectualized. We're presenting the chakras in an Integral Framework with a broad overview of healing lineage teachings that include both healing and awakening. Trust you will receive what you need. Stop trying to understand everything and just receive what comes. Nothing is finally attained, when everything has been let go. Isn't that interesting?

Janel

Can I give everyone a heads up? The firehose is coming. Protect yourself.

Doshin

Yes, that's true. So please don't think you have to remember. Don't even try to take notes. The firehose is coming and it's something so simple, but until it sinks in, which may take years, it might be really confusing. Let it be confusing. That's not a problem. But when it finally does sink in, this is incredibly useful. So just let it be what it is for you, and don't try to understand it. Don't think you need to agree or disagree with it. Just don't. It's not something that will be useful for you to agree or disagree with, that just negates and blocks the value you might receive from it, *in the readiness of time.* Just take it in, if it resonates great. If it doesn't, just let it go.

Wilber-Combs Lattice *from Integral Spirituality by Wilber*

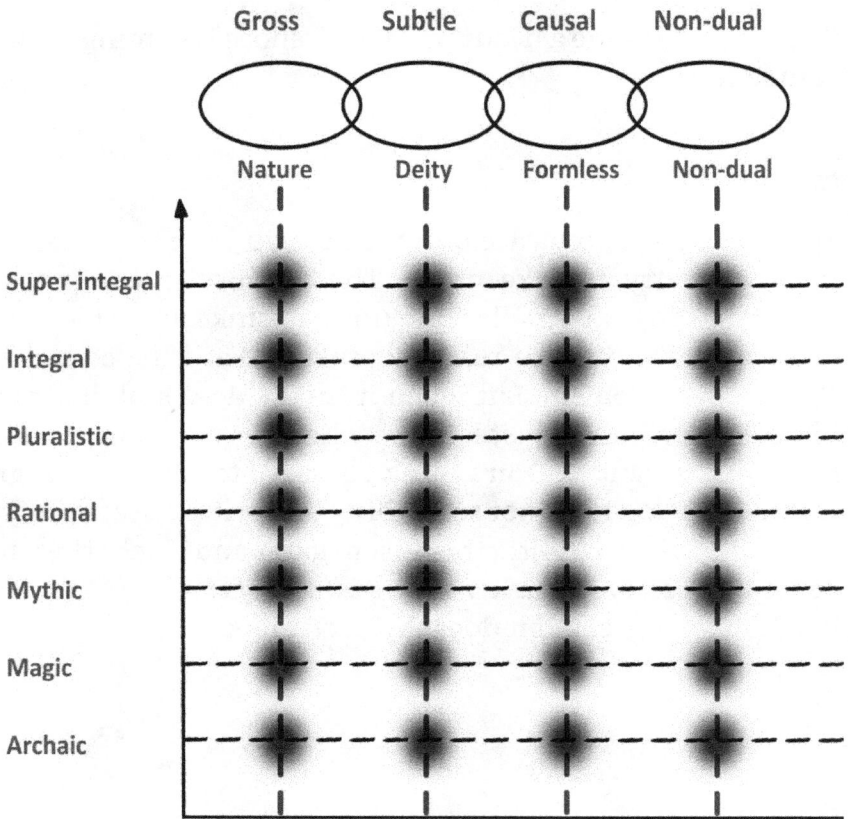

This is the Wilber-Combs lattice he presented in *Integral Spirituality*.[67]

This profound insight of Ken Wilber and Alan Combs emerged prior to 2006. It was published in the book *Integral Spirituality*, where he tells the story of how it came about. So all the people who are only familiar with earlier versions of Ken's work, didn't get this, and it is profoundly important. When this original idea finally soaked in, I slowly began to realize its deep significance, it has profoundly changed the way I look at everything. This idea is the cornerstone of Kosmic Addressing.

(I could write a whole book on the subject of the Wilber Combs Lattice and only scratch the surface.)

So let's take a little deeper look at the Wilber-Combs lattice. In Wilber's version, we have the structures, the levels of consciousness on the left. Archaic, magic, mythic, mythic, rational, pluralistic, integral and super-integral. He is not showing the colors he has assigned to each of the structures in the black and white version. On the horizontal axis across the top, he shows four states. He shows gross, subtle, causal, and nondual states of consciousness.

In presenting this lattice, I found it's very useful to alter his presentation by switching the horizontal and vertical axes. In my inverted version, I'm including all the states and structures that Wilber describes without adding any more or leaving any out. This is the Complete WCL that we use in Integral Zen.

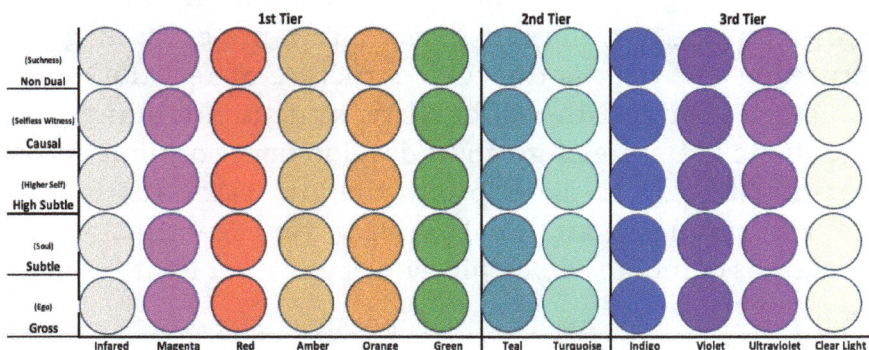

As a Zen teacher, I have more experience and interest in states, so I invert it. From the Integral Zen Perspective, we are turning the W-C Lattice *right side up.* The Integral Zen version puts the developmental structures of consciousness on the horizontal axis to show that it is an evolutionary process. In the individual, the ego structures evolve in a linear progression. The states of consciousness are on the vertical axis to show that with disciplined, dedicated practice, higher states of consciousness can be attained and stabilized. I was surprised to discover that this version is more palatable to groups of people who share postmodern, green values and beliefs. Here are a few examples of these values and beliefs: everyone is equal, all hierarchies are bad, everyone must be nice, we need to rescue all victims, feeling good is very important, we don't need to feel bad, shouldn't make anyone else feel bad, and we are spiritual but not religious.

We won't go into much detail here, but it is important to know that there is a given structure that individual ego development follows. The individual must develop through the ego structures in a linear order. We can't skip any structural level and jump to a more developed one. We each must grow through them in order. We all begin life on ground zero with a Kosmic Address at the infrared structure, the root chakra, and a gross state vantage point. Then, the 2nd chakra comes on line and the self grows into a pre-egoic magenta structure. The next is the egoic structure of red, the ethnic structure of amber, the rationalistic structure of orange and pluralistic structure of green. If development continues, very few might begin to develop into the 2nd-Tier structures of teal and turquoise, and finally a very, very few the 3rd-Tier structures of indigo, violet, ultraviolet and clear light.

That's the whole spectrum of possible structures of ego development at this point in human history at least for those who have been born and indoctrinated into a modern culture. These are the structures that Ken placed on the vertical axis implying that they are "altitudes" or structures of development. He placed the states of consciousness on the horizontal axis.

Here I want to pause and suggest something that I believe Wilber would agree with, but I have never heard anyone else say or even consider. This is where the analogy we are using between chakras and structures of ego development seem to begin to break down somewhat and differ, depending on the culture the individual is born into. The culture, or more specifically the social holon that individuals are born in and indoctrinated into, makes a tremendous difference in the way the upper chakras come alive and the more complex ego structures develop. If we are born in or move into a modern culture, a social holon with orange values and beliefs, then we are more likely to grow into the modern orange and green ego structures at the 5th chakra; perhaps even into teal and turquoise ego structures at roughly the 6th chakra, and a very, very few might even move into indigo, violet, ultraviolet, and clear light ego structures at very loosely the 7th chakra. If the individual is born into a pre-modern culture, the ego development is very different. There is much we have not even begun to explore here, that we will be going into in detail in future books.

As a lineage holder in Zen, I am on much more familiar ground with the states of consciousness than the structures. The practices of Eastern Wisdom Traditions are mainly 1st-person, introspective practices, which have developed over thousands of years in lineages, living streams of teachers who took on students who mastered the teachings and became teachers themselves and who took on students over many, many generations. Given the depth and level of sophistication of these lineage teachings, I find it is helpful to use five states: gross, subtle, high subtle, causal and nondual in order to describe the complexity and different effects of each type of meditative practice.

The levels or structures of ego development are mostly hidden from introspection. Wilber calls them "hidden maps," because like the hidden rules of grammar, they cannot be seen by 1st person introspection. They only become visible with 3rd person observation of many different individuals. The articulation of these hidden rules are derived by using the scientific method. The states of consciousness become visible with introspection, and the structures of consciousness are made visible by 3rd-person formal operational thinking examining the data after studying large groups of individuals. These states and structures are the two components of the WCL.

I haven't seen anyone else in the Integral community invert the WCL like we do in Integral Zen. Let me state again that I found there is a practical benefit of doing this inversion. It seems to ease the bias against hierarchies that most people have who are at a pluralistic stage of ego development. They do not seem to be triggered by this presentation with the states on the vertical axis and the structures on the horizontal axis. We all seem to intuitively know that some people are more awake than others, and higher states of consciousness are earned by practicing introspective meditation methods. In a postmodern-green cultural environment, there is an emotionally charged bias and belief that everybody is equal. So, showing that there is an evolutionary process going on seems to trigger less reactivity than placing the stages of development on the vertical axis where some stages (altitudes) are "higher" than others, the way Wilber does. Postmodern minds seem to interpret the vertical presentation of ego development as a growth hierarchy which triggers an "allergy," an emotionally charged bias against all hierarchies. There is an implicit "green" moral judgment that all hierarchies are bad and disgusting. In this postmodern structure of ego development, the capacity to differentiate between a man-made hierarchy and a natural hierarchy has not yet emerged into consciousness. The capacity to make this distinction between natural and growth hierarchies, Wilber calls "vision logic." It does not emerge and become operational until the individual begins to develop as into 2nd-Tier structures of consciousness.

I know this is a whole lot to take in. Don't get discouraged. Remember: "How do you eat an elephant?" As the saying goes, "One bite at a time." So if your eyes have glazed over that is alright. Just rest, go do something fun. Come back later and take another bite. Take as many bites as you need to. You might even need to go read some Ken Wilber books if you really want to digest some of this. Also consider the possibility that if you are not born and indoctrinated into a modern or postmodern culture with modern and postmodern values and beliefs, then things might be quite different, because of the interconnectivity, interdependence, and interdynamics of both individual and social holons.

Now let's switch our focus from structures to states of consciousness, and show some of these interdependencies and interdynamics. First, there is a big difference between a temporary *peak* state experience and a more permanent state *vantage point*. It is like the difference between visiting Paris and actually living there. Unlike structures of consciousness, anyone can have a peak experience of any state at any time. But actually stabilizing and taking residence in a state of consciousness, means that you are living there full time. This is what Wilber calls a vantage point. You can't just decide to inhabit a state vantage point like you can decide to move to Paris. State vantage points must be earned by maintaining a disciplined, devoted meditation practice. It requires consistent effort, great dedication, and a good teacher to guide you. One that has themselves, earned a higher vantage point through years of devoted practice.

Next is an Integral Zen version of a modern and postmodern Wilber Combs Lattice. We are specificallly describing the ego development of an individual who is indoctrinated into a modern/postmodern culture. As the 4th chakra is energized in the amber structure of ego development, the 2nd person perspective begins to emerge in the individual holon. If held and supported in an amber social holon, it is possible for the individual to develop enough faith, discipline and devotion to practice meditation, contemplation and devotional practices to begin awakening. This involves a process of purification of self-reactivity, beginning with what are known in Buddhism as the *five poisons* also known as the *afflictive or dangerous emotions* of *greed, hatred, ignorance, pride* and *jealousy*.

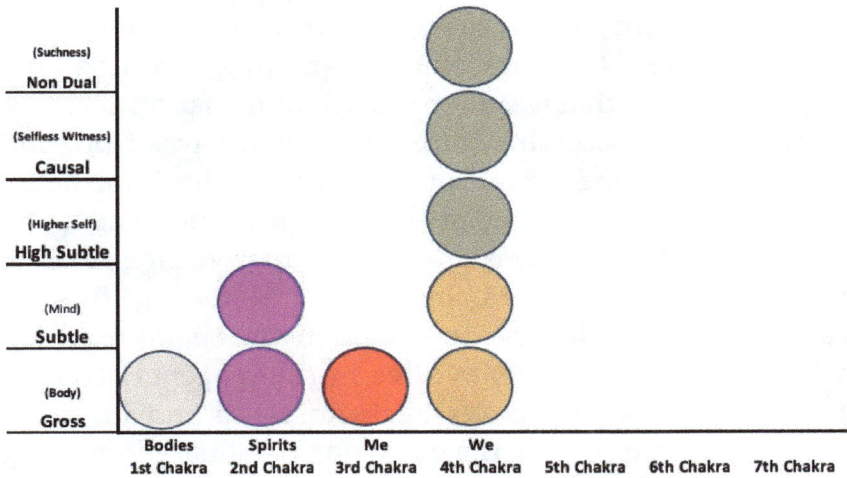

I started seriously studying Jung and practicing mediation the same year, that was over 55 years ago. I encountered my root Zen Teacher, JunPo Denis Kelly Roshi and began reading Ken Wilber over 20 years ago and consider both JunPo and Wilber to be two of the greatest teachers I have had the good fortune to meet and study with. Integral Zen was formed a few years later. I couldn't find any group that would help me integrate the teachings I had received from Jung, JunPo and Wilber, so I founded Integral Zen. It was Wilber's Integral Framework that has allowed me to link together the *five chakras*, the *five poisons*, the *five skandhas*, Jung's Theory of Types, and Wilber's WCL and Kosmic Addressing and integrate them all in an intuitive, radically new and beneficial way that supports the healing and awakening of all beings.

We are all born at ground zero, 1st chakra-infrared structure and gross vantage point. When the 2nd chakra comes alive in the magenta structure of pre-ego development, the *feeling function* comes online. In the Buddhist teachings of the *Five Skandhas*, this is articulated as the *second skandha*. I have come to see that the *second skandha* and what Jung articulates as the

301

Feeling Function in his Theory of Types, are both describing the same territory of magenta pre-ego development, where specific human capacities emerge. For Jung, "feeling" is a rational function that we use to process information and make decisions. It is processing information it receives from both the "sensation" and "intuition" functions. The information being received are both the gross and subtle phenomena that are tetra-arising in all four quadrants. Jung's feeling function is rational, judgmental and binary +/-. This "feeling" function is a "yes or no" decision making function that begins to emerge as the second chakra comes alive in the magenta structure of pre-ego development. We begin to sense and intuit the sense objects, the spirits, the emotions, the first glimmerings of sexuality and magic. We are able to "feel" and differentiate between the helpful and hindering spirits, between the pleasant and unpleasant emotions, and between what feels like black and white magic. This is the beginning of pre-conscious human emotionally charged judgmental reactivity.

As the third chakra begins to energize and we move into the developmental stage of red. Here, we have enough language that the illusion of a separate, permanent sense of self, what we now call an ego, begins to formalize into a more solid form. This form, this sense of "me" is the beginning of the 1st person perspective. From this 1st person perspective, there is only me, and everything is mine. If you have children, you will recognize this stage of development as the "terrible twos."

It is not until the fourth chakra energizes, that we move into an amber structure of ego development. Here the capacity to form a second-person perspective emerges. This enables the individual ego to differentiate between me and you, as well as us and them. The individual ego now has the capacity to be indoctrinated into the "tribe." With the support of the tribe, the social holon, the individual finally has enough of the essential supporting ingredients, such as: personal and collective rituals, ethical values and supporting beliefs to formalize a practice of prayer and meditation. With religious inspiration, it is now possible to rigorously practice prayer and meditation enough to cultivate the virtues of discipline and devotion.

This is where there is a profound difference between a person, an individual holon that has been raised in and indoctrinated into a culture, a social holon that has pre-modern traditional amber "religious" collective ethical values and ideological beliefs, and a modern orange "secular" social holon with religious allergies and secular beliefs. The essence of this profound difference is that the individual human being is indoctrinated into a collective orange belief that the ego is somehow separate from Nature. This modern, orange collective belief has created a spiritual desert and a loss of connection to Nature. When children who are at an amber level of personal development, are indoctrinated into an orange modern collective culture (social holon), they seem to have developed to an orange level of ego development, but they have not. They are still at an amber level of development. This is a source of great confusion in our world, including the Integral Community.

It is the fourth chakra heart centered energy that forms an amber religious foundation which creates the fertile garden where *discipline* and *religious devotion* can develop to support a serious consistent meditation practice. Without this fertile soil, it is highly unlikely or practically impossible for the individual to grow spiritually. If we don't have a serious meditation practice, as the ego develops beyond the early structures of consciousness, we will remain at a gross state vantage point with little or no spiritual development. This is the case from infrared, through magenta, red, amber and orange structures of individual development.

In a postmodern culture, when the individual enters the green structure of ego development, there is a natural shift in the state vantage point. We begin to automatically move from a gross into a subtle state vantage point. This subtle vantage point continues into the 2nd Tier structures. However, at the Amber structure of ego development, if we are supported by an amber "religious" culture that helps us cultivate a serious, consistent meditation practice, it is possible to move past a gross state vantage point into a subtle, causal or non dual state vantage point. Without a serious meditation practice, it is highly unlikely that an individual will move beyond a subtle vantage point into a causal witnessing state vantage point. Wilber suggests that very few naturally begin to move into the rarified air of the 3rd-Tier at the indigo structure of ego development. On the other hand if we have a very serious meditation practice (say 40,000 hours of meditation or more), we are exponentially more likely to reach a causal, witnessing state vantage point and higher. This perspective is likely to upset many true believers who are attached to the belief that they are enlightened.

From my perspective as an Integral Zen Master, the Wilber Combs Lattice is a radically new idea. It is as radically significant today as the Theory of Evolution was in the nineteenth century. I have been shocked how few individuals in the Integral Community seem to have grasped the true significance of the WCL and are actually able to apply it. My theory born out of experience is that the capacity to fully digest the WCL requires a minimal Kosmic Address of a consistent 2nd-tier cognitive perspective and a stable causal, witnessing vantage point. This is likely to be disturbing, even triggering to many who believe they have attained a 2nd-tier center of gravity, but are actually still stuck in a green center of structural gravity with postmodern moral values and ideological beliefs. These are what I call "The True Believers" in Integral Theory.[68]

To summarize and "Zen all this out" for our purposes here, just remember that at the green, postmodern structure of ego development, we begin to automatically move into the subtle realm. Without a *religiously devoted* meditation practice, an individual will remain in the subtle realm even if our ego develops through teal, through turquoise. It is only as an individual moves into the very rare and seldom attained indigo structure of ego development, does it become likely that they will move into the causal state of witnessing-mind, without a serious meditation practice. In the 3rd-tier it is possible to move into violet, ultraviolet and clear light structures. Of course, it is a bit more complex than this Zenned out perspective describes.

Of all the people I have personally met, I only believe one of them is at the indigo level of ego development and that's Ken Wilber himself, and that is because that's where he told me he's at. It doesn't seem like any of us really have the capacity to see levels of ego development much beyond the one that our center of gravity is currently in, certainly very, very few can see indigo. My sense is that I personally am moving into 2nd Tier, but still quite far from moving into turquoise.

This is my perspective and Integral Zen's version of the Wilber-Combs lattice. Like Ken himself we are using chakras, as a useful analogy for structural development. And we are pointing out some significant differences in individual and social holons, before and after the reformation and the unfolding of the age of reason, enlightenment, industrial age and the emergence of science.

Something Very Weird Happened In The West

In what follows we are focusing primarily on ego development in the Western modern and postmodern world, rather than in more traditional amber cultures. *"The WEIRDest People in the World"*[69] is the title of a book that Susanne Cook-Grueter, an expert in the field of Ego Development, sent me for Christmas a few years ago. WEIRD is an acronym: W. Western, E. Educated, I. Industrialized, R. Rich, and D. Democratic. The subtitle is *How the West Became Psychologically Peculiar and Particularly Prosperous.* It is a very scholarly book of over 600 pages, with over two hundred pages of appendices, footnotes, and an extensive bibliography.

I am not going to go into detail here, but the book draws attention to the time of the Protestant Reformation in Western Europe, which was followed by the Age of Enlightenment and Reason, followed by the Industrial Revolution and the Scientific Revolution. This was a time of tremendous changes in the western world. Something very WEIRD emerged in Northwestern Europe that drastically changed everything.

If we have the capacity to use an Integral Framework, we can see that this change was tetra arising in all four quadrants. In the Age of Science, what Wilber calls *scientific absolutism* emerged in the upper right quadrant. A collective bias against everything that was not reasonable and measurable began to grow. This individual and collective bias rejected and ignored much of what exists in the other three quadrants. Religious sentiments, symbols and artifacts were rejected and replaced by scientifically verifiable facts. Personal and collective religious altars were shunned, became culturally unacceptable, and were hidden. It slowly became unfashionable to be "religious." We began to worship in empirical laboratory shrines.

Two of the four functions of Jung's Theory of Types, the *thinking* and *sensation* functions became overly dominant at the expense of the other two functions of *feeling* and *intuition*. In the lower left quadrant, something radically new emerged in the West: modern and then postmodern culture. In the lower right quadrant, the speed of societal changes increased exponentially due to technology. There is a very significant difference between a pre-scientific culture (social holon) and a post-scientific one. With the scientific age came a radical movement toward the head at the expense of the heart. This created a radical change in the culture and has resulted in an imbalance that has scarred many generations since the Protestant Reformation. There was the industrial age with its increasingly more powerful machines and factories. The information age with exponential increase in data collection, storage and now the processing power of artificial intelligence. The emergence of this WEIRD shift in culture has elevated rational thought to the status of the gods, and it has a dark, dark shadow. The pitiful postmodern attempts to be "spiritual but not religious," and reclaim the lost territory of the human soul without violating the religion of scientism have failed and created a false form of spirituality. It is like a line from one of my poems says: "When man's reason rules his spirit dies." It is not possible to worship reason and spirit at the same time. Our hearts are in a collective ethical desert where healthy moral values and virtues cannot even be planted let alone grow and bear fruit.

Now that the stage is set, let's return to the chakras and ego development to articulate another perspective of what self development looked like before the WEIRDest people in the world emerged in the 1600s, 1700s, 1800s and 1900s. At the first chakra the infrared level of development, we have bodies. At the second chakra of development, all of a sudden we begin to experience that not only do we have bodies, but all bodies have a spirit. This is the beginning of human nature. Then at the third chakra, we don't really care about that, we are fascinated with the new first person perspective, the "me" that emerges and the power that accompanies it. This first person perspective begins to emerge in the individual in the upper right quadrant, as well as collectively in the social holons in the lower left quadrant. This is where collectively, the age of empires and kingdoms begin with the emergence of a powerful leader. It is in the 4th chakra, the amber stage of ego development that the individual learns to manage power and the controlling nature of *"me"* in order to fit into whatever the rules are in the collective social holon. In an amber culture, social holon, the *"we"* begins to emerge socially, and the second person perspective begins to dominate. In an individual holon like you and me in the heart chakra, the ME is indoctrinated into a set of moral values and beliefs--a WE. If the "WE" is an amber religious one that supports a dedicated, devoted meditation practice, then each individual can continue their state development through high-subtle, into causal-witnessing and into nondual-suchness. The support of a "religious" community that the individual is indoctrinated into is foundational. A social holon with a nexus of amber "religious" ethical values and religious beliefs provides the foundation for serious spiritual practice with religious devotion and discipline.

The orange structure of ego development correlates to the throat chakra, the 5th chakra. Particularly in a Western modern culture, this stage is where the individual begins to differentiate their own individual moral dogma--their own moral values and ideological beliefs. Some developmental theorists like Robert Kegan don't see this structure of ego development as a separate structure that stands by itself. They see the orange and green structures as connected. This is also how I see it, which fits right into the Integral map, when we use both the wisdom of the older chakra system with the new understanding gleaned from the modern studies of the structures of ego development. In Integral Zen we see that the modern orange and postmodern green structures of ego development are both related to the 5th chakra. I consider postmodernity as a reaction to modernity rather than a separate structure of ego development. This provides the foundation of an Integral Framework where we can begin to explore what I call the *Inter-holonic Inter-dynamics*.

Now, let's examine the 6th Chakra, and the 7th. This is where the third eye begins to open. With a meditation practice, it can open more fully, stabilizing the subtle, high subtle, causal witnessing, and nondual state vantage points. It is in the state of nondual suchness, where all the delusions of *me* and *we* are burned away, and the sensation and intuition have been purified. Then at the 7th chakra, after intuition is pure, in Buddhism in Mahayana and Vajrayana Buddhism, the perfect round mirror turns right side up, and we only see "what is." There is liberation from the illusion of me, all the delusions of me and we, as well as all the negative karma of what we call in Zen Buddhism: the *five poisons* and *five hindrances*. It is now at least possible for suffering to end.

Let me take a deep breath, and remind you that I am using a firehose to give you a sip of water. So please don't be upset if you're not getting all this. Just take in what you can and let the rest go and read as much as you can. You may have to read it a few thousand times and read a few more books. Then you may need to do some deeper work. Perhaps some therapy, work on your shadows, insecure attachment or trauma work. You might need some deeper healing work, and it might be helpful for you to find some religious practices to do even deeper work with Karma, resolving the karmic patterns that came into the root chakra at conception. It is what it is. This is all part of what we're doing in Integral Zen to put the chakras into an Integral Framework, where we can really focus on healing and awakening within an Integral Sangha. This is the type of container that is required for those individuals who were indoctrinated at the amber stage of ego development into the collective moral values and ideological beliefs of modern orange and postmodern green social holons.

So in the Integral Zen framework, the third eye is actually the spiritual line of development. It is the awakening of pure intuition, unpolluted by me or we and all our delusions. And now, due to what Ken Wilber calls the *level line fallacy,* he's pointing to the fact that spiritual development is stuck. I would say that the third eye is stuck, and can't continue to open. In the modern and postmodern social holons, individuals are stuck in an amber, a fundamentalist, orange and green godless realm of the collective secular, modern and postmodern values and beliefs of social holons with anti-religious biases.

This is a profound insight that Ken is presenting with this term *level line fallacy.*

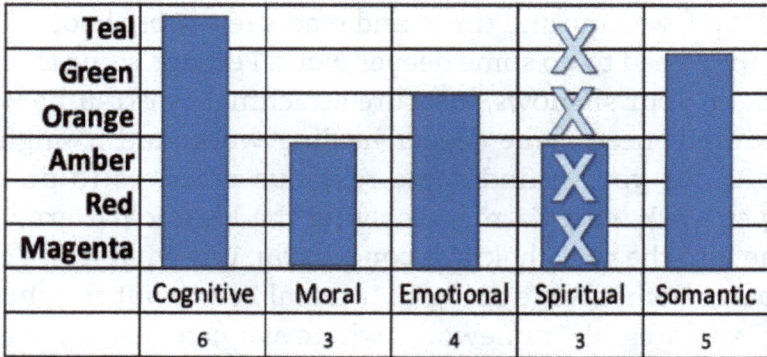

Level Line Fallacy

	Cognitive	Moral	Emotional	Spiritual	Somantic
Teal				X	
Green				X	
Orange			X	X	
Amber				X	
Red				X	
Magenta				X	
	6	3	4	3	5

What it means, is the spiritual line of intelligence, has been stuck with *fundamentalist beliefs of scientific materialism*. This has become a modern political ideology that acts like an amber religious theology.

For Wilber, the level line fallacy is looking at the spiritual line of intelligence. Each of the lines of intelligence that Ken has articulated: the cognitive, moral, emotional, spiritual, and somatic (to name a few of the most important lines of intelligence), develops through the structures of consciousness. Remember, that the lines of intelligence are one of the five AQAL ways of looking at the world in Integral Theory: quadrants, levels, states, lines and types. The lines of intelligence develop through these very clear levels or structures. As the individual develops they can't skip any structure of development and neither can the lines of development. The individual lines can be at different structures. For example, cognition can be at teal, 2nd tier, the moral line can be at amber, the emotional line could actually be exiting orange and entering green. This graph depicts a spiritual line of intelligence that became stuck in amber fundamentalism as the WEIRDest people in the world became the dominant cultural group.

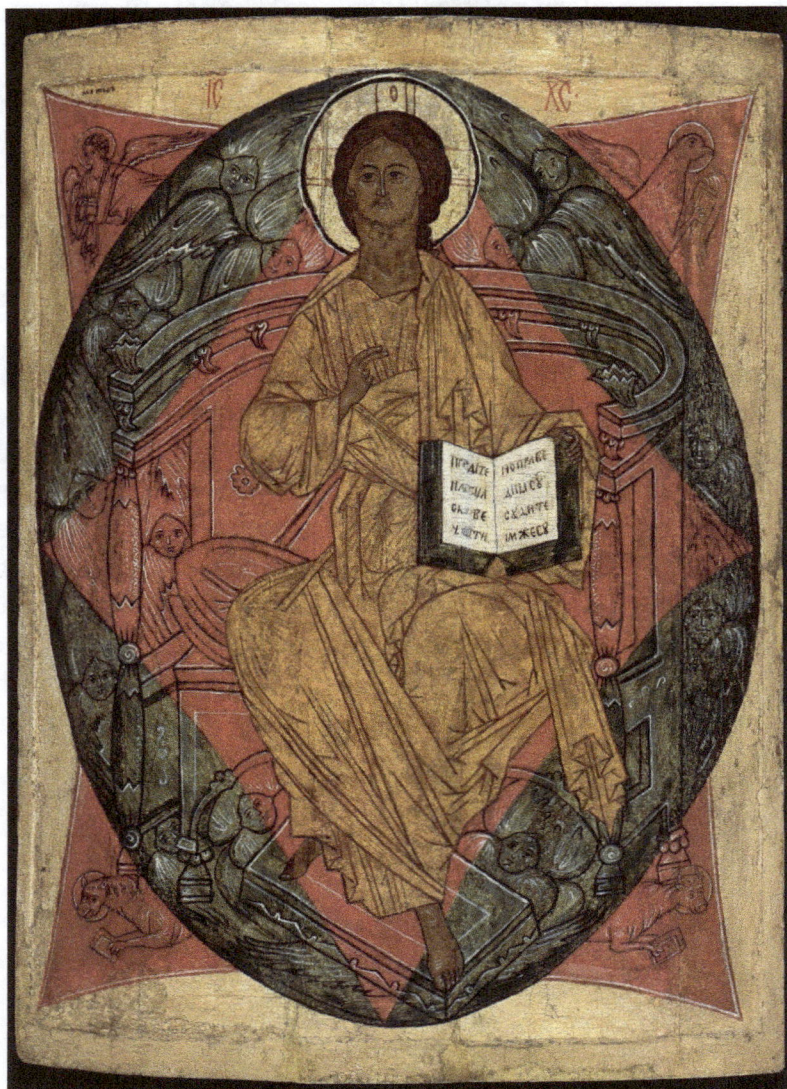

Christ in Glory, Russian Painter (late 15th century), Gift of George R. Hann, 1944, Metropolitan Museum, New York, Public Domain

That's what the level line fallacy is pointing to, the spiritual line of intelligence has hit a ceiling that it cannot go beyond. Consider the fact that there is no orange version of God, no green version of God, or no teal version of God.

I n *Integral Spirituality*, Wilber says: "So horrifying was the mythic level of God—and so extensive were the genuine terrors the Church had inflicted on people in the name of that mythic God—that the Enlightenment threw religion over entirely."[70]

When God was negated in the West, the spiritual line of development was frozen at the amber level of development. In a personal conversation with Ken Wilber and Roger Walsh I asked Ken, "What exactly is the spiritual line of development?" And he said: "It's cognition, directed toward the ultimate concern." When the dirty bathwater of religion was thrown out, so was the baby. The precious baby of ultimate concern.

In Zen, as I'm working with people. I often ask them the koan: *What is the most important thing?* Then I'm very quiet and I listen very carefully to exactly what they say. With the precise words they choose, they reveal what state vantage point they have stabilized, and what level of ego development their center of gravity is usually going to be at. This is the beginning foundation of their Kosmic Address. If they say it's my BMW or something that reflects their status, I know they have a gross vantage point and an orange center of gravity. If they say the most important thing is to lead a meaningful life, then I know that they are moving toward or have a subtle vantage point, and have or are moving toward a green center of gravity. If they say the most important thing is attaining liberation before I die, then I know they have a causal vantage point. And they have moved at least partially into second tier cognition. This is so important, and useful. And don't worry if you don't get it, it takes a long time. So here is another view of the level-line fallacy, it is Integral Zen's full Wilber Combs lattice, after the level-line fallacy in an individual raised in a modern or postmodern social holon.

Looking at this, we have the five states that I like to use. We have the full spectrum

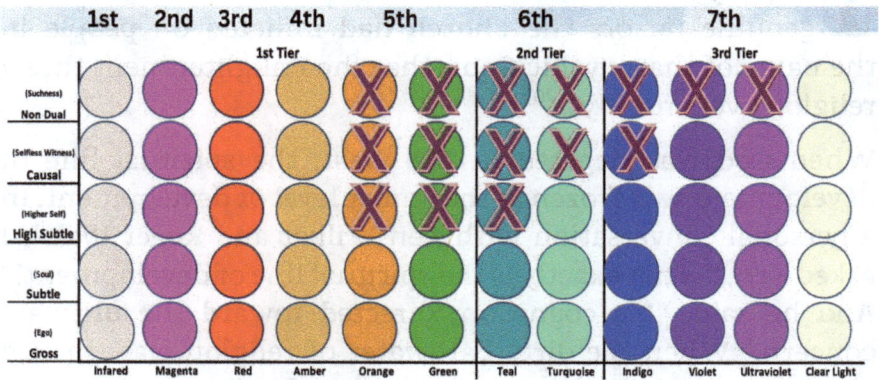

	1st	2nd	3rd	4th	5th		6th		7th			
				1st Tier			2nd Tier		3rd Tier			
(Suchness) Non Dual					X	X	X	X	X	X	X	
(Selfless Witness) Causal					X	X	X	X	X			
(Higher Self) High Subtle					X	X	X					
(Soul) Subtle												
(Ego) Gross												
	Infared	Magenta	Red	Amber	Orange	Green	Teal	Turquoise	Indigo	Violet	Ultraviolet	Clear Light

of evolution of ego development and what happens at orange is everything spiritual is rejected with religion, the baby of spiritual attainment is thrown out with the dirty bath water of religion. And the third eye, the intuitive eye is stuck half closed. There's no movement at orange, green or even at teal. Looking at structural development alone at turquoise, there's some movement into the high, subtle transpersonal realm, the archetypal realm, the realm of gods and goddesses, of hindering and helpful spirits. At orange, spirituality is rejected. At green, because the 5th chakra is connected to the second chakra and the magenta level of development, we have a version of spirituality that is mired in magenta. It's stuck

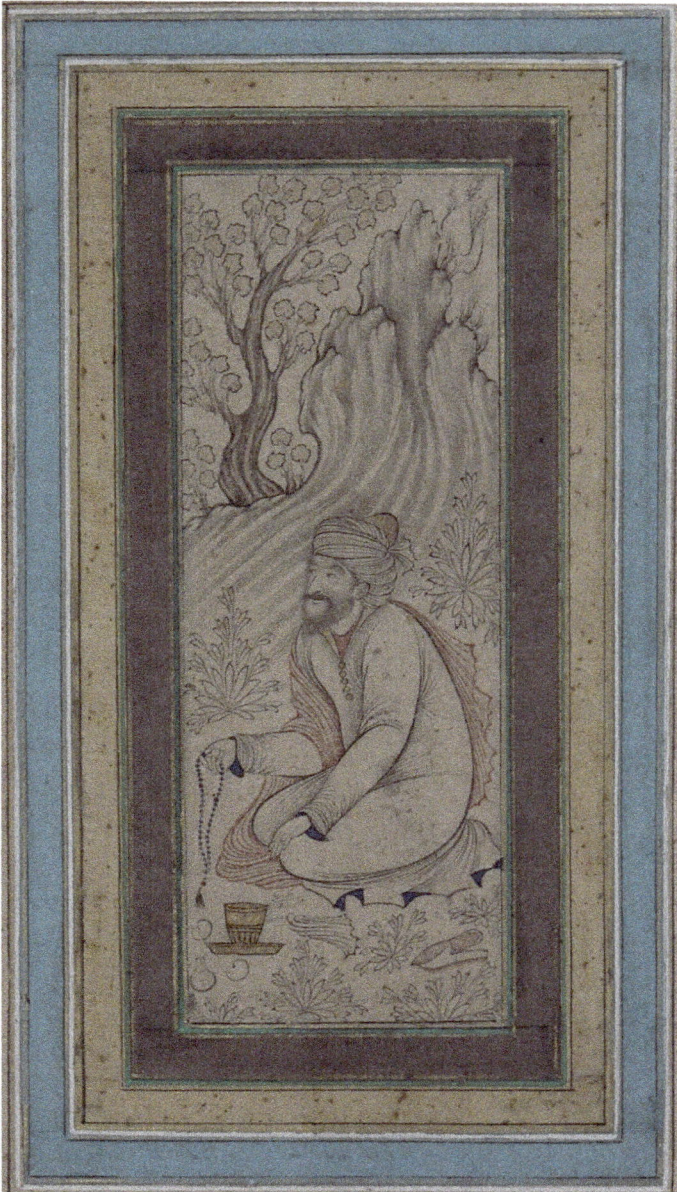

Man with Prayer Beads, Painting by Muhammad `Ali, mid-17th century, Attributed to Iran, Isfahan, Gift of Alexander Smith Cochran, 1913, Metropolitan Museum of Art NY, Open Access at a level of consciousness and social development that is typical of pagan culture. The magenta world is full of spirits, and can't emerge into the archetypal realm of gods and goddesses. The magenta stickiness pollutes the high-subtle realm of transpersonal psychology, and keeps it from developing in a pure, healthy way. The pollution is even worse when it comes to the causal realm of the witnessing mind that is so important, let alone non-dual suchness. At teal, we are intellectually excited about seeing multiple perspectives and being able to hold them at least intellectually. At turquoise, we finally begin to move into the archetypal realm of more sophisticated aspects of transpersonal psychology. But it's not until indigo that things really begin to shake loose, unless you have a serious meditation practice. Sorry to firehose you, but I think this is a perfect time to begin presenting some of the complexities of the Integral Zen Framework so some will be intrigued or perhaps inspired by all of this.

Janel

Thank you Doshin, I really want to appreciate the brilliance with which you lay these frameworks out here. I mean, this is really exciting. I could never present it in that way, obviously, so I just want to appreciate what you shared with us because it's really something extraordinary. Thank you.

The Sixth Chakra, The Third Eye

third eye, Sanskrit Ajna

adolescence to adulthood, Integral 2nd Tier

- Location: Front, center point between eyebrows (the third eye), back, center point at back of the skull
- Essential Functions: Intuition, imagination, connection to energies beyond our 3-D experience, energies connected to dead ancestors and family members, archetypal energies, energy transcending conventional / relative time and space, duality and ordinary life, the experience of merging with environment and transcending physical boundaries, turning ordinary beliefs upside down, spirituality
- Meridians: No meridians associated with the sixth chakra
- Areas of body: Forehead, back of head, temples, eyes and ears
- Developmental needs: Our need for a more spiritual understanding of our world

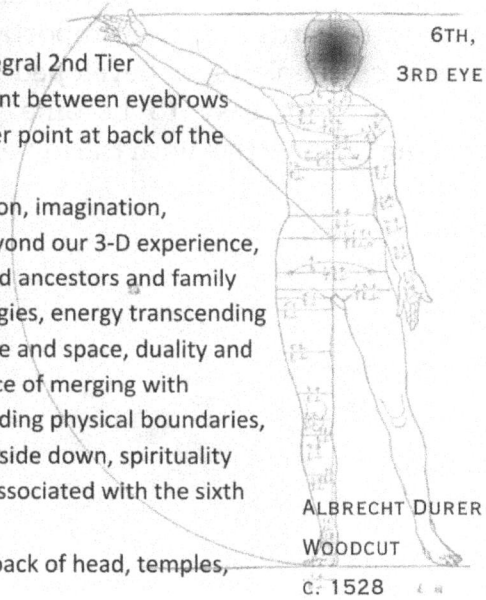

6TH, 3RD EYE

ALBRECHT DURER
WOODCUT
c. 1528

CHAKRAS
SUPERIMPOSED

Third eye themes

Intuition – Perception – Clarity – Creativity – Right View – Inner Guidance – Visualization – Siddhi Powers – Archetypal Realm

We're going to recall here before we dig in, that the third eye is connected to the power chakra. There is a relationship between them, a pairing. Doshin was presenting all of this, but to reiterate, when you're going from the throat to the third eye, you're going from Integral first tier to second tier. Let's also be reminded that most people are going to remain at a gross level of state awareness for the third eye during their life, for both the third eye and crown chakras. To develop these chakras requires, well... Doshin says, one in a 10 million people *suddenly* become enlightened, but generally to evolve structurally and state wise, the upper chakras require you to make an effort, to practice, and then to work on development (healing and awakening). If this is something one has the intention towards, it's also important to get feedback from a person or people more developed and advanced state wise. Otherwise, it is easy to become unbalanced and have a delusional perspective with the upper chakras.

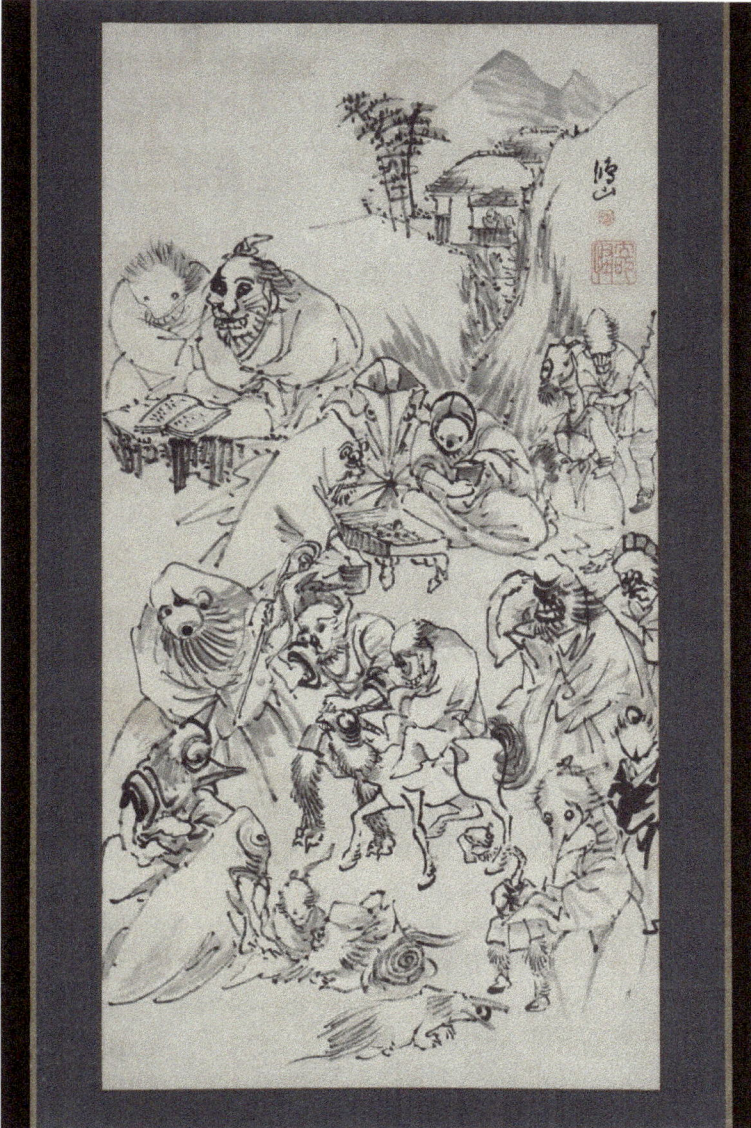

Demons and Monsters, Takai Kōzan 高井鴻山 (Japanese, 1806–1883), ca. 1870s, Japan, Mary and Cheney Cowles Collection, Gift of Mary and Cheney Cowles, 2022, Metropolitan Museum of Art, New York, Public Domain

This period developmentally, is less often happening during adolescence and more likely during adulthood. The location of the third eye is around the middle of the forehead, slightly above the center between the eyebrows. Simply put, the theme, if we could call it that, is purified intuition. A more gross expression might be imagination.

The third eye relates to realms and energies beyond our conventional experience. There are different ways of expressing this, different perspectives one can use in describing this, depending on the framework. It includes energies connected to the dead, ancestors, family members, and the archetypal realms. These are energies transcending conventional relative time and space, beyond going beyond.

So we can imagine there is a developmental *wall* between the throat and above, if we are remembering the integral first and second tiers. If you are entrenched in dualism and dualistic views, you likely will not evolve beyond the throat level developmental structure. The third eye relates to experiences of merging with one's environment, an energetic experience of transcending physical boundaries. The upside down view is a good way to put it. A very relative definition of developmental needs would be our need for a more spiritual understanding of our world. The development and purification of intuition, perception, clarity, creativity. It's a different kind of creativity, not conventional right view, but inner guidance, visualization being connected with this. Siddhi powers and the archetypal realms. So in terms of typology, for example, if you are in the Jungian sense an introverted intuitive for example, if that's your superior function, (that's what Carl Jung was, and that's what Doshin is), your intuition–and it's going to be different person to person, but–images, content, can just arise internally for you in the mind's eye. So when we're talking about visualizations, this will also depend on your dominant typology and individual capacities. This may be more, or less accessible to you.

In terms of the relationship with the power chakra, this seems really important because in observing people, when people experience themselves as disempowered–and there are almost infinite ways people can feel disempowered in this world that we live in–the third eye may go *askew* in all kinds of strange ways. In some sense, we could say, a person can develop a really *distorted third eye*, so for example being vulnerable to conspiracy theories, developing elaborate stories about the world, fixations about "us and them", paranoia, or on the other hand, grand delusions about one's personal influence, megalomania; just a few examples. We've talked about the pairings of chakras before, it seems also that I notice with people who are really disempowered they can tend to project their power and confuse this with archetypal forces in a way that can be very unhealthy. Likewise, there's another way you see examples of this with spiritual teachers, political leaders, with a sense of power very out of balance, and possibly extreme relationships with power.

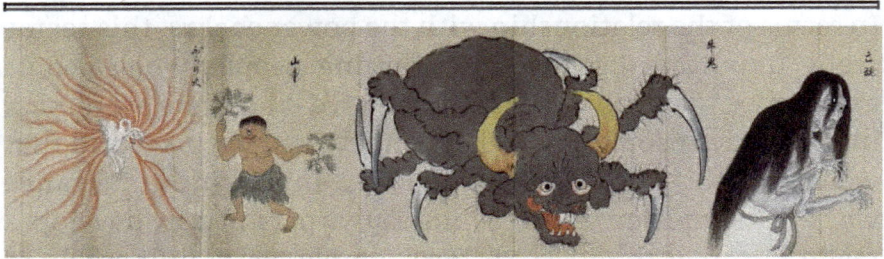

The Bakemono Zukushi "Monster" Scroll (18th–19th century), Artist, Date unknown, Japanese, Public Domain Mark 1.0 Universal

One of the other things that is noticeable is that sometimes when people are young, if their life is relatively difficult, or there is noted trauma, one can observe that higher abilities and upper powers, things like clairvoyance can be unusually advanced. I suspect there is some kind of energetic compensation that happens, although there are other ways to view this.[71]

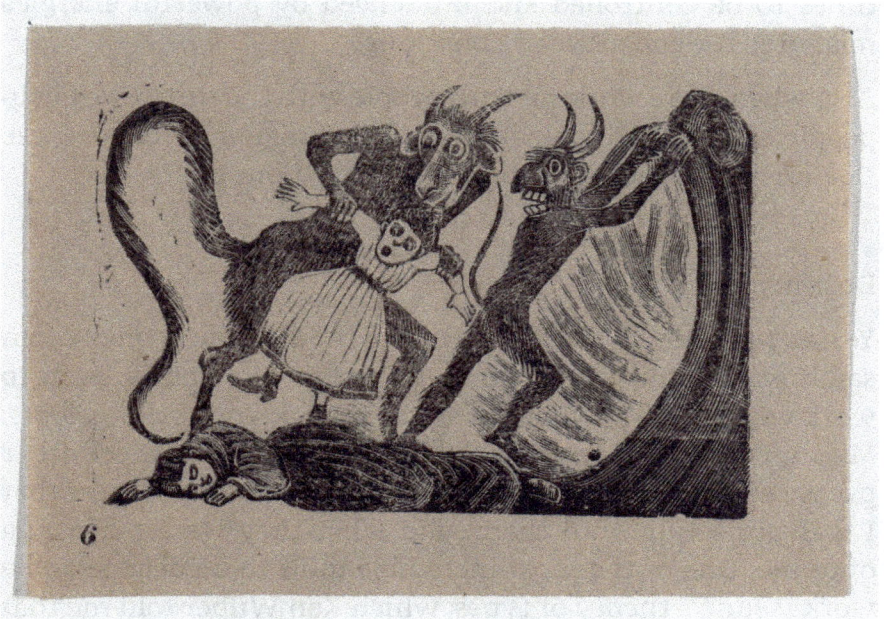

Plate 6: Terrible fate of a young woman who after a calumny was snatched by the devil and dragged to hell, José Guadalupe Posada (Mexican, Aguascalientes 1852–1913 Mexico City), ca. 1896, Prints, Gift of Jean Charlot, 1930, Metropolitan Museum of Art, New York, Public Domain

Meantime if your lower chakra drives aren't balanced, (potent drives, addictions, etc..) and you have some upper chakra abilities that are quite developed, for example powerful clairvoyant, or even magnetizing powers, if the lower chakras remain unbalanced and dysfunctions unhealed, the result can be powerful upper chakras and influence that can potentially cause great harm. I suspect that some of the most powerful fascists and dictators of the world had and have this kind of energetic dysfunction going on. Also I suspect some of these people may have experienced what is considered *archetypal possession* (some could call it demonic possession, which we'll talk about in later courses), where the person can appear at times to be controlled and influenced by powerful energies related to the collective unconscious.

Also when we're working with people with the third eye, I help people explore and look at what their Jungian typologies are. Doshin would you like to talk a little bit about this?

Doshin

Yes, as you know, I have been dubbed the Shadow Roshi. I often say it was because I had so many shadows, I had to learn to work with shadows. I had to learn to work with other people. My super power seems to be able to see the shadows of other people after I had seen them in myself. I could separate what I was projecting onto them, and what they were projecting onto me. One of the most incredible tools to do deep shadow work is Jung's theory of types, which Ken Wilber told me that he studied deeply. He said that he actually loved Jung's theory of types. In Jung's Theory of Types, there are four cognitive types. We have two types of cognitive functions that we use to gather information. They are sensation, "the five senses", and we have intuition, "direct knowing." Then, we have two cognitive functions that we use to process information, and this is what Choan, one of my students, called *the little black box*, the processing box, which in Buddhism is the 6th sense consciousness, the Manovijnana, what Junpo my teacher called fuzzy thinking (feeling) and thinking. Think of the feeling function as "liking and disliking" and think of the thinking function as "categorizing in dualistic ways."

Myers Briggs popularized Jung's theory of types, by focusing on how different types of people get along and interact with each other, but they ignored one of the most valuable parts of Jung's theory. The theory of types is most valuable to help us identify, understand and work with our unconscious shadows. We each have a dominant and inferior function. If I am a primary intuitive type, then intuition is my dominant function. The opposite of that information gathering function of intuition is sensation and that is my inferior function. The dominant function is the one that I trust the most, and is identified with my persona, the part of my ego that I know. The inferior function is identified with my shadow, the part of myself that I have repressed. The inferior function is the one that I keep stumbling over. Once I become aware of which function is dominant and which function is my inferior function, It helps me become conscious of my shadow and better understand myself, the whole self. When you begin to explore from a Jungian perspective, your superior and inferior functions, you begin the journey of seeing the part of yourself that you cannot see, your shadow.

Each one of these four functions: sensation, intuition, feeling and thinking can be primarily directed inwardly or outwardly. For example, my dominant function of intuition is primarily directed inwardly. I am an introverted intuitive type. My inferior function is extraverted sensation. Ken seems to be an extroverted intuitive type. He came up with the four quadrants. Jung seems to be an introverted intuitive, and came up with his theory of the four types. These two typologies really complement one another in the way that we're using them in Integral Zen. This can be a tool and window to learn a lot about yourself, a lot of self knowledge, about both your persona and your shadow. So I think that's all I will say at this point.

Janel

Okay the only other thing, so whatever your dominant function is, the opposite-so it's either intuition and sensing, thinking and feeling–the opposite is your inferior function, and then the two others are auxiliary functions. However, the other thing is and we'll explore this more in the next courses, this is also very much developed in a framework of how you were raised, the time you were raised, the culture. So you know, in orange in the West, if you were raised, say, in the 1950s, if your natural superior function was *introverted feeling* let's say, and your parents were really amber just coming into orange, having very little awareness of their internal feeling world and, it's not like they don't have emotions, but they don't even see them as something substantive, so they may not prioritize nurturing you in your second chakra needs and meet those needs and develop them (this would depend on the inherited attachment style especially along the maternal line). So if you might have the superior function on the one hand, but if you're growing up in a place where there's a cultural bias, and there's always cultural biases, there's always ways that the culture and collectives are influencing us, you know, whatever the trend is, whatever your family's religion is, the economic socioeconomic status, education. All these different factors are greatly going to influence how you develop. So if your superior function is not being supported by your caretakers and environment, then this is really going to not only alter you, but sometimes this can create the seeds of significant shadows. This can be traumatizing to a child, even if the parents are meaning well.

We're going to explore much more of this context that I'm describing, like the historical cultural context, so that people will get a better sense of what their circumstance was in order to understand how they developed, in the next course.

Third Eye Exercise 6

third eye exercise 6

Answer scale 0-5, 0 least / no, 5 most / yes

- presently in my life do I see karmic patterns?
- am I aware of my intuition?
- do I trust my intuition?
- have I explored from a Jungian perspective, my superior and inferior functions, introverted vs extraverted?intuition versus sensing? thinking versus feeling?
- which do I believe is my dominant function? which my inferior function? which are my auxiliary functions?

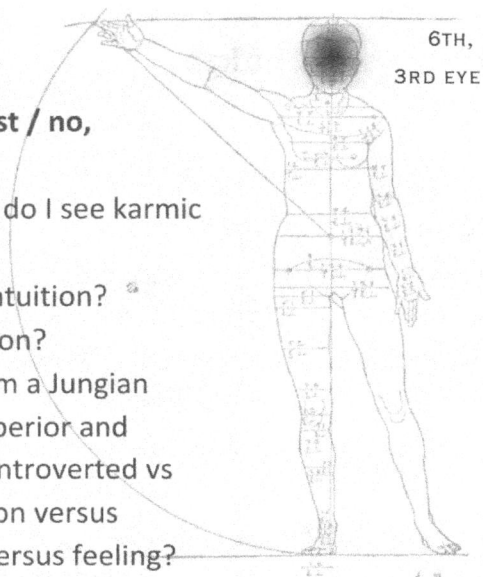

6TH,

3RD EYE

ALBRECHT DURER

WOODCUT

C. 1528

CHAKRAS

SUPERIMPOSED

In case you haven't noticed, we're condensing loads of information today. We're moving on to the crown. I often say to people with these upper chakras; not only should you not be jumping up to develop them prematurely, (remember the heart is at the center); these upper chakras are going to reflect the health of the lower chakras, your health and healing, and they're going to also depend on your own efforts, your own practice, your own good fortune and merit in finding teachers, good teachers who can guide you.

The Crown Chakra

7TH, CROWN

crown, Sanskrit Sahasrara
Integral 3rd Tier
- Location: Beyond physical body, just above crown of the head
- Essential Functions: Awareness, liberation from mind, freedom from thinking and all earthly experiences: mental, emotional, and sense based
- Developmental stage: Die before you die so you can truly live
- Developmental needs: Awakening

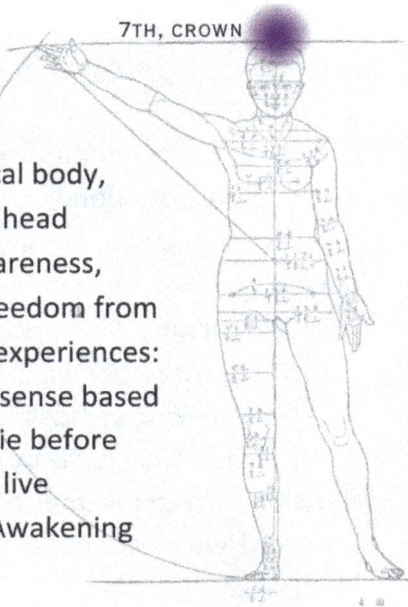

crown themes
Consciousness – Awareness – Spirituality – Presence – Transcendence – Awakening – No-self

ALBRECHT DURER
WOODCUT
C. 1528

CHAKRAS
SUPERIMPOSED

There are many warnings about going straight to develop higher developmental capacities related to these chakras without taking care of so many other factors related to one's basic development, your basic health and healing. Also it's equally dangerous if one has not been on a path of introspection. This is increasingly problematic in terms of psychedelic and plant medicine use these days, people wanting state experiences and not having established an internal foundation to ground or hold this within. It's considered dangerous to try to shoot up into the stratosphere, without being rooted in all senses of the word, and people, I mean, I would say looking out to the spiritual world now, people are really messing with all kinds of things, thinking there are shortcuts (*a hard earned mantra of mine, there are no shortcuts*) and I will not be surprised to see a lot of psychological trouble and breakdown among a lot of you know, well-intentioned but not well informed, people in their 20s, 30s and 40s eager to evolve, but just not getting the right context or feedback to know that you you can't skip, can't bypass, what must be addressed, one way or another, without risking psychic chaos, breakdown, some of which is more recoverable than others. Unfortunately it seems we are on the precipice of many individual and societal problems resulting from this, as first time plant medicine and psychedelic use is dramatically on the rise.[72]

The crown is the area connected with (also working with the root and heart) spiritual development, evolution, potential for awakening; the specific location is at the top of the head, at the crown and beyond the physical body. The potential of experiencing and even stabilizing pure awareness, liberation, freedom from thinking and all earthly experiences, mental, emotional and sense based freedom, no self. In Zen this is called *dying before you die*, so you can truly live. Also a reminder these higher chakras have great potential for reception to the highest levels of consciousness transcending relative individual awareness. Again, these higher chakras we will explore in more detail in future courses, remember, this is an introduction. Would you like to add anything Doshin?

Doshin

One thing, don't forget the crown chakra is connected to the heart chakra and the

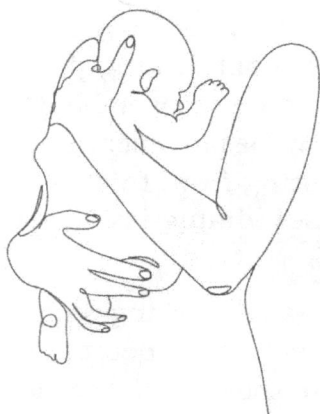

Babies and children need to be safe, need to be seen, need to be taken care of, and those needs developmentally met in each stage / chakra

If these needs are not met healthily in a child's development in the lower chakras (1-3), there is a high likelihood that imbalances in any and all chakras, starting at the lower three will act as drivers of unmet needs and contribute to personality disorders and split off shadow subpersonalities in adult life, unless the root causes are addressed and healed

root chakra. If you don't feel safe, then your heart remains closed and can't begin to open. The root chakra is the first stage of attachment and development. If you physically were not safe and you continue to feel not safe, you will continue to feel that way until the insecure attachment is repaired in attachment theory. In our view Integral Zen is that since we're not machines, we are not going to be repaired. We are human beings, therefore we heal. So when you begin to heal your root chakra issues, your heart naturally begins to open. And, if your heart doesn't fully heal and break open, you will never find liberation. The root chakra is connected to the heart chakra, and the heart chakra is connected to the crown chakra. Swaha.

Crown Exercise 7

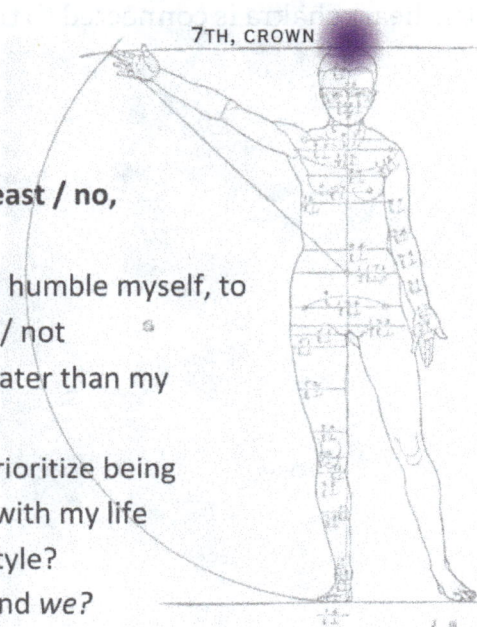

7TH, CROWN

crown exercise 7

**Answer scale 0-5, 0 least / no,
5 most/ yes**

- Do I connect, and humble myself, to a source / power / not knowingness, greater than my "self" (be honest)
- How much do I prioritize being present "NOW", with my life choices and life style?
- Am I free of *me* and *we?*

ALBRECHT DURER
WOODCUT
C. 1528

CHAKRAS
SUPERIMPOSED

Janel

Thank you so here's another exercise for us. The critical part of development beyond the throat chakra, for self reflection, do I connect and humble myself to a source of power, not-knowingness, greater than myself? How much do I prioritize being present, within how I live my life? Is presence a priority? Then, am I free of both me, and we?

So summarizing this course. Let's recall the importance of attachment, and how babies and children need to be safe. They need to be seen, need to be taken care of and those needs developmentally met in each stage. So I hope all of you see this at least see this in what we've reviewed. If these needs are not met healthily in a child's development in the lower chakra developmental periods, there's a high likelihood that imbalances in any and all chakras starting at the lower three, will act as *drivers of unmet needs* and potentially contribute to personality disorders, and split-off shadows or sub-personalities in adult life. Unless the *root causes* are addressed and healed, and one of the things I really want to point to here is that there's so much out in the therapeutic world that I don't think really identifies nor addresses root causes- especially karma. I think it's like a Band-Aid, that falls off at least once a day, on the mere manifestations, symptoms of the deeper problems.

Doshin

Yes, and I'd like to add something to that. I would go so far as to say that as wonderful as psychotherapy and the many different variations of psychotherapy are, there is nothing in Western psychology that can get beyond the psychology into the root causes that are karmic. Western psychology has no tools to get into karma, and this is where the deepest disturbances are both individually and collectively. When we're working with people, we find that you can't really get to the healing, until you start digging into your family, karma and your ethnic karma and the karma of what it means to be human that seems buried in the deepest, most hideous darkness. Only when this territory is brought into consciousness into the light of day, can the deep healing really begin. I want to say that very clearly. This is why you need the ancient wisdom of the religious lineage traditions that have been around for a long time. To dig into this territory, you need psychotherapists who have a high enough Kosmic Address that they can see this and have practiced meditation religiously. In my experience, these are rare and far between in this current age.

Janel

Yes, since the likelihood of finding psychotherapists with a high Kosmic Address is very slim, you work on your understanding of Kosmic Address to know you know, to really discern, oh, I can get this (structural level) help from this person and this is their kind of limited capacity, and then get something else from other people, which is probably the more realistic way.

Doshin

Thank you Janel, thank you for adding that.

Janel

Sure. So continuing, just a reminder, of what secure attachment health in the lower chakras in an individual might look like. Attuning to one's own emotions and needs. Developing a healthy, or healthier, self. This is critical and this cannot be skipped. First just knowing one's needs, preferences, limits, etcetera, you know we are in the present world which means being conditioned to just exist and delusionally expecting everything will be met externally. And it's just a horrible lie. So be real with oneself, and others, regarding this.

We can attune to the emotions and needs of others, we can become a secure attachment base for one's own environment and others, and practice what the trauma expert Bessel Van der Kolk[73] calls, *safe reciprocity* in relationships. For those with early trauma and insecure attachment, Van der Kolk summarizes similar conclusions that we see in our work in Integral Zen. The conclusion being that talk therapy focused on insight is generally often not effective. I think Doshin added not effective *enough*. Preverbal trauma and I would posit that also ancestral and karmic as well as collective trauma tends to be unconsciously acted out, not just once, but over and over and over again, and will not stop unless it is brought into consciousness, and then able to be disrupted. This is exactly what we are seeing in the world now. Somatic and preverbal approaches in treatment are more effective as a first step, so again, until the 3rd chakra, it's preverbal. We don't have the language for our experience, therefore most of the time (there are always exceptions), we can't remember it. It's in our body, so we need other ways to work with it. So bodywork, yoga, internal martial arts, massage, singing, dancing, meditation can all be effective. It's going to vary person to person. For certain kinds of insecure attachment and trauma, healing will take years, and potentially and depending on your view, I would say, a lifetime. The focus is on you regaining trust internally (to start) and building a healthy self or sense self.

Doshin

A healthy sense of self and a healthy relationship to power.

Janel

In order to develop and establish secure attachment, it's good to remember that our brains have neuroplasticity, so we can change and heal, and also that attachment styles are not genetic.[74] Generally it is said to keep a minimum of healthy social connection, people need at least one person from whom they can have some type of secure relationship for basic psychological health. Also to know, that at any time in life, one can develop and heal insecure attachment.

G etting back to karma, so I'm going to present some Buddhist perspectives. If it works for you, great, but you don't have to believe any of this. The Sowa Rigpa tradition teaches that families, parents and children come together due to karma. I see how this perspective is actually very helpful for healing. The concept of collective and family karma is called *Chi le* in Tibetan, which can make it easier to accept difficult family situations, limitations, the size of your family, still birth, etcetera when one accepts this as due to karma. Also from the East, is a context and framework of duty and connection to family that tends to be lacking in the West. There's a really strong familial sense of attachment that's quite different in Tibet for one, although depending on the province, some of the areas are matriarchal, where it's not unusual for women to have different fathers for their children, and they can keep this private.

I want to emphasize the importance, again from a Buddhist perspective, of *mind protection*. I'd mentioned before the secondary causes of illness and disease within Sowa Rigpa, and *provocations* can result from cause and effect/karma. COVID is a provocation, as is global climate change. Things like spirit possession, illnesses from such things. In the view of general health, a discursive mind can become extremely damaging for people. You may have noticed that we're frequently reminding you to meditate as a practice for awakening, but it's also for your basic physical and mental health, all of your well-being. Discursive mind, discursive thought, including fear, left unrestrained, invites the conditions for disease, and opens up all kinds of gateways to all kinds of physical and psychological illness. This may be a perspective that seems strange, but for the view of protecting your own mind, I would really really encourage being open to this. We talked before, you know, about being mindful of all the sense stimuli we let in, what we see, what we hear, the impact of hateful words. We talk about self care so often in the West these days, but true self care starts with realizing and being proactive in protecting your own mind. And if you need to get help, seek it. People have much more power to help your body and mind heal than they often realize.

Doshin

I'd like to say something here.

Janel

Sure.

Doshin

This is a perfect opportunity to use Integral semiotics. Discursive is such an interesting word and the meaning has begun to change. I looked it up in the dictionary. The word has two very different definitions. The first definition for discursive is *wandering,* so you're telling a discursive story, you're telling a story that wanders all over the place and doesn't really get to the point. That's one meaning of discursive. The second meaning of discursive, is *not intuitive.* Now these two different meanings can seem quite different, or they can seem complementary, if I'm at an orange level of development and I have rational thinking and empiricism on my altar, and I don't even know that I have an altar. But that's what I'm worshipping in an unconscious amber way. Discursive is *not intuitive,* which means that intuition will be negated by an extroverted thinking sensation type. If I'm an introverted intuitive type, then I'm going to see the value of intuition. It is possible to both be deeply intuitive and not wander around, but that intuition is not going to be recognized or valued by somebody with a Kosmic Address that is emphasizing orange rational thinking and outward sensation. Anything intuitive is going to be rejected or interpreted as wandering around talking about nothing that is important or real. Especially the things that are in the internal left hand quadrants in Integral Theory. It is these internal things in the left hand quadrants that need the precision of language. The precision of measurement works very well in the external right hand quadrants, but not so well in the internal left hand quadrants. This can be a little confusing and it doesn't need to be. Jung's theory of types is most valuable here. We really need to understand and communicate about exactly what the word discursive means, and understand how it is being interpreted in order to truly communicate with each other. Which definition is appropriate for the circumstances? If you're just locked onto one definition and so that I say that because this is so important. Non-intuitive thoughts can be really misunderstood by intuitive people, as can wandering rational thoughts. Protecting your own mind from both the positive and negative biases of the different individual and collective holons is really important. There's so much more I could say about all this, but not now, this is just an introduction.

Janel

Gampopa

Let's look at Gampopa, a 12th century doctor and great Buddhist tantric master (founder of the Kagyu school). In the 12th century he wrote this advice for remedying mental afflictions. This is related to the topic of discursive thought, and keep in mind this was written for monks.

Gampopa's (12c) advice for remedying Mental Afflictions (especially for monks)

"The antidote for desire-attachment is meditating on ugliness

The antidote for anger-hatred is meditating on loving-kindness

The antidote for confusion is meditation on interdependent origination

The antidote for jealousy is meditating on equalizing yourself and others

The antidote for pride or egotism is meditating on exchanging yourself and others

When you experience the kleshas or afflictive emotions coarsely and in equal measure or when you have a lot of discursive thoughts, meditate on the breath"

-GAMPOPA, SUMMARY OF THE SUTRIC APPROACH
TO REMEDYING MENTAL AFFLICTIONS, THE JEWEL
ORNAMENT OF LIBERATION[75]

So these were the antidotes for what you should meditate on, and some may find this helpful now. The antidote for desire, attachment, is meditating on ugliness. The antidote for anger, hatred, is meditating on loving kindness. The antidote for confusion is meditating on interdependence. I'm going to talk about that in a minute. The antidote for jealousy? Meditating on equalizing yourself and others. The antidote for pride or egotism is meditating on exchanging yourself and others. And then lastly, this is just such great advice when you experience the kleshas or afflictive emotions coarsely and in equal measure, or when you have a lot of discursive thoughts, meditate on the breath, just going back to shamatha. Some of this is some really traditional advice here. So if this speaks to you, then you know, look into it more. You've heard Doshin talk about it before.

12 links of Dependent Origination
Samsara, or "we are little hamsters running in a wheel"-Dr. Nida

- Ignorance, Not knowing / seeing
- Mental Imprint, Formation
- Consciousness
- Name and Form
- The Six Sensory Fields or Bases
- Contact
- Sensation, Feeling
- Craving
- Grasping
- Becoming
- Rebirth
- Old Age and Death

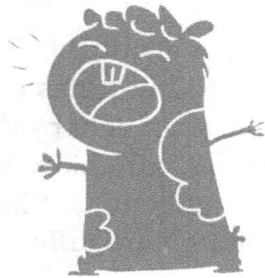

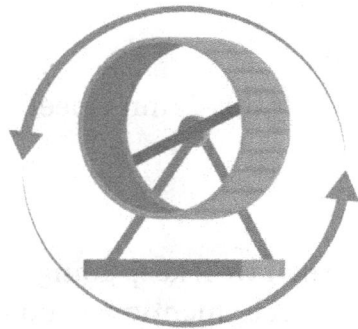

The 12 Links of Dependent Origination

Moving onto another essential Buddhist teaching, are the *12 links of dependent origination.* Basically the wheel of life, birth, sickness, old age and death, samsara or as Dr. Nida says, how "we are little hamsters running in a wheel." So this is an outline of Samsaric existence, that supposedly the night when the Buddha awoke, he saw Karma, which is he saw his past lives, and as a result he came up with 12 links. And this was part of a great teaching of the links, or that, you know, one thing leading to another, the stages of samsara. It is said, I don't know if you've heard, but there's a type of Buddha called the *lonely Buddha* called *pratyekabuddha*. These are people who were born in times where there's no Buddha Dharma around, no Dharma teachings, and so they awaken on their own ultimately through insight.

In talking about this, he says that 12 specific links should be understood in terms of three groups. The links of dependent origination taught by the sage are encompassed in these three categories, Affliction, Karma and suffering. The 1st, 8th and 9th are afflictions. The 2nd and 10th are Karma, while the remaining 7 are suffering. Doshin, anything to add?

Doshin

Get me off this damn wheel.

Janel

Okay, then we'll keep going. So here's another thing. I think it's important to mention a quote by Garchen Rinpoche, who lives in Arizona, an extraordinary teacher. He spent many years in a Chinese Communist prison. He actively teaches and you can still study with him. Not that I am qualified to judge, but he seems like an awakened being. So he writes about the ripening of Karma,

> "After entering the path of Dharma and practicing
> for many years, some people fall under the power of
> inner obstacles and adverse conditions..sometimes they
> experience various physical illnesses and the like..it is
> said that however profound one's practice is, there will be
> correspondingly great obstacles to the path... Throughout

*this and former lives, one has accumulated negative
actions that have not yet ripened into suffering. ..if one
can bring illness, affliction and other obstacles onto the
path through recognizing provocation and liberating it in
the moment, one will attain a great, high ground."[76]*

KYABJE GARCHEN RINPOCHE

There is illness and you know, with it, all kinds of challenges that can arise. From a Buddhist view this happens due to the ripening of karma, so that the seeds of illness may have been planted lifetimes ago, and it is taught that we never know when it's going to ripen. So while we're presenting certain relative frameworks around chakras and what you need to work on, there's this. From the Buddhist view, this is an extraordinary opportunity to awaken. From whatever is on your plate, as Doshin might say, whatever comes and shows up on your plate (which Junpo said, "Eat what's on your plate").

I like to remind people that we can't really talk about healing if we don't include death, and preparation for death. A healthy relationship with the fact that we will all die, and some of us will die sooner than others, and sooner than we expect. Preparing for this, from a Buddhist view, makes perfect sense. At the same time, we don't want to demonize illness. We don't want to stigmatize illness. Illness is just like death, a natural part of life. For me, I have found Buddhist teachings extremely helpful and have allowed me to make peace with so many things, that until I was presented with this view, really, caused a lot of mental emotional internal confusion, and so I would say these views can be very liberating.

Next, we don't want to forget, we want to always remember. I think that's what Rabjam Rinpoche told Doshin when they met on a retreat, "Always start with Bodhicitta." And what actually is Bodhicitta?..it is the mind that is aimed at awakening with wisdom and compassion for the benefit of all sentient beings.

"Precious bodhicitta protects the mind from afflictions. ..one should begin to nurture conventional bodhicitta first by contemplating the kindness of loved ones, then by cultivating patience for those enemies who despise one."[77]

GARCHEN RINPOCHE

Garchen Rinpoche mentions protecting your mind. Bodhicitta will protect your mind. One first begins to nurture what is called *conventional bodhicitta*, and then can work towards developing *ultimate bodhicitta* or *absolute bodhicitta*, which is awakening. To work simply in this way, first, we can contemplate the kindness of loved ones. Then, we can cultivate patience for those enemies who we may despise. Practices like *The Four Immeasurables* are a perfect tool for starting to generate conventional bodhicitta.

Doshin

Does anybody have any questions that you've written down and are dying to ask? Questions that will contribute to the group and the container we have built.

Question

Something I didn't understand and I realized as time passed, maybe I probably don't need to understand it, but. I was a little stuck on the concept that certain stages get stuck. One can't go any further in spiritual development like the modern orange stage. I was thinking of somebody like Einstein.

Doshin

What I want to really caution you is not to make a theology or a dogma out of this. You know, the Buddha said: *Do not trust teachers. Do not trust teachings, only trust your own direct experience.* So, the minute I say anything about what's really important, the most important things, I'm lying. Because the most important things cannot fit into dualistic language, and the minute somebody believes one of my lies, then they've created a barrier to healing and awakening for themselves. They've created a dogma, a "sacred lie" that they need to liberate themselves from, but that sacred lie, that dogma can become a path, that they walk and practice and will lead them to a deeper awakening and a broader healing. Einstein, you know, I would say based on things I've read of his, he is way into second-tier on the development scale, and he had a deep level of awakening.

We're creating an Integral Framework out of Integral Theory, and there's one thing to remember about any theory; it's just a theory. Don't believe it, it's not the truth. It's a theory which automatically means it's wrong. So there are many exceptions to what we're presenting. This is a general framework to follow, not dogmatize. Do not try to understand it as gospel. I would give you an example of Byron Katie. I've met Byron Katie. In my view, she's one in 10 million that actually just woke up without any meditation or religious practice. One in 10 million people will spontaneously wake up. How would a Buddhist describe her? Well, we have no idea of what her karma is from previous lifetimes. I don't know if that's true, but I would acknowledge that she is very awake and she never meditated in this life at all. So, take what we're saying, the framework we're representing, with a grain of salt. It is extremely useful and it can really help you, but don't believe it. Don't make a dogma out of it. And when we try to understand something, that's what we often do. So is that helpful?

Questioner

Yes. Thank you.

Doshin

Great.

Questioner

Well, it's interesting what is being said. I can relate to it most, let's say on an individual level. But at the same time I'm struggling with all the suffering in the world, and all the traumas that each day, violent situations, new traumas again and again and again. It's like a circle.

Doshin

So let me interrupt you and ask you a question so that I can understand what you're saying. You said you're understanding it individually. But only individuals suffer. Do groups suffer?

Questioner

Yes.

Doshin

Only individuals. There is no suffering outside of individuals.

Questioner

Let's say what I mean is that the tools for healing and so on in general are for the individual.

Doshin

That's because only individuals suffer.

Questioner

Okay.

Doshin

Only individuals can awaken; groups of people, cultures, social holons cannot awaken.

Questioner

Yes, okay, but what I mean is let's say maybe I can pay for healing for myself, yes, but. There are so many individuals, individuals with trauma in the world, how can they heal?

Doshin

Well, the same way that you can heal, there is no way to heal everybody.

Janel

There are religious practices to practice and support others.

Questioner

Yes, okay, okay, yes.

Janel

There are many.

Doshin

But only individuals can do something. Only individuals have agency. Anything we do collectively often creates *more* suffering. Because we create a belief system; this is where it gets so tricky, and this is where the moment we all get together and believe something, we're creating an us, and a them. There are those that believe what we do, and those that don't believe what we do. In that us and them, we've created a war. If that polarization increases, we're turning up the knob of the intensity of suffering. You know what happened in Israel is horrible. What's happening in Gaza is horrible. The minute you start talking to anybody about it, the conversation itself is going to polarize, and yes, war is always completely horrible. That's just true. I don't need to polarize and take sides to see that.

Janel

To step back a minute, if we take a Sowa Rigpa, Tibetan Buddhist framework, I would recall *provocations*, so there's cause and effect on an individual level, and when human beings don't respect the smaller systems, you know, like local systems, of which they're a part of, these provocations can grow and get worse. So these systems kind of get more complicated and grow bigger and the problems grow bigger and bigger, like climate change, war. Ultimately, I mean, if you look at this kind of five element balance that all of form existence is in, this elemental balance is constantly going in and out of, constantly seeking balance. Eventually, if it's too out of balance, you have, you know for example, a massive ecosystem collapse. Cause and effect. So, in some sense, stepping back, looking at everything, cause and effect. Really, on a personal level, clarifying what you have power over, what you don't have power over. Then practicing, for the benefit of all beings. How much can be done?

Doshin

As Rohab Rinpoche once told me, Always start with Bodhicitta, and I would add, just notice when the bodhicitta is interrupted, by *me*. And then return to Bodhicitta, and balance. Balancing the opposites, the five elements, the types. Doing the best we can possibly do. If you find yourself in a war, in Israel or Ukraine? Practice dying. It's an incredible opportunity. It is the dharma gate which is wide open. Let your heart break open with Bodhicitta, with clarity and compassion we can rest in absolute equanimity, zero reactivity, unconditional love, compassion, and boundless joy, no matter what. That is Buddha Nature. To get to Buddha Nature, you have to experience every aspect of human nature, and there's no place that you can see the worst of human nature more clearly, than war.

Janel

I saw a lovely quote by the Buddhist teacher Robert Thurman, which was something like the more along you get in your practice, the more fear you have of hatred, than of dying. For me, that sums up a lot.

Questioner

Hi, thank you, you talked about clairvoyance, and I don't want to let that go because I want to ask you if you're talking about. So if I understood you right, some people you're saying some people talk to dead people. That's related in the context of having the Crown chakra function? Is that what you're talking about?

Janel

I don't recall what the exact definition of clairvoyance is, but we're talking about siddhi powers, so...

Doshin

So I'd like to interrupt here.

Doshin

When we're talking about clairvoyance, we're talking mainly about intuition about direct knowing. This is where the Wilber Combs lattice becomes extremely useful. Because at every level of consciousness, each one of these colors has a different interpretation of what is clairvoyance and what isn't. And every state of consciousness, every vantage point, every stabilized state of consciousness has a different degree of how clairvoyant, how open that third eye is. So when we open a conversation about something like clairvoyance in a group of people there are going to be so many different opinions about what clairvoyance is. They are going to be all over the place. It's not actually a helpful conversation to have in a group in my experience.

Questioner

It means different things to different people you're saying?

Doshin

Well, to me it means knowing something directly immediately, but it has different interpretations at every level of consciousness. So somebody that's at a magenta level of consciousness is going to have a very different view, interpretation of what direct knowing is. Somebody at an amber level of consciousness is going to use it to see who's following the rules and who isn't and who we should kill. Somebody at an orange level of consciousness is likely to deny that there is such a thing, and unconsciously use this direct knowing to improve their status and make money. Somebody at a green level of consciousness is going to use their interpretation of what to do with clairvoyance, with direct knowing, to be meaningful and to improve their status by being seen as being more meaningful. Somebody at teal is going to use that clairvoyance to improve their ability to hold multiple perspectives, and so on. There is no real fully open pure complete clairvoyance until clear, light nondual suchness all the way at the upper right hand part of that Wilber Combs lattice. So that's why it's really difficult to have a meaningful conversation that produces anything useful when people are all over the board at different Kosmic Addresses.

"The Way is perfect like great space,
Without lack, without excess.
Because of grasping and rejecting,
You cannot attain it.
Do not pursue conditioned existence;
Do not abide in acceptance of emptiness.
In oneness and equality,
Confusion vanishes of itself.
Stop activity and return to stillness,
And that stillness will be even more active.
Merely stagnating in duality,
How can you recognize oneness?"

excerpt, Faith in Mind - "Hsin Hsin Ming"
the Third Patriarch Seng Can, 6th Century
Translated by Chan Master Shen-yen

Questioner

Yes. Thank you Janel and Doshin for this course. I'm still a bit confused between the cleaning up and healing dimensions as I grew up in Wilber, you know, waking up, growing up, cleaning up and showing up, then Doshin added healing.

Doshin

Yes, I did. It was actually. You can blame Janel for that, by helping me see how much healing I still need to do, and how important it is for all of us.

Questioner

OK, I'll blame Janel.

Doshin

I just brought my Zen disease to the table and decided I needed to heal.

Questioner

Yeah. So thank you for speaking today about the limits of Western psychotherapy in this. And I believe that a large part of the healing area cannot be addressed or cannot be solved by only Western approaches. But still, can you talk a little bit more about this borderline between cleaning up a shadow work and does it ensure that there will be allergies and addictions?

Doshin

Yes. Western psychotherapy does a wonderful job at dealing with personality disorders in the context of a social holon, and the social holon that they're working with is a modern or postmodern culture with all its benefits and drawbacks. You can't fit in perfectly to an orange culture unless you're suffering from the insanity of being driven by greed, which is one of the poisons. You don't fit into a green, postmodern culture driven by social justice and democracy for all unless you're not infected by the poison of hating everybody that is not green, everyone that doesn't share your postmodern beliefs and values. So, what psychotherapy is doing is trying to make people fit into a culture that to some extent has gone insane.

Final assessment, solo or group exercise
- Which chakra or chakras feel more balanced? which chakra or chakras feel unbalanced?
- What are your lingering "themes" ?
- What are your biggest insights from the course?
- What did you learn that most surprised you?
- What do you wish to learn more about, or an activity or practice wish to explore further?
- How have your views around health and balance changed, if at all?

I personally, don't want to be sane in an insane culture. I mean, I don't want to be insane, like the culture is insane. Janel was quoting a Zen master, Dogen. She sent me a text, she said "The only person that can remain sane in an insane world is a Zen master" of course that made me laugh. And it's partially true. For me, it's true unless I'm attacked. Somebody's very likely to take a position if they are being shot at, it seems guaranteed. So let me go back to your original question, I wanted to really make it simple. I saw something that was not being addressed by focusing on just two simple things: healing and awakening. These two simple things that are extremely interrelated, have gotten lost in the integral confusion of with the focus on growing up, cleaning up, waking up, and showing up. That just kind of created confusion where too many people were thinking way too much, and the more they think about it, the more confusing it becomes. So healing and awakening is really simple. You can't heal, without getting to the early chakra dysfunctions and the karma, which are at the root, in my experience of the later chakra neuroses, the shadows and split off sub-personalities.

When Wilber says shadows are addictions and allergies in states and structures, and what drives them. The addictions and allergies are the poisons. Greed, hatred, ignorance are the main 3 poisons. Addictions are greed, allergies are hatred, and integral ignorance is not realizing the significance of the Wilber Combs lattice and using it to benefit all beings. This is all healing and awakening. And it's using Buddhist wisdom which Ken is intimately familiar with through his own practice. It's all about using Integral Theory. So I like to think of a triangle. You know, we have the polarity of healing and awakening, which is very useful, and then we add an apex which is becoming a better person. The spiritual line of development, the *sila* practices of early Buddhism, all religions have some sort of *sila* practices where we practice becoming a more moral and a better person. We stop sinning and we start acting like a saint. This is what I call spiritual development. Now that's not healing or awakening, but all three of these are interrelated. I'm kind of stirring up the muddy soup of waking up, growing up, cleaning up because it got too muddy. So I'd like to think of healing and awakening, which are really fundamental, and then don't forget about becoming a better person, having more integrity and then in order to do all of this, you really have to cultivate witnessing mind. And always start with Bodhicitta. Then stop poisoning yourself. You know, if you keep poisoning yourself, you're going to die. If you poison other people, they're going to die. So when you stop poisoning yourself with the *five poisons*, you still are left with *the hindrances*. The way you get rid of the hindrances is you practice being a better person, you practice *the paramitas,* and you keep practicing the paramitas until you arrive at what I consider the pure emotions of a Buddha: zero reactivity, unconditional love, selfless compassion, and unreasonable joy. Practicing these not just today, but always. And there's a teaching that I received from Junpo, his teacher Eido Roshi translated it from Japanese into English. JunPo cleaned up the English a bit. It is from the Sutra Book. It is the first chant in our morning service:

> Atta Dipa! You are this light. Pure selfless awareness.
> Rely upon selfless awareness. Do not rely upon concepts
> of self and other that appear. Do not depend upon beliefs,
> sensations and emotions which arise and fall away.
> Meditative awareness. Clear intention, acting wisely,
> compassionately, and skillfully, are this practice. Rely
> upon this only. Rely upon this ceaselessly.

To awaken we each must ceaselessly become this light, with no exceptions. Don't let anything disturb this practice of being this light and you will be a Buddha. Accept nothing less.

Is that helpful?

Questioner

That's a firehose. Thank you, Doshin

Janel

And while we're doing that, we're probably not going to get to it, but at the end of the materials, there is an old image of Green Tara. Now Green Tara practice is a practice you can do for healing of the self and for all beings. It is also a protector practice. You can get the practice and prayer *Praise to 21 Taras* online (Lotsawa House is a good source). You don't have to have taken refuge or have had an empowerment to do this practice. I know the world, current times are intense now, so anyone who's interested, might find this helpful. Also remember the *Faith in Mind* poem translated by Master Sheng Yen.[78] That living teaching that Doshin loves so much.

For the end of our teaching, let's look at a question that looks good to you. After all of this exploration, which chakra or chakras feel most more balanced? Which feel unbalanced? What are your biggest insights from the course? What did you learn that most surprised you? What do you wish to learn more about or an activity or practice you wish to explore further? How have your views around health and balance changed, if at all?

Janel

And if people want to say something different, it doesn't have to be. Of those questions. Please go ahead.

Questioner

Hi, so two days ago, I was in an accident, and broke 3 vertebrae in my back. And I nearly died, and so many of the things that have been discussed during these weeks were powerfully with me during those intense moments that I was laying there wondering what was going to happen. And I had such peace come over me. Thinking about, really the things your own, your voices, were running through my mind, from some of the stuff that was said. And since then, I've just felt such an amazing appreciation for everything. For every bite of food, for every breath, for all the love in my life and. And yet, I also acknowledge that there's this really big healing that needs to occur that makes total sense along the chakras. What you have taught, because my big issue was my third chakra, and my sense of personal power. I would always put other people, their needs ahead of mine, and play small and then, you know, maybe put down my anger and not express when I didn't like something. And that behavior actually led to this accident. Then having to now be in a place of receiving so much love and help.. and being quiet, and going within and just laying down and meditating and the connection between the third chakra and my and my third eye is really clear and the opportunity that I've been asking the universe for just hey, give me any space to just meditate. Well, it's been answered, so I really just wanted to express my appreciation. This course has been extremely profound for me, and will continue to have lasting effects as I move forward. So thank you.

Doshin

You've just broken our hearts all open; thank you. And deepest condolences. And congratulations. Wow.

Janel

I'm speechless. Feel free to contact us, we'd like to support you.

Questioner

Thank you. Thank you so much.

Janel

Thank you so much.

Doshin

Swaha. So let's just hold her in our hearts, for a bit, okay?

Janel

Thank you. Anybody else have anything?

Doshin

You always say the most brilliant things when you're muted.

Questioner

Right. I should stay muted. But anyway, I think that was incredibly deep and amazing sessions, which I can't even comment on, because it needs a lot of time to sink in and to reflect. But to thank you both, Janel and you for the incredible work you put into this course I think it is absolutely wonderful. What I realized is that the only thing that I can say now is that, each stage, even if you go to the top, carries a shadow.

Doshin

Swaha..

Questioner

But thank you from the depths of my heart for your work and for your dedication. And we are very lucky to have this. It is absolutely priceless. Thank you.

Janel

Thank you. It was so wonderful to have you here.

Questioner

Is it better to have one big shadow than lots of little ones? There's a question for Doshin.

Doshin

The answer is. Both are true. There's one big one and. Lots of little ones.

Questioner

So I hope that we can continue on that road because this was really an introduction, a beginning of reflection. It needs time for me, I feel I need time to digest most of the things, look at them. There is so much more that can be done together and I think I hope you continue.

Doshin

Thank you. That's our plan. Well, I think it's time, Janel.

Janel

Is it? Oh, we didn't hear from so many people, so.

Doshin

Yeah. I know there's just never enough time.

Janel

So one thing the next time is we will do the next course the first three chakras more in depth.

Doshin

So next time we'll roll up our sleeves and get in the muck. Mud slinging. So our next course, our intention is to begin with the early chakras and really dig into them. Healing the early chakras, from my perspective, is very important. The only place to start is where you are. But you really have to have a healthy little child, to develop a healthy adult, and you have to have a healthy self to get out of the prison of self. Start with where you are. But man, let's go play in the mud because it's a great place to start. Janel, thank you for what you've done and you really brought a feminine heart, compassion to my firehose. Swaha.

Janel

Thank you, Doshin. Thank you everyone. It was wonderful. Thank you.

Atta Dipa

You are This Light

Leader:

(You are this light) pure selfless awareness.

Rely upon selfless awareness.

Do not rely upon concepts of self and other that appear.

Do not depend upon beliefs, sensations, and emotions, which arise and fall away.

Meditative awareness, clear intention, acting wisely, compassionately and skillfully are this practice.

Rely upon this only!

Rely upon this ceaselessly!

Everyone:

I am this light, pure selfless awareness.

I rely upon selfless awareness.

I do not rely upon concepts of self and other that appear.

I do not depend upon beliefs, sensations, and emotions, which arise and fall away.

Meditative awareness, clear intention, acting wisely, compassionately and skillfully are this practice.

I rely upon this only!

I rely upon this ceaselessly!

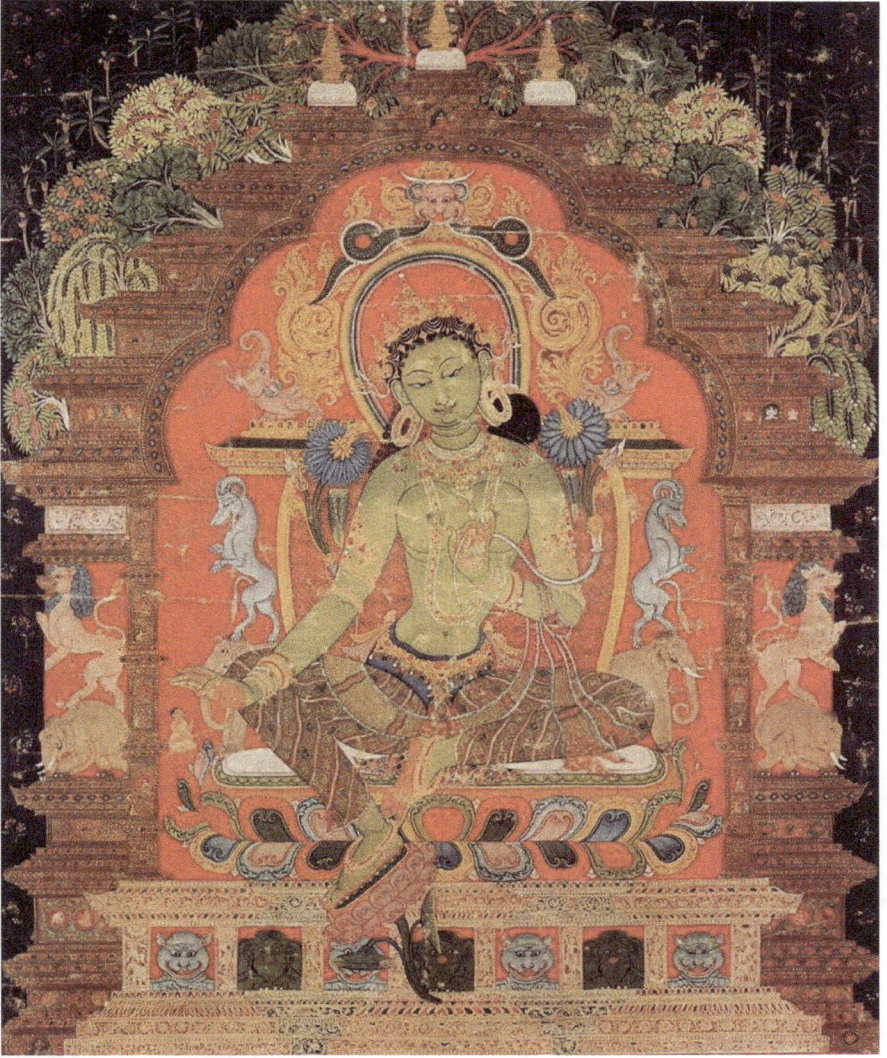

13th century Tibetan thangka painting of Green Tara, Araniko, 13th century, Public Domain

BIBLIOGRAPHY

Books

Barrett, L. F. (2017). How emotions are made: The Secret Life of the Brain. HarperCollins.

Brennan, B. A. (1987). Hands of light: A Guide to Healing Through the Human Energy Field : a New Paradigm for the Human Being in Health, Relationship, and Disease.

Bstan-'dzin-Rgya-Mtsho, D. L. X. (1997). Healing anger: The Power of Patience from a Buddhist Perspective. Motilal Banarsidass Publisher.

Chai, C., & Chai, W. (1967). Li Chi: Book of Rites: An Encyclopedia of Ancient Ceremonial Usages, Religious Creeds, and Social Institutions.

Chenagtsang, Foundations of Sowa Rigpa: A Guide to the Root Tantra of Tibetan Medicine, 2024, SKY Press

Chenagtsang, N. (2017). The Tibetan Book of Health: Sowa Rigpa, the Science of Healing.

Coberly, M., PhD RN. (2003). Sacred Passage: How to Provide Fearless, Compassionate Care for the Dying. Shambhala Publications.

Collective, B. W. H. B. (1976). Our bodies, ourselves: A Book by and for Women. Simon & Schuster.

Darwin, C. (1902). On the Origin of Species by Means of Natural

Selection, Or, The Preservation of Favoured Races in the Struggle for Life. New York: P.F. Collier.

Darwin, C. (2023). *The expression of the emotions in man and animals.* BoD – Books on Demand.

De Bary, W. T. (1999). *Sources of Chinese tradition.* Columbia University Press.

De Bary, W. T. (2001). *Sources of Japanese Tradition: From earliest times to 1600.* Columbia University Press.

Ekaku, H. (2010a). T*he Essential Teachings of Zen Master Hakuin: A Translation of the Sokko-roku Kaien-fusetsu.* Shambhala Publications.

Ekaku, H. (2010). *Wild Ivy: The Spiritual Autobiography of Zen Master Hakuin.* Shambhala Publications.

Fisher, J., & Durante, E. (2019). *Healing the fragmented selves of trauma survivors: Overcoming internal self-alienation.* Tantor Media.

Gonpo, Y. Y. (2011). *The Root Tantra and The Explanatory Tantra from the Secret Quintessential Instructions on the Eight Branches of the Ambrosia Essence Tantra* [Men-Tsee-Khang]. Mentseekhang Documentation & Publication.

Haidt, J. (2013). *The righteous mind: Why Good People Are Divided by Politics and Religion.* Vintage.

Henderson, R. (2015). *Emotion and healing in the energy body: A Handbook of Subtle Energies in Massage and Yoga.* Simon and Schuster.

Henrich, J. (2020). *The weirdest people in the world: How the West Became Psychologically Peculiar and Particularly Prosperous.* Penguin UK.

Hildegard, S., & Throop, P. (1998). *Hildegard von Bingen's Physica : the complete translation of her classic work on health and healing.* Healing Arts Press, C.

Judith, A. (2017). *Eastern body, western mind.* Jaico Publishing

House.

Jung, C. (1973). *Collected works of C.G. Jung: The First Complete English Edition of the Works of C.G. Jung.* Routledge.

Jung, C. (2016). *Psychological types.* Taylor & Francis.

Jung, C. G., & Hull, R. F. C. (1959). *The archetypes and the collective unconscious* C. G. Jung. transl. by R. F. C. Hull. Pantheon Books.

Lama, H. H. T. D. (2010). *Mind of clear light: And Living a Better Life.* Simon and Schuster.

Lama, H. H. T. D. (2005). *The World of Tibetan Buddhism.* Simon and Schuster.

Laozi. (1972). *Tao Te Ching.*

Masterson, J. F. (2011). *Search for the real self: Unmasking the personality disorders of our age.* Free Press.

Nan, H., & Allen, K. (1984). *Tao and Longevity: Mind-body Transformation: an Original Discussion about Meditation and the Cultivation of Tao* by Huai-Chin Nan.

Ni, M. (n.d.). *The Yellow Emperor's Classic of Medicine: A New Translation of the Neijing Suwen with Commentary.* Shambhala Publications.

Padma, J. H. (2021). *Field of blessings: Ritual & Consciousness in the Work of Buddhist Healers.* John Hunt Publishing.

Saunders, E. D. (1985). *Mudrā: A study of the symbolic gestures in Japanese Buddhist sculpture.* Princeton University Press.

Sgam-Po-Pa. (1998). *The jewel ornament of liberation: The Wish-Fulfilling Gem of the Noble Teachings.* Snow Lion.

Sheng-Yen. (2006). *Faith in mind: A Commentary on Seng Ts'an's Classic.* Shambhala Publications.

Vāgbhaṭa. (1995). *Astanga Samgraha of Vagbhata.*

Van Der Kolk, B., MD. (2014). *The body keeps the score: Brain, Mind, and Body in the Healing of Trauma.* Penguin.

Von Franz, M., & Hillman, J. (1971). *Lectures on Jung's typology.* Spring Publications.

Von Franz, M. (n.d.). *The Problem of the Puer Aeternus.* Inner City Books.

Wilber, K. (2007). *Integral Spirituality: A Startling New Role for Religion in the Modern and Postmodern World.* Shambhala Publications.

Wilber, K. (2017). *The religion of tomorrow: A Vision for the Future of the Great Traditions-More Inclusive, More Comprehensive, More Complete.* Shambhala Publications.

Wilber, K. (2001). *Sex, ecology, spirituality: The Spirit of Evolution, Second Edition.* Shambhala Publications.

Wilhelm, R., & Baynes, C. F. (1989). *I Ching, or, Book of changes.* Penguin Books, Limited (UK).

Yeshi Donden. (1997). *Health through balance : an introduction to Tibetan medicine.* Delhi Motilal Banarsidass.

Articles

Abbott, Geoff "In search of new medicines from plants.", https://communities.springernature.com/posts/in-search-of-new-medicines-from-plants, 2025

Bateson, G., Jackson, D.D., Haley, J. and Weakland, J. (1956), Toward a theory of schizophrenia. Syst. Res., 1: 251-264. https://doi.org/10.1002/bs.3830010402

Divine, Laura. "Looking AT and Looking AS the Client: The Quadrants as a Type Structure Lens" Journal of Integral Theory and Practice, 4.1 (Spring 2009): 21-40

Singh J, Desai M S, Pandav C S, Desai S P. Contributions of ancient Indian physicians - Implications for modern times. J Postgrad Med 2012;58:73-8

Vågerö, D., Pinger, P.R., Aronsson, V. et al. Paternal grandfather's access to food predicts all-cause and cancer mortality in grandsons. Nat Commun 9, 5124 (2018). https://doi.org/10.1038/s41467-018-07617-9

─────────────

[1]John Bowlby's (British, b1907) experience with his nanny inspired his pioneering research on childhood attachment which formed the basis of much of contemporary understanding and research of childhood attachment today. For people who were cared for by a nanny or other non-parental caretakers, attachment dynamics can be more complicated. The Western idea of "nuclear family" is relatively recent and there are still many people and places in the world where people live with extended family, which can greatly help support and in relatively healthier settings provide a more ideal attachment setting (Integral Magenta countries). However in the West it can become more complicated, as well as factoring the increase in daycare of babies and young children, both of which have not been well researched.

[2]A collage was presented in the original course, which included photos of Doshin Roshi, JunPo Kelly Roshi, Dr. Daniel P. Brown, Chogyam Trungpa, the 16th Karmapa, Father Thomas Keating, Marie Louis Von Franz, Eido Shimano Roshi, Carl Jung, Dr. Nida Chenagtsang, Vidyadhara Acharya Mahayogi Sridhar Rana Rinpoche, Rev Kapya Kaoma, Soen Nakagawa Roshi, Mary Lang, Ken Wilber, Dr. James Bae

[3] Divine, Laura. "Looking AT and Looking AS the Client: The Quadrants as a Type Structure Lens" *Journal of Integral Theory and Practice*, 4.1 (Spring 2009): 21-40

[4] From what I've read which is far from exhaustive, the first solid reference to a seven chakra system comes from about the 15th century, and it wasn't until the late 19th century that this started to become presented and reinvented in the West, which a lot has been, and could be said about, all of which is not really relevant to how we are presenting or working with the chakras. The best framework that we are aligning ourselves with is that presented by Ken Wilber in *The Religion of Tomorrow*.

[5] Some say there are front and rear chakras, but to avoid further complication we are using ones centrally located.

[6] There are many published variations of interpretations of each of the chakras in the seven chakra system. Other than Wilber's *The Religion of Tomorrow,* a book by Robert Henderson called *Emotion and Healing in the Energy Body* is a valuable resource for working with the chakras from a healer's perspective, and should be credited for some of the definitions we provide here in our illustrations and definitions.

[7] Vågerö, D., Pinger, P.R., Aronsson, V. *et al.* Paternal grandfather's access to food predicts all-cause and cancer mortality in grandsons. *Nat Commun* 9, 5124 (2018). https://doi.org/10.1038/s41467-018-07617-9

[8] This is also connected to your Jungian typology, whether you are introverted or extraverted, more tuned in internally versus externally.

[9] What is a mudra? A mudra is a ritualistic or symbolic gesture, or pose in Buddhism, Hinduism, and Jainism, usually made with the hands and fingers but sometimes with the body. In Sanskrit मुद्रा, translating to mudrā, seal, mark or gesture, in Tibetan: ཕྱག་རྒྱ་, chakgya. Prajwal Ratna Vajracharya is a priest of one of the Vajrayana Buddhist lineages

of Nepal and a ritual master both of the Charya Nritya dance tradition and other ritual forms performed by the Newar Vajracharya lineage, in a course on traditional mudras I attended he told us that each person has their own unique mudra, for them to discover. -JH. See also Saunders, E. D. (1985). Mudrā: A study of the symbolic gestures in Japanese Buddhist sculpture. Princeton University Press.

[10] I mention periodically, this is different in different systems even within Tibetan Buddhism.

[11] Nāgārjuna (c. 150 – c. 250 CE) is considered one of the most important Mahayana philosophers and Buddhist teachers in the Madyamaka school of Mahayana Buddhism. His texts are considered foundational and include Mūlamadhyamakakārika is revered as the most important text on the Madhyamaka view of emptiness. He is also credited with the Prajnaparamita sutras, revealed scriptures of treasure teachings (terma), having recovered them from nāgas (serpent spirits that inhabit the underworld).

[12] Bodhidharma was a Buddhist monk who lived during the 5th or 6th century. Traditionally he is credited as having introduced and transmitted Chan Buddhism to China. He is regarded as the first Chinese patriarch, and is also said to have begun physical training of monks at Shaolin Monastery, which was the birth of Shaolin kungfu. In Japan, Bodhidharma is known as Daruma. With little biographical accounts available most of the information has come from legend.

[13] Lecture on Marma points from Dr. Eric Rosenbush, Dr. James Bae course,"Buddhist Yoga, from Sutra to Tantra" 2023

[14] Instruction from Dr. Nida Chenagtsang

[15] "lunatic: late 13c., "affected with periodic insanity dependent on the changes of the moon," from Old French *lunatique* "insane," or directly from Late Latin *lunaticus* "moon-struck," from Latin *luna* "moon" see etymonline.com

[16] These developments don't start as a hard line time wise, and different frameworks will describe the process differently.

[17] For practical purposes we'll say at the spine, but some people say there are front and back chakras at each location (Barbara Brennan I believe talks about this in *Hands of Light.*) Again there are so many systems and many many energy locations in the body, so most systems reduce them to one of the numbers we've presented.

[18] For example a mother who is greatly traumatized and goes about in frequent fear and anxiety, will transmit this to the baby, just as a mother who is more generally peaceful, will transmit a state of peace.

[19] Haidt, J. (2013). *The righteous mind: Why Good People Are Divided by Politics and Religion.* Vintage.

[20] Barrett, L. F. (2017). *How emotions are made: The Secret Life of the Brain.* HarperCollins.

[21] Ālayavijñāna translates to "storehouse consciousness" or "all-ground consciousness." It is the eighth of the eight consciousnesses as described in the Yogacara school. A subtle level of consciousness, it holds traces of past actions, which are stored as (karmic) 'seeds' with the potential to ripen into future experience. The ālayavijñāna is explained and described in treaties by Asanga (4thc CE) and half-brother Vasubandhu (4th to 5thc CE) influential teachers and philosophers in Mahayana Buddhism.

[22] We explore trauma more in the next course. One sign of a trigger being more

likely connected to trauma is when you recognize a response to a trigger is far more intense than merits, is not reasonable, for a present situation. In extreme cases a person can feel a high level of personal reactivity, threat, fear, withdrawal, intense emotions, which are reflecting parts of ourselves that were deeply wounded in the past, triggered by something present that is reminiscent of prior events. Ordinary life can provide reminders of what is called implicit trauma that may be presently evoked and can in a sense trick the brain back into animal instinct survival mechanisms and reactions (lethal level fear despite the fact there is not anything lethally threatening present), which we may not understand or recognize, and find quite distressing and confusing, in the present. See Fisher, J., & Durante, E. (2019). *Healing the fragmented selves of trauma survivors: Overcoming internal self-alienation*. Tantor Media.

[23] This is very clearly articulated in Buddhism with the teaching of the five skandhas, the five aggregates, the five heaps of grasping and aversion due to ignorance. These ancient teachings are a profound pre-modern way of understanding the human mind and how it develops in relation to the three poisons of greed, hatred, and ignorance. Integrating them with Jung's 4 types and Wilber's four quadrants, can exponentially increase their usefulness. We will not go into greater detail about this in the more advanced courses and books. -Doshin Roshi

[24] From the Tibetan view the zygote forms and builds a spinal column at first from the naval area where it develops from the umbilical cord, so technically the spinal cord forms from the middle and then from the root upward, so this is a bit of a technical point to consider (again different frameworks provide different lenses on all of this), and also just reminds us that the gut area is so important energetically, spiritually, in different eastern systems, it is increasingly considered our "second brain". For the purposes of metaphor and developmental stages we begin with the root.

[25] Vāgbhaṭa. (1995). Astanga Samgraha of Vagbhata. Tibet was flooded by Indian culture in the 11th and 12th centuries, and numerous Indian medical texts were transmitted and translated, including the Ayurvedic Astāngahrdayasamhitā (Heart of Medicine Compendium) which was attributed to Vagbhata, and translated into Tibetan by Rinchen Zangpo (957-1055). See https://encyclopediaofbuddhism.org/wiki/Sowa_Rigpa_(Traditional_Tibetan_medicine)

[26] Lecture, Dr. Eric Rosenbush, Dr. James Bae course,"Buddhist Yoga, from Sutra to Tantra" 2023

[27] instruction from Dr. Nida Chenagtsang

[28] Lama, D. (2005). The World of Tibetan Buddhism. Simon and Schuster

[29] Account described in Singh J, Desai M S, Pandav C S, Desai S P. Contributions of ancient Indian physicians - Implications for modern times. J Postgrad Med 2012;58:73-8

[30] "The Yuthok Nyingthig, the 'Heart Essence of Yuthok' is a unique and comprehensive set of Tibetan Buddhist practices transmitted by Yuthok Yönten Gönpo the Younger, the great 12th century Tibetan physician and meditation adept who is considered to be an emanation of Medicine Buddha. It is a complete system of practice from the Anuttarayogatantra (Highest Yoga Tantra) class of teachings, beginning with Ngöndro (the preliminaries) and progressing through Kyerim and Dzogrim (Creation and Completion Stage practices) to the highest practices of Mahamudra and Dzogchen.

The tradition includes concise and essential methods perfectly suited for busy contemporary practitioners that offer both worldly benefits including improved health and longevity for oneself and others, as well as the ultimate benefit of complete spiritual liberation. The Yuthok Nyingthig is the main spiritual tradition connected with Sowa Rigpa (Tibetan medicine), and it contains many unique methods to heighten the intuitive, diagnostic, and healing capacities of doctors. It is the only complete cycle of Vajrayana teachings in which Medicine Buddha as a yidam (personal meditative deity)." see www.purelandfarms.com

[31] https://encyclopediaofbuddhism.org/wiki/Yuthok_Nyingthig

[32] Chenagtsang, *Foundations of Sowa Rigpa: A Guide to the Root Tantra of Tibetan Medicine*, 2024, SKY Press, p. 14

[33] Gonpo, Y. Y. (2011). The Root Tantra and The Explanatory Tantra from the Secret Quintessential Instructions on the Eight Branches of the Ambrosia Essence Tantra [Men-Tsee-Khang - ☐☐☐☐☐☐☐☐☐☐☐☐]. Mentseekhang Documentation & Publication.

[34]The information here on Sowa Rigpa is both from instruction from Dr. Nida Chenagtsang, much of which can be referred to in his book Chenagtsang, Foundations of Sowa Rigpa: A Guide to the Root Tantra of Tibetan Medicine, 2024, SKY Press

[35] Yeshi Donden. (1997). *Health through balance : an introduction to Tibetan medicine*. Delhi Motilal Banarsidass, pp. 16-17

[36]Chenagtsang, *Foundations of Sowa Rigpa: A Guide to the Root Tantra of Tibetan Medicine*, 2024, SKY Press

[37] Hildegard, S., & Throop, P. (1998). *Hildegard von Bingen's Physica : the complete translation of her classic work on health and healing.* Healing Arts Press, C.

[38] "Plants have been used as medicine since before the emergence of our species, by early hominids, non-human primates, and even other animals. *Homo sapiens* has taken this natural apothecary to another level of organization and scale, with perhaps 40% of modern medicines being derived in some form from plants. Our ancestors discovered the medicinal effects of plants by accident, trial and error, and/or learning from effects of similar plants and then experimented with the optimal methods of extraction, combination and application. Bitter plants, for example, were sought after by shamans in the Amazonian rain forests because of previous experience of beneficial effects of other bitter plants (due to the presence of alkaloids). An extraordinary wealth of knowledge in the medicinal properties of plants has been accrued by generations of shamans and their pupils, and much of it tragically has been lost due to the combination of destruction of indigenous peoples and their cultures, the lack of a written record of many traditional medicine approaches (many cultures transmitted information solely via oral tradition) and loss of the medicinal plants' habitat due to logging, farming, expansion of towns and cities, and more recently climate change." Geoff Abbott, "In search of new medicines from plants.",https://communities.springernature.com/posts/in-search-of-new-medicines-from-plants, 2025

[39]Adapted, 84000 Translation Team, trans., The Vaiḍūryaprabha Dhāraṇī, Toh 505 (84000: Translating the Words of the Buddha, 2024).

[40] You can find recordings of this online, and this translation is from Sowa Rigpa.

[41]realm beyond conceptuality

[42]Excess wind causes varieties of mental and emotional instability, from the manageable to extreme (psychosis, depletion of life force energies, etc..), this perspective and the frameworks from Sowa Rigpa and other Eastern systems is very important for all around health and well being, and it is a perspective that is absent in Western Medicine which doesn't present a corresponding typological framework, although the symptoms of these problems are observed, and described within a completely different Western Biomedical context. -Janel

[43]All of this is instruction from Dr. Nida Chenagtsang.

[44] In Tibetan, anger essentially arises from ignorance of who we are, notions of the self, ignorance of the inherent emptiness of self, ignorance around the impermanence of things, states of being - Janel

[45] In Tibetan "marigpa" is delusion, a fundamental lack of awareness, lack of understanding of true reality, our true nature, true wakefulness - Janel

[46] In the Tibetan Buddhist view desire, attachment, wanting to hold onto things, is driven by the confusion again related to notions of the self, rooted in ignorance of the illusion of a permanent self.

[47]Gregory Bateson, British, 1904-1980, was a pioneer who made significant contributions to the fields of anthropology, cybernetics, psychiatry, and, most important of all, to the new interdisciplinary field of cognitive science, thinking in terms of relationships, connections, patterns, and context. He is known for his Double-Bind Theory, "first stated by Gregory Bateson and his colleagues in the 1950s, in a theory on the origins of schizophrenia and post-traumatic stress disorder. Double binds are often utilized as a form of control without open coercion— the use of confusion makes them difficult both to respond to and to resist." (see Wikipedia, www.thebatesoninstitute.org)also see Bateson, G., Jackson, D.D., Haley, J. and Weakland, J. (1956), Toward a theory of schizophrenia. Syst. Res., 1: 251-264. https://doi.org/10.1002/bs.3830010402

[48]A developmental view more common today posits that humans as a natural part of development split into many varied parts, which is an approach worked with in the therapeutic model Internal Family Systems. Jung differentiated between people having a conscious persona, with different conscious components also creating unconscious split off shadow selves. The current view in terms of trauma and development suggests that it actually seems natural that splits occur normally throughout development and life, with some parts conscious and favored by the individual, and other parts rejected and exiled, or completely unconscious. Relative psychic health can integrate that we are all a mix of many varied components, conscious and unconscious, favored and unfavored, malleable and workable, with room for a spectrum of being without rigid fixation that any aspect of our being is solid, inflexible, a whole that is nuanced versus black and white. -Janel

[49]Also parents can model this in a more healthy way, so if a parent is feeling quite angry around a child, communicating about it "Everything is okay but Mommy got a phone call and got some news, and she feels angry and disappointed right now. It will pass soon, but she's going to take a walk, calm herself and do some settling breathing for five minutes", versus denying it, since children can already sense the anger anyways, and if we model avoiding it, the children will learn exactly what we model. - Janel

[50]E Dale Saunders. (1960). *Mudra*. Pantheon Books For The Bollingen Foundation, p. 66.

[51]Wilhelm Reich (1897-1957) was an Austrian doctor of medicine and a

psychoanalyst, a member of the second generation of analysts after Sigmund Freud.

[52]Dr. James Masterson posited that in these cases people often develop a false self, versus an authentic self. See Masterson, J. F. (2011). *Search for the real self: Unmasking the personality disorders of our age.* Free Press.

[53]Instruction from Dr. Nida Chenagtsang

[54]Instruction from Dr. Nida Chenagtsang

[55]Instruction from Dr. James Bae, *Buddhist Yoga* Coursework, 2022-2024

[56] In a medical context *dön* refers to "various invisible influences which can trigger disease in patients. The traditional Tibetan view of the world is an animist one. In this view, the landscapes and eco-systems through which we live and move as human beings are understood to be populated by a host of non-human beings, with their own lives, priorities, and points of view." p201, Chenagtsang, Foundations of Sowa Rigpa: A Guide to the Root Tantra of Tibetan Medicine, 2024, SKY Press

[57] From the Tibetan Buddhist view the optimal location it is said for the consciousness to leave the body is at the crown, otherwise the closer to the crown, the better potential for liberation or a favorable rebirth.

[58] The Six Yogas of Nāropa 𐖙𐖙𐖙𐖙𐖙𐖙𐖙𐖙𐖙𐖙𐖙𐖙 are a group of tantric practices in Tibetan Buddhism attributed to the the Indian mahasiddha Nāropa. Naropa transmitted these practices to the Tibetan translator-yogi Marpa, who then brought these practices back to Tibet and transmitted them to his students there. Marpa's most prominent student was the great yogi Milarepa. The six yogas are fundamental to the meditative training of the Kagyu school, but are also practiced by other schools of Tibetan Buddhism. The six yogas are: inner heat/ Tummo, illusory body, clear light, dream, transference of consciousness /Phowa. Info credit www.encyclopediaofbuddhism.org

[59] "In Bon, the kunzui is the basis of all that exists, including the individual. It is not synonymous with the alaya vijnana of Yogacara" p 142, Rinpoche, T. W. (2014). *Healing with form, energy, and light: The five elements in Tibetan shamanism, Tantra, and dzogchen.* Snow Lion Publications.

[60] I ching / Book of Changes, Shu ching / Book of History, Shih ching / Book of Poetry, Li chi / Book of Rites (Ritual), Ch'un-ch'iu Spring and Autumn Annals

[61] De Bary, W. T. (1960). *Sources of Chinese Tradition.*

[62] pp 53-54, De Bary, W. T. (1960). *Sources of Chinese Tradition.*

[63] pp 192-193, from Huai-nan Tzu, De Bary, W. T. (1960). *Sources of Chinese Tradition.*

[64] There seem to be treasure troves of documents, sutras, teachings, archives, in temples that are less openly shared publicly, that have been traditionally given limited access to monastics and priests versus the public. I say this meantime from what I've observed from some written accounts of monastics in Japan, and also looking at the fact that literary language is not accessible to the public, so even with access to materials, most contemporary Japanese people will not have the training to read archaic text, which would be limited to understanding generally by specialists and scholars. Then there is the gulf between Japanese writing and English translation, which despite

software improvements, still remains a significant gulf, which presumes that a text has been translated to English in the first place, which most are not.

[65] Not having explored this in great depth, there are books in English about this, but generally it seems to be concluded that an individual named *Hakuyu* did not actually exist, that a *story* was derived from Hakuin's experiences, his autobiography, the book *Wild Ivy* includes an account of this.

[66] Henrich, J. (2020). *The weirdest people in the world: How the West Became Psychologically Peculiar and Particularly Prosperous*. Penguin UK.

[67] Wilber, K. (2007). *Integral Spirituality: A Startling New Role for Religion in the Modern and Postmodern World*. Shambhala Publications.

[68] I'm going to say something that will be even more triggering to other True Believers. Once the significance of the WLC is realized and fully digested, it also becomes clear that most traditional Spiritual Teachers, Zen Masters and Rinpoches who may have attained enlightenment, a causal or nondual state vantage point, are structurally still at the amber level of ego development. Wilber and I have had this discussion and we both agree with this perspective. In fact, I have heard Wilber even suggest that the Buddha himself was at an orange level of ego development. This of course was vastly superior to the level of ego development anyone else had attained 2500 years ago in a culture where only a few individuals had reached an amber structure of development.-Doshin

[69] Henrich, J. (2020). *The weirdest people in the world: How the West Became Psychologically Peculiar and Particularly Prosperous*. Penguin UK.

[70]Wilber, K. (2006). *Integral Spirituality: A Startling New Role for Religion in the Modern and Postmodern World*. Integral Books; Boston, p 186.

[71] For example, when young children grow up in an atmosphere of threat, they often become hypervigilant observationally as a means of self protection, survival mechanism. As they become adults they may appear more developed in these ways than those who experienced less stressful environments. This often goes hand in hand with trauma. On the other hand, some children will dissociate in highly stressful situations, which will have a completely different line of development as they become adults, so there are a variety of ways childhood trauma impacts development that will vary individual to individual. -Janel

[72]This is not to say there aren't very promising opportunities to work in healing with plant medicines, however without guidance and without a healthy ground to do so, people may be unwittingly putting themselves at significant risk. One needs not just individual guidance when working in these areas but I would say they need a wider support system for both physical health, emotional and mental health, and spiritual guidance on top of professionals or lineage based shamans who will support an individual long term. - Janel

[73] Van Der Kolk, B., MD. (2014). *The body keeps the score: Brain, Mind, and Body in the Healing of Trauma*. Penguin.

[74]Attachment style is not technically genetic, however there is a strong evidence based correlation between maternal attachment and her child's attachment. It is absolutely possible to develop secure attachment but it is generally not easily done without healing, therapeutic support, and development. -Janel

[75] Sgam-Po-Pa. (1998). *The jewel ornament of liberation: The Wish-Fulfilling Gem of the Noble Teachings.* Snow Lion.

[76] www.garchen.net

[77] www.garchen.net

[78] Sheng-Yen. (2006). *Faith in mind: A Commentary on Seng Ts'an's Classic.* Shambhala Publications.

ACKNOWLEDGEMENT

Deep gratitude to those who contributed money, time, effort, resources, blood sweat and tears; to all who have chosen to be open, honest, vulnerable and real as they have freely given their support, bringing their gifts, karma, wounds and shadows into the cauldron of Integral Zen.

Daicho, Shikyo, Choan, Hozo, KoShin, Kodo, Guruma, Daiden, Jeremy, Ryushin, Maitri, Melita, Jitsujo, Jakusan, Jakob, GoShin, Kaku, David, George, Chiso, Gozan, Genyo, Shigetsu, Zenho, Ani Lodro, all the communities in Europe: Sacred Mirror, Venwoude, Findhorn and Doshin-ji, and many more who remain unnamed.

ABOUT THE AUTHOR

Zen Master Doshin Michael Nelson

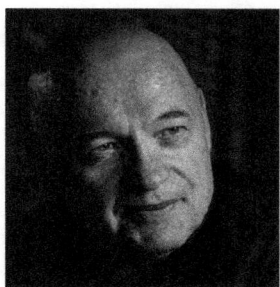

Doshin Roshi is a poet, teacher, and troublemaker—a Zen Master of no rank. He is the founder of Integral Zen. He met his first great teacher at 17 in the late 1960s, who introduced him to the works of Carl Jung, Joseph Campbell, Krishnamurti, and D.T. Suzuki. The same year he started meditating, but without the direct guidance of a good teacher, he was confused and discouraged by the obscurity of Zen teachings. It wasn't until he met Zen Master Jun Po Kelly Roshi that the disciplined practice and eloquent simplicity of Zen suddenly took root and began to penetrate the dense clouds of his stubborn conditioned mind, revealing the ordinary, openness of vast empty sky. About the same time, Doshin also began studying Ken Wilber's Integral Framework and studied directly with him. Integral Zen was born and the Integral Zen Framework began to emerge. Doshin's teachings integrate Jung, Wilber and Zen in an Integral Framework that focuses on both healing and awakening. It is not possible to fully awaken without healing and it is also not possible to fully heal without awakening.

Zen Master Dōshin Michael Nelson

ABOUT THE AUTHOR

Reverend Shikyo Jiryu Janel Houton

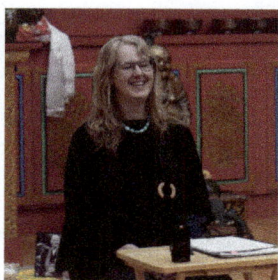

Rev Shikyo Jiryu, Janel Houton, has been working under the guidance of Doshin Roshi since 2019, forming a more Integral understanding of several Chakra systems, including traditional Tibetan Medicine and healing, with the intention of bringing these ancient methodologies into the 21st century, in a way that is helpful.

Studying with Dr. Nida Chenagtsang, head of the Yuthok Nyinthig Medicine Buddha lineage, and Dr. Caroline Van Damme, a Belgian Psychiatrist, she completed the Sowa Rigpa Institute for Tibetan Medicine Counseling Program in 2024. She was ordained Minister in Integral Zen in the fall of 2023 and has been developing and teaching courses and healing retreats since.

After spending a decade in Japan, and prior studies of Art History, Historic Research, and working as an Asian Antique dealer, Janel returned to live near her parents north of Boston, Massachusetts to raise her young daughter around 2008, when she then met her husband. Janel then returned to school to study Clinical Massage Therapy at Cortiva Institute in Watertown, MA in 2009, and offered therapeutic massage in the Boston area, designing treatments combining Eastern Five Element theory, hot stone and aromatherapy. She also was active as an artist (landscape painting) for several years. Combining experience in bodywork and study with Doshin Roshi, she brings together Zen, Integral Theory, Carl Jung, Buddhist energy healing, Yuthok Nyinthig, and Tibetan Medicine study to customize a unique path for each individual.